CLOTHING MATTERS

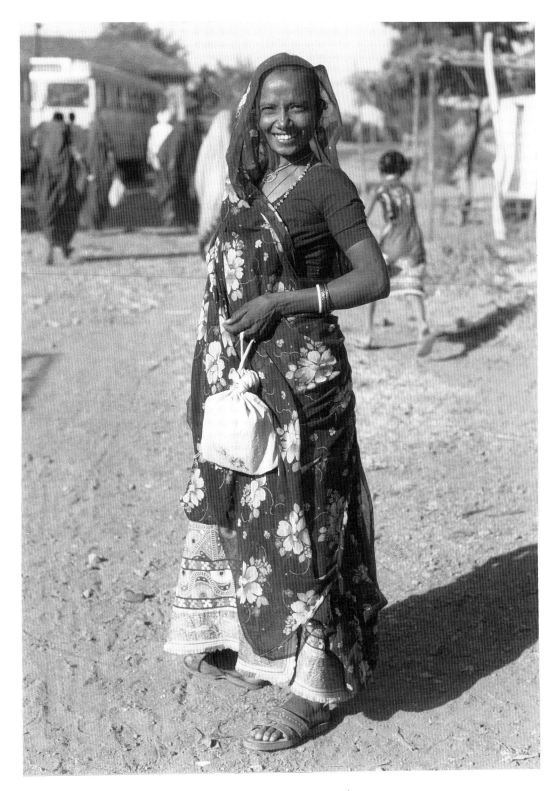

Jalia woman going to market

Clothing Matters

DRESS AND IDENTITY
IN INDIA

Emma Tarlo

The University of Chicago Press

EMMA TARLO is British Academy Post-Doctoral Research Fellow in Anthropology at the School of Oriental and African Studies, University of London.

The University of Chicago Press, Chicago 60637

C. Hurst & Co. (Publishers) Ltd., London

Printed in Hong Kong

04 03 02 01 00 99 98 97 96 1 2 3 4 5 6

ISBN: 0–226–78975–6 (cloth); 0–226–78976–4 (paper)

Library of Congress Cataloging-in-Publication Data
Tarlo, Emma.
    Clothing matters: dress and identity in India / Emma
Tarlo.
        p.   cm.
    Includes bibliographical references (p.   ) and index.
    1. Costume — India — History.   2. Costume — India — Symbolic aspects.
    3. Costume — India — Psychological aspects.   4. India — Social life and
    customs.   I. Title.
    GT1460.T37   1996
    391′.00954–dc20.   95–31464
                                                               CIP

This book is printed on acid-free paper.
Page lay-out by Janet Allen.

IN MEMORY OF RAMESHBHAI

Acknowledgements

This book is based on my Ph.D dissertation, submitted to the University of London in 1991 and examined in 1992. Neither the thesis, nor its conversion into a book, would have been possible without the support, both moral and academic, of a number of different people. First I would like to thank the people of Jalia village for accepting me into their midst so warmly and making my stay in their village not only possible, but also enjoyable. Secondly I must acknowledge my debt to the late Professor Rameshbhai Shroff for his constant encouragement and enthusiasm. His unexpected death while I was completing my fieldwork was a great loss not only for me but also for all those scholars who might have experienced his special welcome to Gujarat.

One of the most difficult aspects of doing fieldwork in a rural area is the absence of people who share an interest in one's research. Here I was fortunate to be in frequent contact with the artist and folklorist Khodidasbhai Parmar and the lecturer in Fine Arts, Sureshbhai Seth, both of whom were always willing to discuss points and share their rich knowledge of the region. In Gujarat, I extend my thanks to Raymond Parmar, Jignaben Dave, Sumanben and Bhagwanbhai Chaudhuri, Bindiben and Dilipbhai Trevedi and especially Yogeshbhai Vyas and his family. In Delhi my thanks go to the villagers and boutique-owners of Hauz Khas village, who were surprised to have an anthropologist in their midst but remarkably tolerant none the less.

In England I am much indebted to my research supervisor Professor Lionel Caplan for the time he spent wading through the letters and chapters which formed my doctoral dissertation on which this book is based. Others who have offered instructive comments include Brian Moeran, Christopher Pinney, Peter Robb, Deborah Swallow, Audrey Cantlie, Christopher Bayly, David Arnold and Giles Tillotson. For help over linguistic terms my thanks to Rachel Dwyer and Jagdesh Dave, and for their multifaceted support I thank especially Len, Helen, Jane and Harriet Tarlo, Mary Davies and, most of all, Denis Vidal.

This publication would not have been possible without a three-year studentship from the Economic and Social Research Council, which enabled me to carry out the initial research, and a Post-doctoral Fellowship from the British Academy which has supported me during the period of revising the text for publication. I am also indebted to the Central Research Fund and the School of Oriental and African Studies Research and Publications Committee for their contributions towards the cost of photographic reproductions. For photographic assistance of a more practical kind, I thank Paul Fox of SOAS. Finally, I am greatly indebted to those individuals and institutions who have supplied me with illustrative material. Of particular help were the library staff of the Oriental and India Office Collections, the National Gandhi Museum, the Nehru Memorial Museum and Library, and the School of Oriental and African Studies. I would also like to thank all the contemporary cartoonists whose satirical drawings have made such an important contribution to the text: Ravi Laxman, Mario Miranda, Sapre, Jaspal Bhatti, Crowquill, Manjula Padmanabhan and Prakash. Great efforts have been made to trace the copyright holders of all the illustrations included in this book for permission to reproduce them; their names are cited in the text alongside the illustrations as they occur. The author and publisher hereby acknowledge permissions duly sought in good time but not yet officially granted. Last, but by no means least, I would like to thank my publisher, Christopher Hurst, for deciding to embark on this venture some four years ago, and for seeing it through.

December 1995   E. T.

Contents

Glossary of Foreign Words

It is difficult to write on the subject of Indian dress without including large numbers of specialist foreign words – a difficulty compounded in this book by the fact that my fieldwork took place both in Hindi-speaking Delhi and in Gujarati-speaking Saurashtra. Furthermore, the regional dialect of Saurashtra, known as Kathiawadi, differs considerably from mainstream Gujarati in both vocabulary and pronunciation. Added to this, many of the historical examples I discuss enter other linguistic territories such as Bengali and Sinhalese. In anticipation of the confusion that leaping from language to language might cause, I have tried to keep foreign words to a minimum and would like to apologise to all those Hindi- and Gujarati-speakers who find this policy frustrating.

Foreign words are written as closely as possible to the way they are pronounced. Most words are written in the singular, with the English plural 's' being added where appropriate. An exception is made only in those cases where Gujarati-speakers use only the plural form, as when referring to names of designs. In such cases the Gujarati plural form is retained and the English plural omitted. Again, my apologies to the Indian reader. Listed below are those words which appear several times in the text. Roughly speaking, Hindi words are used in chapters 2–4, Gujarati words in chapters 5–8 and a mixture of the two languages in chapters 9 and 10. These headings refer to the usage of words rather than their origins, which may be Persian, Arabic, Sanskrit etc. Those words spoken in both Hindi and Gujarati have been listed only once, according to the first context in which they appear in the text. Diacritical marks have been added in brackets below for the benefit of those who know how to read them, but are not used in the text itself.

HINDI

angarkha (angarkhā) Long-sleeved long coat worn by men
bharat (bhārat) India
chadar (cādar) Shawl or wrap
chapkan (capkan) Type of long tunic particularly popular among Muslim men

charkha (carkhā) Spinning-wheel

choli (colī) Blouse, usually with a short body and short-sleeve

deshi (desī) Indigenous, of the local place

dharma (dharma) Religious duty

dhoti (dhotī) Men's waist-cloth, worn by draping, folding and tucking

dupatta (dupaṭṭā) Scarf, often worn with the *shalwar kamiz*

(ghagra (ghāghrā) Full skirt

kacha (kacca) Raw. The term is used to refer to foods cooked in water as opposed to oil, and may be used for anything that is in a raw state, such as a mud track as opposed to a concrete road

kamiz (kamīz) Tunic, worn by women, usually in conjunction with *shalwar*-type trousers

khadi (khādī) Hand-woven cloth. The term was used by Gandhi to refer to cloth that had been hand-woven using hand-spun yarn. In North India the word *khaddar* is more common

kurta (kurtā) Knee-length men's tunic

langoti (laṃgoṭī) Loincloth

lehnga (lehṃgā) Full gathered skirt

lungi (luṃgī) Waist-cloth, often stitched to form a large tube of cloth

odhni (oḍhnī) Veil-cloth, worn by being wrapped around the body and over the head

pakka (pakkā) Ripe, well-cooked, durable

phenta (pheṃṭā) Type of turban

pugri (pagarī) Turban worn by men

pyjama (pāyjāmā) Type of Indian trousers, often worn with a *kurta*

shalwar (salvār) Loose trousers worn by women, usually with a *kamiz*

sherwani (servānī) Men's long coat, usually collarless

sola topi (solā ṭopī) Pith helmet, worn primarily by the British and Eurasians

swadeshi (svadesī) Home produce, literally 'of own country'

swaraj (svarāj) Self-rule

topi (ṭopī) Cap or hat

GUJARATI

adadiya (aḍadiya) Sweets made from black adad pulses

akhi laj (ākhī lāj) Total veiling

anu (āṇuṃ) Ceremonial departure of a daughter to her conjugal home

ardhi (ardhī) Half

boloya (boloyā) Thick ivory bangles, worn by married women

chandlo (cāṃdlo) Auspicious mark on the forehead, usually made with vermilion powder or paste

Glossary of Foreign Words

chaniyo (caṇiyo) Skirt

chorni (corṇī) Pantaloon-type trousers, loose at the top and tight from the knee down

chundadi (cumdaḍī) Veil-cloth, usually tie-dyed

dori (dorī) Thread or chain-sticth

gam (gām) Village

ghaghro (ghāghro) Thick skirt. The term is used here to refer to the thick wrap-around skirts worn by many Saurashtran women.

ghaghri (ghāghrī) Skirt or petticoat made from thin cloth

gharcholu (gharcholum) Special veil-cloth worn by the bride in marriage

ghunghut (ghūmghaṭ) Veiling

hirawala (hīrāvālā) Someone involved in the diamond business

jada (jāḍum) Thick, coarse, rough

jianu (jīṇum) Ceremonial departure of a daughter to her conjugal home after giving birth to her first child in her natal home

jimi (jīmī) Waist-cloth worn by *Bharwad* women

kapdu (kāpaḍum) Open-backed bodice

(keḍiyum) Smock top worn mainly by farming men in Saurashtra

khetiwala (khetīvalā) Farmer

laj (lāj) Shame and the practice of veiling associated with it

mangalsutra (mamgalsūtra) Necklace worn by married Hindu women

najar (najar) The 'evil eye', an envious or malevolent look capable of causing harm

nath (nath) Nose-ring

paneter (pānetar) Special wedding sari, usually red and white

pardo (paḍḍo) Curtain

polka (polkum) Short button-down blouse

sadlo (sāḍlo) Half-sari, worn by being wrapped around the body and over the head. It is also used for veiling the face and body

sarawala (sārāvālā) Well-to-do person

saubhagya (saubhāgya) The auspicious state of a woman whose husband is living (known in Hindi as *sohag*)

shalwar kamiz (salvār kamīz) Outfit consisting of a long tunic worn with loose trousers, generally worn with a *dupatta*

sharum (saram) Modesty, shyness, respect

sikul (sīkal) Used here to refer to circular stitch formation

sudharo (sudhāro) Progressive, developed, advanced, reformed

tajvu (tājvum) Tattoo

toran (toraṇ) Auspicious hanging above a doorway

vau (vahu) Wife; daughter-in-law

videshi (videsī) Foreign, referring to all that is not *deshi*

Abbreviations

CAVA   Creative Arts Village Association

CWMG   Collected Works of Mahatma Gandhi

ILM   *Indian Ladies' Magazine*

NGM   National Gandhi Museum

NMML   Nehru Memorial Museum and Library

NRI   Non-resident Indian

OIOC   Oriental and India Office Collections, British Library

SOAS   School of Oriental and African Studies

SWJN   Selected Works of Jawaharlal Nehru

SWMN   Selected Works of Motilal Nehru

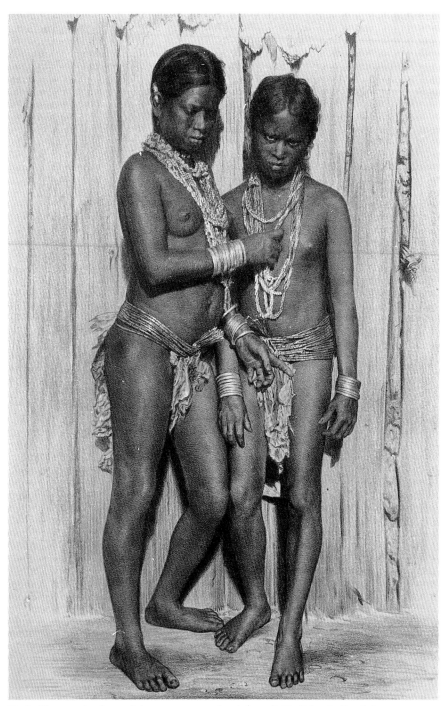

Pl. 1 Photograph of two *Juáng* women reproduced from E. T. Dalton's *Descriptive Ethnology of Bengal*, 1872. Courtesy of SOAS.

Preface: Reflections on a Portrait

This lithograph portrait of two young women, based on a photograph taken by Tosco Peppe, was used by the British administrator Colonel E. T. Dalton to illustrate his *Descriptive Ethnology of Bengal* (1872). Dalton, then Commissioner of Chutia Nagpur, stumbled across these women in the forests of the Juang hills and was much impressed by the scanty nature of their clothes. He recalls:

> The *Juángs* are in habits and customs the most primitive people I have met with or read of. . . .
>
> Adam and Eve sewed fig leaves and made themselves aprons. The *Juángs* are not so far advanced; they take young shoots of the Asan (*terminalia tomentosa*) or any tree with long soft leaves, and arranging them so as to form a flat and scale like surface of the required size, the sprigs are simply stuck in the girdle fore and aft and the toilet is complete. . . .
>
> The beads that form the girdle are small tubes of burnt earthen ware made by the wearers. They also wore a profusion of necklaces of glass beads, and brass ornaments in their ears and on their wrists, and it was not till they saw that I had a considerable stock of such articles to dispose of, that they got over their shyness and ventured to approach us. They made their first appearance at night and danced by torch light; it was a wild weird-like sight. . . .
>
> At Gonasika I saw them in their more normal state, when they returned from their work in the evening with dishevelled hair, dusty bodies, and disordered attire, ie somewhat withered leaves, and it was truly like a dream of the stone age (Dalton 1872: 153–6).

The lithograph has attracted the attention of a number of ethnologists and historians. Not only was it used to illustrate Dalton's work; it was also published, along with some of Peppe's other photographs, in Risley's *The People of India* (1908). By that time the image was over thirty years old, but Risley justified his decision to include it partly on the grounds that many of Dalton's lithographs had been destroyed. In the introduction to his book, he stated:

It seemed ... to my publishers worthwhile, and to myself as a lover of Chutia Nagpur and its people, a pious duty, to preserve from oblivion these fine pictures, one of which, the study of *Juang* female attire ... is, I believe, absolutely unique. (Risley 1908: vi)

More recently the historical significance of the image has been reconfirmed by its inclusion in the encyclopaedic exhibition catalogue *The Raj* (ed. Bayly 1990). There we are reminded of the circumstances in which the original photograph was taken:

Mr. Peppe had immense difficulty in inducing these wild timid creatures to pose before him, and it was not without many a tear that they resigned themselves to the ordeal (Dalton, cited in Pinney 1990: 282).

But it is not merely the nakedness of the women or the disturbing account of their unwilling subjection to Mr Peppe's camera that accounts for the photograph's popularity. Another reason is simply that by the early twentieth century it was probably already difficult to find young *Juáng* women still dressed in leaf clothes. Risley's assertion that the portrait is 'absolutely unique' seems to be confirmed by Dalton's footnote suggesting that 'when the *Juáng* girls posed themselves for the photographs ... it was almost their last appearance in leaves' (Dalton 1872: 156, footnote). It is not insignificant that the *Juángs*' first-ever subjection to the camera should have coincided closely with the apparent demise of their customary attire (although ironically anthropologists and photographers have since been accused of trying to get the *Juángs* to dress up in leaves for photo sessions). But it was neither Colonel Dalton nor the enthusiastic Mr Peppe with his camera who actively strove to stamp out traditional *Juáng* dress. This was left to a 'Political Agent' of whom we read: 'Captain Johnstone, with his usual liberty and tact, has clothed two thousand naked savages, and has succeeded in inducing them to wear the garments' (Ravenshaw, preface to Johnstone 1896: xxiv).

Details of this momentous achievement and of the origins of *Juáng* clothing are found in another footnote, this time in Risley's volume. The information is revealing, as is the fact that such blatant cases of direct intervention by the authorities should have been relegated to mere footnotes in ethnographic accounts. The note reads:

The origin of *Juang* millinery is obscure. According to one legend the goddess of the Baitarni river caught a party of *Juangs* dancing naked, and ordained for the women, on pain of divine displeasure, the costume shown in the illustration. ... The *Juang* ladies, according to Colonel Dalton, repudiated this scandalous tale and alleged that their attire expressed their genuine conviction that women's dress should be cheap and simple, and that fashions should never change. How much this was worth was seen a year or so later when a sympathetic Political Agent took the prevailing fashion in hand. An open air darbar, fitted out with a tent and a bonfire, was held in the *Juang* hills. One by one the women of the tribe filed into the tent and were robed by a female attendant in Manchester *saris* provided at the Agent's expense. As they came out they cast their discarded *Swadeshi* [home-made] attire into the bonfire. Thus ended a picturesque survival. (Risley 1908: pl. xx, footnote).

The lithograph of the *Juáng* women tells us little about them, except of course that they were the reluctant victims of colonial administrators, photographers and ethnographers. It tells us even less about the clothes of the people of India, most of whom have far stricter codes of modesty than any European. It is included here not for its undoubted iconic value but for the debate that surrounds it. For it is in the writings of men like Dalton, Risley, Johnstone and Crooke that we encounter a series of attitudes and presuppositions that have permeated not only colonial discourse but also anthropological literature and perceptions on the subject of dress.

Let us examine Risley's footnote in detail. First, there is the question of the origins of *Juáng* dress. Here we encounter a classic conflict, familiar to all ethnographers: the conflict between outsider and insider explanations. Usually this takes the form of the outsider (in this case, Dalton and later Risley) searching for magical and symbolic explanations of phenomena which the insiders (in this case, the *Juáng*) consider the ordinary everyday aspects of life. The desire for interesting information often leads the outsider to impute symbolic significance where it is inappropriate or unrecognised by the insider. Such treatment is all too common in the literature about Indian dress. Risley tried to avoid the trap by at least including the *Juángs'* denial of the mythic origins of their sartorial heritage. Yet by revealing how willingly the women accepted Johnstone's Manchester saris, he showed how little he valued their explanation.

We have already seen how Colonel Dalton coaxed the *Juáng* into a sense of security with offers of jewellery. Once they had advanced, they were then made tearful at the prospect of being photographed. Their will was ignored and the photograph was not only taken but published and later republished, out of Risley's sense of 'pious duty to preserve'. These were but the first stages in a series of acts which served to rid the *Juáng* completely of their right to express themselves as they wished. The next stage involved stifling their own explanations of their attire; their simple and practical considerations were discarded in favour of the more exotic, indeed erotic story of naked dancing women and angry goddesses. Finally, there was the abolition of their sartorial identity altogether. Captain Johnstone, assuming that he knew best how these 'wild timid creatures' should be dressed, persuaded them to submit their native clothing to the flames and accept his generous offer of saris, woven in Manchester. From Crooke we learn the final detail: 'The girls were marked with vermilion as a sign that they had entered civilized society and the men promised not to allow the women to resume their primitive dress' (Crooke 1906: 157).

It is no small paradox that, despite trying to put an end to the *Juáng* tradition of dressing in leaves, the British simultaneously preserved the image of the *Juáng* as 'naked savages'. By the time Risley's treatise on the peoples of India was published, they may well have been wearing saris or some other apparel for more than thirty years. Yet no attempt was made to provide a photograph of *Juáng* women in Manchester saris. Rather, they were caught and exposed forever in their 'primitive' nakedness where they fulfilled the reader's expectations of 'wild timid creatures'.

But what of such timidity and such passivity? Can we assume that Captain Johnstone's magnanimous act was the end of the story? Were the *Juáng* to wear Manchester saris for the rest of their lives now that a British Political Agent had shown them the way? We can assume nothing. For even subjugated tribals are not without the powers to act, despite being pinned like entomological specimens to the ethnographer's page. Writing of one of the *Juángs*' neighbouring tribes, Colonel Dalton makes a remark that is not without its resonance: 'The *Singhúm Kols* have a tradition that they were once similarly attired, and during the American war, when cotton was so dear, they told the cloth merchants that they would revert to their leaves if cloth was not sold cheaper! Manchester beware!' (Dalton 1872: 157). He realised what many writers on Indian dress have failed to acknowledge: that even within the constraints of a given tradition, whether ancient or modern, there is room for individuals to negotiate and to act. The clothes of the peoples of India are not so indelibly fixed to labels as our museums and photographs would sometimes have them. And if clothes are badges of identity, they can, like badges, be removed and replaced. Some *Juáng* women did in fact return to their leaves, at least for a time (Crooke 1906: 157), although by the 1920s they were reported to be wearing saris (cf. Bose 1973: 33). The British, meanwhile, were forced increasingly to heed Dalton's prophetic warning: 'Manchester beware!' For, during the struggle for Indian independence, India resurrected the bonfires of clothes that were once kindled by 'sympathetic agents' such as Captain Johnstone in the remote corners of the *Juáng* hills. In these new bonfires, Gandhi and other nationalist leaders encouraged Indians to strip off their European apparel and cast it into 'sacrificial flames', replacing it with Indian hand-spun and hand-woven cloth (*khadi*).

The curious relationship between Indian- and European-manufactured clothes continues today. Before I left for India in 1988, a woman in Delhi wrote me a letter requesting me to bring a bottle of whisky, some Paco Raban aftershave and two London saris. At the time it seemed strange that I should be expected to carry saris from London to Delhi. I also felt entirely unqualified to choose the appropriate designs and left the choice to an Indian friend who had spent her childhood with the woman in Delhi. She selected synthetic saris with floral patterns in subtle blues and browns. These were received with pleasure in Delhi and I was left wondering how, with all the choice of different saris available there, these two that seemed to me so dreary could possibly be admired. The research which has resulted in this book at least enabled me to begin to understand.

1 Introduction: The Problem of What to Wear

The aim of this book is to examine an apparently mundane dilemma as it manifests itself in India. It is one which most of us face every day, but which we seldom treat with any degree of intellectual seriousness. That is the problem of what to wear. It is generally considered a rather trivial problem, more suitable for discussion in women's magazines than anthropological treatises. From time to time newspaper articles and films expose our secret dithering at the wardrobe, and elicit a smile. However, if this problem is examined more widely and with greater intensity, it can reveal much about society, history, politics, culture and, above all, the way in which people seek to manage and express their own identity.

To speak of clothes as if they present a dilemma in the Indian context is to challenge the conventional academic view that Indian identity was, till recently, neatly prescribed by caste or religious tradition, and that people dressed in the clothes dictated to them over generations. In fact much of this book concerns those often controversial moments when individuals and groups choose to change their clothes or combine one type of clothing with another. In analysing specific historical and contemporary sartorial dilemmas the aim is to reveal the active role that clothing has played in the identity construction of individuals, families, castes, regions and nations.

A theme which runs throughout is that of 'dress and undress': the building up and casting aside of different identities by means of clothes. To this may be added the theme of 're-dress': the choosing of alternative images, with the rediscovery of self that this sometimes implies. But the book is also concerned with another form of redress, namely redressing an absence in the anthropological literature about India which, despite its emphasis on social behaviour, has largely ignored clothes. Some of the reasons for this neglect, along with the strengths and weaknesses of less neglectful disciplines, are explored in this introduction.

But first, a word about terminology. The word 'costume' has been systematically avoided on the assumption that to use it would be to contribute to the process whereby we analytically separate clothes from the people who wear them. Since present-day English-speakers do not refer to their own clothes as 'costume', there seems little reason why they should classify Indian dress in that way. The words 'clothes' and 'dress' are therefore used throughout, as reminders that the central theme is the significance of clothes as people wear them, not as they are arranged in museums and catalogues.

Indian anthropology without clothes
The famous story of the emperor who had no clothes is, of course, a lesson in perception. Until the intervention of the little boy who exposed the monarch's nakedness, an entire crowd was willing to assume that its ruler was really magnificently dressed. The crowd of anthropologists that has spread itself about the Indian subcontinent appears to have the opposite problem. Confronted by continual visual evidence of people wearing clothes, most anthropologists treat these as somehow insignificant, little to do with the 'real people' underneath. Yet clothes were not always so marginal to Indian anthropology. Their marginalisation was part of the historical development of the discipline which, during the twentieth century, became increasingly separate both from the museum and from earlier imperial concerns.[1]

In his discussion of the relationship between material cultural studies and anthropology, Daniel Miller shows how, before the emergence of mass photography, objects played a vital role in symbolising strange and exotic places (Miller 1983: 5). Clothes, weapons and curiosities were collected and arranged for the purpose of portraying other cultures, and displayed in museums, exhibitions and trade fairs, thereby making different races visible to the public. These representations not only presented other cultures to the public but also framed the public's perception of those cultures (cf. Breckenridge 1989). In India the role of the museum, with its overriding emphasis on the classification of types, was to have a profound influence on the perception of clothes. They became divorced from the contexts in which they were made, exchanged and worn, and instead were seen as part of a wider system of classification which enabled the museum visitor to identify the multifarious 'types' of peoples that made up the Indian population. In the Victoria and Albert Museum[2] in Bombay, for example, human types were displayed in the form of small clay models, and different styles of headwear were presented in ordered rows to aid the process of identification (cf. Pinney 1990: 256).

1   The following account is restricted to the role of clothes in anthropological literature relating to India. For comparative material see R. Barnes and J. Eicher's *Dress and Gender* (1993), especially Eicher and Higgins's introduction. It is interesting that Indian material is conspicuously absent in their historical survey of ethnographic literature on dress, although the volume itself does contain some Indian examples. Unfortunately, owing to the timing of its publication, it is impossible to make more than footnote references to this volume.
2   Now the Dr Bhau Daji Lad Museum.

Introduction: The Problem of What to Wear

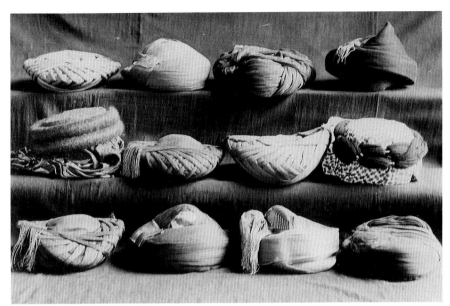

Fig. 1.1 Late 19th-century display of headwear at the Victoria and Albert Museum in Bombay (now the Dr Bhau Daji Lad Museum). Courtesy of Chris Pinney.

This emphasis on classification was not, of course, unique to museums, but characteristic of a whole framework through which Victorian intellectuals codified information about the world around them. The quest for systematic knowledge of the unknown was, in turn, linked to the idea of mastering the social and natural environment, and it is no coincidence that many of the early ethnographies on Indian dress were collated by men, like Colonel Dalton, heavily involved in the colonial administration. Using the new 'objective' medium of photography to record their findings (cf. Pinney 1990), such ethnographers put together large volumes which classified native peoples according to their physical appearance, including their dress (cf. Johnson 1863–6, Watson and Kaye 1868–75, Dalton 1872). This assumption that 'knowledge' could be 'gained through visibility' (Pinney 1990: 254) was still current in Indian anthropology in the first decade of the twentieth century when Risley published his famous book *The People of India* (1908), which included lithographs and descriptions of dress taken from Dalton's *Descriptive Ethnology of Bengal* (1872).

As the century progressed, however, a new form of anthropology emerged in which fieldwork was to play an increasingly important role. By the 1950s functionalist and structuralist models of society had shifted the focus away from imperial and evolutionary trends towards an understanding of the functions of Indian social institutions. To study such phenomena, anthropologists lived among Indian peoples, usually in small communities such as tribes or villages. Their insights did much to dispel

Western myths of the exoticism and strangeness of Indian peoples; customs, lifestyles, kinship systems and rituals were shown to be functionally interrelated in a rational system. At a theoretical level, the influential French sociologist Louis Dumont encouraged a school of thought which interpreted Indian society as a socio-religious caste-bound world in which each element served to maintain the fundamental principle of hierarchy that governed the whole (cf. Dumont 1970). This interpretation opened up a series of debates about the nature of the caste system, culminating in the suggestion that the two concepts of 'caste' and 'tradition' do not provide the exclusive keys to understanding Indian social life. Advocates of this view argue that continual emphasis on these concepts has skewed analysis in favour of all things social, to the detriment of the thinking, acting subject who has always existed in India as elsewhere (cf. Inden 1990).

What, one might ask, have the familiar old debates about 'caste' and 'tradition' to do with clothes? The answer is: very little. Anthropology's overriding emphasis on social relationships seemed to make clothes largely invisible in ethnographic accounts. If they were discussed at all, they were analysed mainly in terms of production and design (cf. Fischer and Shah 1970, Swallow 1982). The birth of fieldwork therefore coincided with the marginalisation of dress in Indian anthropology, because at the precise moment when anthropologists developed close personal contact with the people they studied, they ceased to pay attention to their clothes.[3] This was no doubt partly because the 'functions' of clothes as markers of social identity in India seemed so obvious and so natural as to obviate the need for discussing them. But perhaps it also reflected the fact that early ethnographers were largely men, who despite showing considerable interest in nakedness showed much less in clothes.[4] Clothes were considered a 'feminine' issue, and little to do with serious academic pursuit.[5] It was only with the multiplication of women anthropologists in the early 1970s that dress began to reappear in ethnographic accounts. These were usually restricted either to discussions about the significance of the veil (cf. Jacobson 1970, Sharma 1978b, Nanda 1976, C. Thompson 1981) or to those about women's rituals, where clothes, though not the central focus, were inevitably mentioned (cf. Luschinsky 1962, Fruzzetti 1982). So, even with the advent of female anthropologists writing about Indian women, very

3   For exceptions see V. Elwin 1959 and Ehreufals 1948.
4   Early ethnographic titles such as C. von Fürer-Haimendorff's *The Naked Nagas* (1939) and *Return to the Naked Nagas* (1976), or N. Watts's *The Half-clad Tribals of Eastern India* (1970) are perhaps indicative of a certain male vision.
5   For a discussion of the hierarchical division of the arts into serious activities pursued by men, and 'feminine' ones pursued by women, cf. Pollock and Parker 1981, also Parker 1986.

Introduction: The Problem of What to Wear

little attention was directed towards the subject of dress, although for many Indian women it is a topic of great importance.[6]

In short, clothes, like many other social phenomena, became subject to academic partition. They were discussed *either* in terms of social institutions and rituals in the village *or* in terms of production, design and trade in the museum. In the former case little attention was paid to the artefacts themselves, and in the latter the artefacts and their classification were the primary focus. In Ahmedabad the Shreyas Museum houses a permanent display of 'folk costumes', neatly arranged by caste and occupational group. Similarly Elson's exhibition catalogue *Dowries from Kutch* (1979) emphasises the overriding importance of classification: 'The cut, the material and ornamentation of a costume reveal the age, occupation, origin, caste and marital status of the wearer' (Elson 1979: 19). If this way of viewing Indian clothes has barely changed since the late nineteenth century, it has none the less provided some valuable insights into the importance of clothing differences in India. So too has the abundant museum literature on textile production and design (cf. Buhler and Fischer 1979, Nabholz-Kartaschoff 1986, Mohanty and Mohanty 1983, Irwin and Hall 1971, 1973, Crill 1985, Murphey and Crill 1991, Nicholson 1988, J. Jain 1980, 1982). But museum-generated knowledge tends to be constrained by certain factors which have served to conceal the existence of the problem of what to wear. First, there is the fact that most museums are to some extent answerable to their public, which means that they are expected to display clothes and objects of 'public interest'. This inevitably restricts the museum curator's choice of artefacts. Faced with the range of clothes worn in India today, curators will usually select those that are classified as 'traditional' and which fulfil the public's notion of 'authenticity'. This inevitably leads to a sifting out of many contemporary forms of dress, such as trousers, shirts and plastic flipflops, all of which may have important social significance.[7]

A second limitation of the museum approach is that curators 'collect' and 'display' clothes, and in so doing take them out of their social, political and economic context. In other words, they rob clothes of much of their usual 'social life' (cf. Appadurai 1986). During this process of sartorial

---

6 A. Grodzins Gold has pointed out the inordinate amount of time that Rajasthani women spend discussing clothing, and the rigorous attention they pay to matters of beauty and adornment, but Gold herself does not expand upon the subject (Gold 1988: 15).

7 An example of this weeding-out process is Julia Nicholson's exhibition catalogue, *Traditional Indian Arts of Gujarat* (1988), where in accordance with her title she displayed only so-called 'traditional' artefacts and dress. This was an understandable choice; if she had displayed too many flipflops and synthetic trousers, she would no doubt have lost her public.

kidnapping, clothes usually become reclassified as 'costume', a word more associated with history and theatre than everyday living. Clothes, which in the normal course of events are exchanged, purchased, worn, stored and discarded, become ossified in the museum display case where their meaning often appears static and rigid. Instead of playing an active role in the making of identities, they become mere labels which do little more than *reveal* identities to the museum public.[8] The very notion of identity itself becomes fixed and constrained in the process. And when identities are so neatly prescribed, the problem of what to wear goes unnoticed and unquestioned. For it seems that there is no problem.

Towards an anthropology of the problem of what to wear in India
During my stay in an Indian village in Gujarat I realised that anthropologists and museum curators were not the only people who made classificatory assumptions about the other. At Diwali time (the business new year), one of my neighbour's sons returned to the village for the celebrations. Seeing me for the first time, he scrutinised my appearance and asked the proverbial question of where I was from. When I replied that I came from England, he looked at me in disbelief. He had seen white people often because he worked on the railway and, he assured me, they never dressed like me. They wore brief shorts, both men *and even the women*, and had naked arms, and you could always recognise them by the huge plastic sacks they carried on their backs and, of course, by their cameras. Why wasn't I dressed like that if I was from England? Having conveyed his esoteric knowledge of white people, he began demonstrating to his family just how brief the typical white person's shorts actually were. And I was left contemplating what he might write if he were required to give an ethnographic description of my people: an exotic tribe of backpackers, obscenely dressed, largely nomadic, migrating through India with cameras. Distinctive features: style of bag and bare legs, *even the women*.

My neighbour's account of white people perhaps reconfirms the idea that in village India behaviour is socially prescribed and that people wear badges of identity, neatly fixed. For he seemed to attribute some kind of generality

8 A notable exception is B. N. Goswamy's recent catalogue of Indian Dress at the Calico Museum of Textiles in Ahmedabad (1993). Goswamy brings his subject to life through a fascinating discussion of some of the problems of classification. But he too is struck by the sterilising effect of museum catalogues in general, pointing out that the clothes he describes have to be 'seen worn and used . . . for then alone do they begin to breathe a life of their own' (Goswamy 1993: 2). Regrettably, the present work was finished before the publication of Goswamy's catalogue, thus it can only be referred to in footnotes.

Introduction: The Problem of What to Wear

to the few white people he had seen, and now described their characteristic features as if they constituted something akin to a caste. But clothes and classifications are not that simple. Amid the sartorial silence of ethnographic accounts, small incidents have crept in which suggest that a person's clothes are not so easily determined in India as one might expect. We read, for example, of a low-caste man in Gujarat who imitated the turban style of high-caste landowners and was beaten for so doing (Pocock 1972: 28); of local élites in the Ramnad district of South India who tried to impose consumptuary restrictions on their social 'inferiors', including prohibitions on certain types of ornament and dress (Hutton 1946: 74–5); of Muslim women in northern India who veiled their faces within their home-towns but not when they travelled to other towns and cities (Sharma 1980: 232), and of a Nayar man who claimed that when he put on his shirt for work, he literally 'took off' his caste (cited in Srinivas 1968: 123). These incidents, brief and scattered though they are, hint at the fact that clothes can be a controversial issue in India and that classifications, though they exist, are open to manipulation and dispute. More recently, Alfred Gell's account of how the Muria Gonds of Madhya Pradesh invent their own uniforms for public occasions reveals the dynamism of what he calls 'collective styles' (Gell 1986: 120). In other words, people are involved in *making* classifications as well as in simply following them (cf. Parkin 1982, Douglas and Isherwood 1980).

It is noteworthy that some of the most dynamic accounts of people's attitudes to their clothes in village India appear in books written outside the institutions of anthropology and the museum. A fine example of such an account is found in *Behind Mud Walls* (1930), written by the two American missionaries Charlotte and William Wiser. They had been living in a village in Uttar Pradesh and wished to record certain events which seemed inappropriate to their official documentation: 'Many of our experiences along the way have been too personal to have a place in the survey. And yet they are too revealing to be discarded' (Wiser and Wiser 1930: vii). One such 'revealing' experience was their conversation with a villager in which he described how local people deliberately dressed in shabby clothes in front of government and hospital officials:

> When we are to deal with strangers we suit our dress to the occasion, not to our means. And most occasions call for poor clothes. You have heard them complain in the hospital that they are at a loss to know who should be charity patients and who should pay. We would be foolish to bring ourselves big bills, when the simple matter of dressing will

give us charity rates. The Memsahiba let appearances influence her that first year when she picked out what she thought were the ten poorest among our children. She did the choosing so we did not interfere. They [the children] had learned the most effective way of appealing to her sympathies, by word and dress. And their reward was a ride in the motor and new clothes from the landlords' wives in Mainpuri. Later she learnt how mistaken her choice had been. And the next winter she came much nearer to the poverty line. What a joke we had on the accountant when the new Deputy came on tour! There sits friend Accountant, looking very smart, all ready for the Deputy's arrival. At the last moment someone breaks in with the news that the Deputy rebukes well-dressed accountants. Tells them they cannot live within their income honestly and have fine clothes. Off comes the new turban, off comes the yellow silk waistcoat. Friend Accountant rushes about and borrows a shirt and loincloth that look neat but old. In these he bows humbly before the Deputy Sahib. And some of us who were absent during the rapid change, did not at first recognise our grand Accountant in his shabby clothes. The visiting Deputy was properly impressed (Wiser and Wiser 1930: 158).

What such incidents provide is a picture of people making decisions, choosing to some extent their own self-image, playing with identities and recognising the role of clothes in image construction and interpretation. In other words, clothes are not merely defining but they are also self-consciously *used* to define, to present, to deceive, to enjoy, to communicate, to reveal and conceal (cf. Schneider and Weiner 1989, Lurie 1992).[9] If we shift the focus away from the garments themselves to the wider issue of the relationship between clothing and its wearer, we are faced with a number of questions. What do clothes mean to the people who wear them? Why do certain individuals and groups choose to dress in a particular way? What are the various constraints within which they formulate these choices? And what are the consequences of their choosing one particular image over another? We arrive, at last, at a theory of dress in which clothes are central to a person's identity, but not in any rigid and deterministic way. We arrive in other words at a theory which takes as its central theme the problem of what to wear rather than the description of what is worn. This enables us not only to see beyond classifications, but also to avoid

---

9   There are a few articles which highlight the dynamic nature of dress in non-Western societies. See, in particular, I. Hodder's ethno-archaelogical study (1982) and H. Kuper's historical study (1973) – both concerned with African dress – and P. Baker's historical analysis of clothing reforms in Turkey (1985). All of these make highly recommended reading.

Introduction: The Problem of What to Wear

some of the highly subjective value judgements characteristic of the modern literature which takes an aesthetic and moralistic approach.

Aesthetic and moral approaches to Indian dress
Literature concerning the aesthetics and morality of Indian dress dates back to the pre-Christian era when socio-religious clothing presciptions were recorded in the *dharmasastra* (Sanskrit religious laws).[10] But to privilege ancient dress prescriptions in a discussion of contemporary clothing issues would be to fall prey to the very essentialism this exploration seeks to avoid. The following account is therefore restricted to what might be termed the 'modern aesthetic approach' to Indian dress, an approach formulated principally in the late nineteenth century. This was a period when some professional Indian men were adopting Western-style clothes and when a significant proportion of the Indian population were buying machine-made cloth imported from Europe. The modern aesthetic approach to Indian dress was therefore linked to the more general idea that Indian textiles and crafts were under 'threat' and required 'revival'. So while anthropologists tended to project an over-static image of Indian society and traditions, advocates of the aesthetic approach claimed, on the contrary, that local traditions would be obliterated if conscious efforts were not made to preserve them.

One of the early exponents of this view was George Birdwood, founder of the Victoria and Albert Museum in Bombay and Art Referee for the Indian Section of the South Kensington Museum. In 1880 he assembled his famous work, *The Industrial Arts of India*, in which he praised the skill of Indian craftspeople and discussed the need for craft preservation. He was disturbed by the decline in the Indian handloom industry and by the popularity of Manchester cottons. Arguing on both economic and aesthetic grounds, he called on British and Indian peoples to return to hand-woven clothes. Speaking of Indian cottons, he wrote:

> Nothing could be more distinguished for the ball room, nothing simpler for a cottage, than these cloths of unbleached cotton, with their exquisitely ornamented narrow borders in red, blue, or green silk. Indian native gentlemen and ladies should make it a point of culture never to wear any clothing or ornaments but of native manufacture and strictly native design.... (Birdwood 1880: 244)

Of course Birdwood was not alone in his appreciation of Indian dress.

---

10 These prescriptions included details of the clothing appropriate to different social groups (white for priests, red for warriors, yellow for merchants and cultivators, and dark colours for the service castes) as well as details of the dress deemed suitable for different stages of the life-cycle and for specific rituals. For further discussion of these, see J. Leslie (1993) and O. P. Joshi (1993).

There were a number of leading figures both in India[11] and England who were deeply concerned about the decline not only in traditional textiles but also more generally in the whole realm of hand-made artistic production.[12] In England William Morris, founder of the Arts and Crafts Movement, can perhaps be considered the figure most influential in trying to elevate the notion of craftsmanship to an aesthetic and moral ideal. He saw craft as part of a whole conception, 'the good life', which he felt had existed in Europe in the Middle Ages and which still existed in distant village-based societies. This life, he argued, was being destroyed by industrial development:

> So far reaching is this commercial war that no country is safe from its ravages: traditions of thousands of years fall before it in a month: it over-runs a weak semi-barbarous country, and whatever romance or pleasure existed there, is down trodden into a mire of sordidness and ugliness; the Indian or Japanese craftsman may no longer ply his craft leisurely, working a few hours a day, in producing a maze of strange beauty on a piece of cloth: a steam engine is set a-going at Manchester (cited in Lipsey 1977: 262).

Morris's attitude to crafts embodied a number of value-laden moral dichotomies. Just as beauty was opposed to ugliness, so the hand-made product was opposed to the machine-made, the rural to the urban, the past to the present, the non-Western to the Western and the domestic to the commercial. These dichotomies, which typically emerge in rapidly industrialising societies (cf. Moeran 1984, Dewey 1972, Appasamy 1968), were later to become a sort of blueprint for both Indian and British writers on the aesthetic aspects of Indian dress.

They were first given wide credence by the Anglo-Ceylonese geologist, art critic and philosopher Ananda Coomaraswamy. Brought up in rural Kent by his English mother, owing to the premature death of his Ceylonese father, he received a thoroughly British education. When, at the age of twenty-five, he returned to Ceylon for field research, he was horrified by what he termed the 'vulgar imitation' of the West. In 1905 he published a book entitled *Borrowed Plumes*, where he denounced the adoption of European dress, which he described as part of 'the continual

---

11   In India the primary exponents of these ideas were men like E. B. Havell, Lockwood Kipling and members of the Tagore family.

12   The founding of the *Journal of Indian Art* in 1886 marked a decisive step in favour of documenting, reviving and adapting Indian arts with a view to increasing both quality and commerce. Indian dress, however, featured comparatively little in these impressive volumes, perhaps because it was less suitable for trade than other 'art manufactures'.

destruction of national character and individuality and art' (cited in Lipsey 1977: 18). That same year, he founded the Ceylon Social Reform Society, which aimed to encourage the retention or readoption of national dress along with vegetarianism and other social customs (*ibid.*: 24).

Coomaraswamy recognised that he had an outsider's viewpoint when he criticised 'natives' for wearing European dress. He told an audience in Jaffna: 'I believe it is difficult for any of us who have not been brought up in England to realise the hopeless inadequacy of any attempts at imitation; to Englishmen the absurdity is obvious, but to us it is not revealed. Coming freshly to the East and starting from the ordinary English point of view, I have been struck' (*ibid.*: 18). The 'ordinary English point of view' was, of course, the ideological view of the Victorian romantics. The subjective nature of Coomaraswamy's attitude, spoken from a standpoint of superior judgement, is perhaps best revealed by his own actions. He soon put aside his European suits and adopted a *dhoti* (waist-cloth), *kurta* (long shirt) and turban (cf. Mohan 1979). Logically this could have been interpreted as a 'vulgar imitation of the native'. Yet he saw his own actions as an aesthetic and moral example to the Ceylonese, despite (or perhaps, more accurately, because of) his 'ordinary English point of view'.

The recurrent themes of the destruction of 'Indian tradition', the futility of 'Western imitation' and the need for a revival of local textiles were expounded in a number of different forms in India in the late nineteenth and early twentieth centuries. Some early nationalist leaders such as Dadabhai Naoroji, Justice Ranade, B. G. Tilak and G. K. Gokhale advocated the need to buy *swadeshi* (Indian-made) cloth in order to restore a declining Indian economy (cf. Bean 1989). In Bengal, the call to *swadeshi* was most vigorously propounded from 1905 to 1910, following Lord Curzon's announcement of his intended partition of Bengal; there it was not merely an economic revival but a political protest and national ideal (cf. Bayly 1986). The Nationalist Movement was later to weave together political, economic, aesthetic and moral arguments under the leadership of M. K. Gandhi, who tried to encourage all Indians to revert to 'Indian' dress. But for men like Coomaraswamy beauty was the key to a clothing revival. In 1910 he wrote: 'Swadeshi must be something more than a political weapon. It must be a religious-artistic ideal' (Coomaraswamy, 1911: 8).

This aesthetic and moral approach to Indian dress flourished immediately after independence with the formation of the Indian Handicrafts Board (1952) which aimed to stimulate the appreciation, support and revival of Indian handmade cloth, clothes and craft. It was accompanied by a flurry of literature on the subject, most of which embodied the aesthetic and moral judgements listed above. Urbanisation was interpreted as an 'onslaught' (Nanavati *et al.* 1966: 9), commercialisation as a 'blight' (Chattopadhyaya 1964: 4). Factory-made articles were described as 'humdrum commercial' products, as opposed to the colourful variety of India's 'ancient costume traditions' (cf. Mangaldas's preface to J. Jain 1980). The arrival of machine-manufactured goods was thus perceived as the destruction of a more beautiful Indian heritage which was being steamrollered by the powerful forces of industrialisation.

Implicit within these aesthetic judgements is a deep moral overtone and an implication that those Indians who adopt European dress are either innocent victims or lack good judgement. S. N. Dar exemplifies this viewpoint:

> In India we sometimes come across recalcitrant rebels who exult in disparaging oriental ways indiscriminately. They affect foreign manners and so camouflage themselves that, whereas had they followed the modes of their country, they could with their superior mental culture have made themselves an excellent model for their countrymen, they have now to be content with becoming at their best a mediocre 'half caste' type of youth. A modernity which is achieved by an intellectual serfdom of this type would not be a mark of real progressiveness (Dar 1969: 207).

One of the major disadvantages of this aesthetic and moral approach to Indian dress is that it fails to consider the perspective of the person who is wearing the clothes. Instead, Indians who adopt Western dress are perceived as weak or immoral,[13] while villagers who adopt commercial products are seen as the passive victims of industrialisation. In this book I hope to provide an alternative framework for comprehending the clothing choices that people make. By focusing on the problem of what to wear, I try to examine *why* people make certain choices of dress and what these choices mean to them. This involves recognition of the idea that buying and wearing a certain type of dress is in fact a creative act (cf. Wilson 1987, Hodder 1982, Gell 1986, Lurie 1992). It is one of the ways in which people participate in the formulation of their own self-image. While the creative element of all clothing choices is rarely recognised in the ethnographic and moral literature about Indian dress, it *has* featured in historical literature.

Historical approaches to Indian dress
Historical literature on Indian dress is, on the whole, more dynamic than the literature generated through anthropology and museum

13 For years this idea was also perpetuated in Hindi cinema, where women of low repute tended to wear European styles while virtuous wives and heroines wore Indian styles. However, this situation has changed somewhat more recently.

catalogues,[14] not least because historians and art historians recognise the temporary nature of different types of dress. This is evident from the number of impressive volumes which have documented clothing changes over time, using a mixture of literary and artistic sources (cf. Fabri 1960, Chandra 1973, Alkazi 1983, Ghurye 1951). Focusing less on the visual properties of the garments than on the political contexts in which they are used, a few writers and scholars turned their attention instead to the symbolic aspects of historical developments in Indian dress (cf. Chaudhuri 1976, Bayly 1986, Bean 1989, Cohn 1989). In particular Bernard Cohn, who describes himself as 'an anthropologist among the historians',[15] has provided some fascinating insights into developments in Indian dress in the nineteenth century. He sees dress as part of a wider issue concerning the nature of the relationship between the British ruler and the Indian ruled during the colonial period. Taking the example of the distinctive style of Sikh turban, nowadays interpreted as a badge of Sikh identity, he suggests that it became standardised largely as a result of British attempts to classify Sikhs in the army.

By shifting the focus away from the simple act of reading classifications, Cohn shows how classifications were actually created in official and public intercourse between Indian and British men. In particular, he demonstrates how the British sought to reinforce their separateness from the Indian population by rigorously adhering to British standards of dress and by encouraging Indians to dress in an 'oriental manner'. A second essential point made by Cohn is that dress codes are often at the centre of a number of wider issues concerning modesty, honour and respect, and that a clash between different styles of clothing is often symbolic of a wider conflict between different cultural and social values and norms. He goes on to argue that in India clothes have a special meaning since they are considered capable of retaining the very essence of the people who wear them. This point has also been widely discussed by Christopher Bayly, who outlines what he calls a distinctively pre-colonial Indian view of cloth 'as a thing that can transmit spirit and substance' (Bayly 1986: 286). Having defined a number of Indian beliefs about the 'moral' and 'transformative' properties of cloth, Bayly reveals how Gandhi rekindled these essentially dormant beliefs when he encouraged Indians to reject British dress and return to Indian clothes.

But the problem with defining an 'Indian view' of cloth is that it encour-

14 There is of course a certain overlap between the types of literature produced by different disciplines and institutions, especially since contemporary museums may employ a mixture of historians, anthropologists and art historians. None the less, it is still possible to isolate tendencies which characterise the different approaches.
15 This phrase is also the title of his book (1987).

ages a deterministic approach. Yet it is impossible to judge the extent to which such a view was actually adhered to by the Indian population. While some Indians today might argue in favour of the transformative aspect of cloth, others might deny it. But can we assume that there was ever a past age when everybody shared the same point of view? As is shown above (Preface: xix), outsiders are often more inclined to read 'magical' beliefs into Indian clothes than the people who actually wear them. When this process occurs in reverse, and an Indian scholar expounds the magical aspects of Western dress, we are perhaps less willing to accept too many suppositions. Certainly I felt a strange lack of recognition when I read S. N. Dar's analysis of sartorial customs in Europe:

> In Europe, a cultural refinement of a primitive form of sex-worship requires men to keep their hats off and their shoes on, when in the presence of ladies. The removal of the hat is an act of homage to the eternal feminine, while the injunction against bare feet is a symbolic acknowledgement of woman's monopoly in the field of corporeal display (Dar 1969: 138).

While the belief that cloth is capable of transmitting and retaining the moral properties of its wearer is stressed in certain contexts in India, it is underplayed in others. For, as Arjun Appadurai has pointed out in relation to contemporary food habits, ideas of purity and pollution are often context-specific (Appadurai 1988: 9).

Of all the approaches to the subject of Indian dress, Nirad Chaudhuri's is perhaps the most dynamic and ambitious, if at times outrageous.[16] He sees the evolution of clothes in India as part of 'the historical evolution of the peoples of India, possessing similar features, following similar lines, and producing similar results' (Chaudhuri 1976: xi). After defining what he calls the 'generic types' of dress available in India, he discusses the historical development of clothing traditions in terms of a series of battles (Hindu vs. Muslim, Indian vs. British). Finally he describes the 'decline and fall of clothing' (*ibid.*: 97) as all types degenerate into what he terms 'bad taste and ugliness' (*ibid.*: 133). While it is advisable to reject Chaudhuri's moral judgements and 'generic types', it must be recognised that his book provides the most valuable and indeed entertaining documentation of the problem of what to wear, for it is crammed with personal observations and historical detail as well as

---

16   Chaudhuri, who claims at the beginning of *Culture in the Vanity Bag* (1976) that 'a man who has lost interest in clothing and adornment has also lost interest in life', is adamant that his book is not a scholarly work. Yet again, the most interesting approaches to Indian dress seem to be coming from outside the confines of academic disciplines.

interesting, though at times contradictory, analysis. It is refreshing in assuming that Indian clothes can be explained as much in terms of conflict as of consensus. Chaudhuri's sensitivity to this point stems perhaps from his own personal experience of the problem of what to wear; brought up in a Bengali village, settling in Calcutta and finally Oxford, living through the rise of nationalism, the attainment of independence and after, he has had ample experience of it. Although he does not focus on his personal dilemma, he refers in his introduction to the troublesome range of clothes in India and suggests that it is the discomfort they inflict which has motivated him 'to seek their cause, and to find peace if [not] in anything else at least in understanding' (*ibid.*: xii).

Why is the problem of what to wear a problem?
It has become clear that the problem of what to wear in India is, or at least can be, a difficult one; but it remains to be seen where the complications lie. Below are three theoretical issues which seem to be at the heart of the problem as it manifests itself in India. These do, of course, combine and interact with other practical considerations such as price and the availability of choice.

The first theoretical issue concerns classification. How can we reconcile Elson's orderly museum classification of clothes and identities with Chaudhuri's perception of clothes as a series of battles? The two arguments are in fact reconcilable for they are but aspects of the same debate. It is precisely because the social classification of clothes is so important that the conflict exists. Museums have been right to stress the importance of clothes as markers of social identity, but their weakness lies in their often favouring one criterion of identity over another. But identities, like classifications themselves, may be multiple and conflicting.

Classification is about the dual processes of identification and differentiation, and choosing a certain type of clothing is one of the means whereby individuals participate in these processes. Yet classification is problematic when a person's identification with one group conflicts with his or her identification with another group. In India, a country that is highly stratified on a number of different levels (social, sexual, religious, political, economic, cultural, regional), the likelihood of wishing to identify with more than one group simultaneously is considerable. At times a certain type of clothing may coincide with a person's religious, regional, social and political beliefs, but at other times these may be at sartorial loggerheads.

An example serves to illustrate the point. A Hindu man living in Delhi might dress in a cotton *kurta pyjama* (tunic and trousers). To most foreigners, he looks 'Indian' but if he wishes to attend a particularly auspicious Hindu ceremony, he may find his stitched clothes associated with impurity, and even with foreignness in certain traditional regional contexts. Then again, if he returns to his home village his family may rebuke him for deserting his caste dress. Other villagers may think he looks too modern (deserting local regional styles) or conversely too old-fashioned (he is dressed in cotton when they are dressed in synthetics). In other words there are a number of different criteria by which a person's clothes may be judged, and the clothes appropriate to one set of classifications are not necessarily appropriate to another. When individuals have to decide what to wear they have to consider the problem of their audience, but they may, like the man in Delhi, have multiple audiences with multiple expectations. Historically this has been the case particularly with Indian men's dress, since men have travelled more widely and participated in a more diverse range of public activities. Women, whose movements are generally considerably more restricted than men's, have till recently had fewer alternative audiences with which to contend.

Thus part of the problem of what to wear hinges on deciding where one's sartorial affiliations lie at any given moment, and this of course means risking the consequences of offending those who do not agree with one's choice. This leads to the second issue. Why should clothes be treated so seriously? What does it matter if a person is 'wrongly' dressed according to his or her family, friends and associates? It matters because of the unique and peculiar role that clothing plays in perceptions of identity. For clothes are frequently perceived as expressions and even extensions of the people who wear them (cf. Wilson 1987). Anthony Trollope recognised this when he wrote of one of his characters: 'Never at any moment ... was he dressed otherwise than with perfect care. Money and time did it, but folk thought it grew with him, as did his hair and fingernails' (cited in Douglas and Isherwood 1980: 47).

Like other social phenomena, clothes are often dehistoricised, naturalised, converted to myth (cf. Barthes 1973). Yet at the same time they are detachable,[17] thereby denying the very permanence they sometimes seem to suggest. They are both part of us and superfluous to us. What this suggests is not that clothes have any particular meaning, but that their peculiar proximity to our bodies gives them a special potential for symbolic elaboration:

> A part of this strangeness of dress is that it links the biological body to the social being, and public to private. This makes it uneasy territory, since it forces us to recognise that the human body is more than a

---

17 The word 'clothes' is used to refer only to those items of adornment or protection that are detachable; 'dress' has a wider application and, following Eicher and Roach-Higgins, may be used to include not only 'body supplements', but also 'body modifications' such as make-up and tattoos (1993: 15–21).

biological entity. It is an organism in culture, a cultural artefact even, and its own boundaries are unclear.... Dress is the frontier between the self and the not self (Wilson 1987: 2–3).

While India has a highly developed philosophy concerning the inseparability of spirit and matter, most cultures view clothes within this framework at least to some extent (cf. Schneider and Weiner 1989, Lurie 1992). In Europe and America people are often reluctant to buy secondhand clothes, as if the previous wearer somehow adheres to the cloth, yet precisely because of the close proximity between people and clothes, pop fans will clamber on stage to touch the T-shirts of their heroes and heroines.[18] We even try on new clothes in shops and ask the question: 'Is it really me?' These incidents suggest that people interpret the ambiguous boundary between their biological and social selves at a number of different levels.

One consequence of the common idea that clothes are part of the human being is that a change of clothes is regarded as a desertion of the former self. Where the concept of fashion introduces a wide range of constantly changing images to be aspired to, we are no longer expected to define ourselves in too permanent or consistent a way. Change, according to Roland Barthes and indeed any women's magazine, is built into the fashion system. But in India, where social, religious and regional stratifications are still strongly expressed and where the fashion industry is still relatively young, a change of clothes is likely to be interpreted as an act of desertion or a change of affiliation. Speaking of dress in the Indian vs. British sartorial battle, Chaudhuri argues:

> Like language and other features of life which distinguish one human group from another, it is part of the national personality, it is one expression among others of a distinctive culture. Therefore no one can change his clothes until there has been, in part or whole, a transfer of cultural allegiance (Chaudhuri 1976: 73).

But this leads to a third theoretical problem. While clothes may at times express 'cultural allegiance', this depends on the attitude of the wearer to his or her clothes. Just as clothes can challenge social and political norms as much as they uphold them (cf. Hebdige 1979, Bean 1989, Baker 1985), so they can conceal identities as much as they reveal them (cf. Lurie 1992, Schneider and Weiner 1989). Alison Lurie's witty and observant book *The Language of Clothes* (1992) reveals much about the complex ways in which people communicate and miscommunicate through dress. She leads the way

---

18 Marilyn Monroe's swimsuit was selling at Christie's for £13,200 on the very day that I happened to be writing this passage (in 1991).

to the minefield of communication theory, with its complex debates about problems of intention and interpretation. Many communications analysts have, like Lurie, addressed this problem in relation to clothing in the West (Hoffman 1984, Phelan 1984). It is a problem intimately linked with the problems of classification and identification already discussed. People may *seek* to communicate their identity or beliefs through wearing certain clothes, but they cannot guarantee that their message will be understood in the way they intend. As Hoffman puts it, 'The communicative offer made by means of one's costume is frequently understood, but rarely coincides with what the wearer wants to express' (Hoffman 1984: 7).

Two scholars have recently discussed the communicative aspect of clothes in India (cf. Ramanujan 1984, Bean 1989), but both fail to address the problems of intention and interpretation. Susan Bean describes Mahatma Gandhi as a semiotician who used 'his appearance to communicate his most important messages in a form comprehensible to all Indians' (Bean 1989: 368), and claims that the communicative power of Gandhi's loincloth 'transcended the limitations of language' itself (*ibid.*). But much of Gandhi's difficulty lay in the imperfect nature of his communication through clothes. Throughout his political career he was constantly trying to define the meaning of his dress through verbal explanation, but was never able to control the multifarious interpretations which proliferated around him. While clothes, like language, communicate, they are, like language, capable of communicating anything from truth to lies, from the intelligible to the unintelligible (cf. Lurie 1992). Their meaning, like meaning itself, is open to interpretation and debate:

> But what is meaning? It flows and drifts; it is hard to grasp. Meaning tacked to one set of clues transforms itself. One person gets one pattern and another a quite different one from the same events; seen a year later they take a different aspect again. The main problem of social life is to pin down meanings so that they stay still for a little time (Douglas and Isherwood 1980: 64).

Deciding what to wear is one of the ways in which people try to 'pin down meanings' and control both presentations and interpretations of the self. But since, as we have seen, the problem of what to wear addresses a whole range of issues about classification, identification and communication, it is a very real and sometimes highly complex problem.

How this book evolved
Trained in the anthropological tradition, and equipped with the usual intellectual baggage that encourages one's gaze in certain directions and not

Introduction: The Problem of What to Wear

in others, I had not intended to study, nor had I seriously considered, the problem of what to wear before setting out for fieldwork in India in 1988. The intention at the time was to study the social and cultural significance of women's embroidery traditions in a Gujarati village. With this in mind I selected a large multi-caste village in Saurashtra, an area renowned for the persistence of its artistic traditions. It was one of the few regions where a substantial proportion of peasant women still wore and made embroidery entirely for domestic use, although the craft was clearly in a phase of rapid decline. I was immediately welcomed into the village and shown the contents of many dowry chests containing embroidered clothes, hangings and animal regalia. For some months I concentrated earnestly and sometimes exasperatedly on the subject of embroidery and anything that might conceivably be related to it. But there was one major problem. There was I, showing inordinate interest in embroidery, when the women who actually made it were largely uninspired. Some had given up wearing it altogether, while others, who still did, confessed that they were embarrassed by its backward connotations and were keen to be rid of it.

There was something slightly farcical about the anthropologist trying to uncover the vital significance of a textile tradition that the villagers themselves were keen to put behind them. It was also rather depressing that there was more information about embroidery designs in museums and books than in the village. Yet the attitudes of village women to their textile heritage interested me. I became increasingly aware of how and why they no longer wanted to wear embroidered clothes. I also became more generally aware of a number of different clothing controversies that were brewing in the village. While the idea that each caste had its own dress was often propounded, what this dress actually consisted of was frequently in dispute. Furthermore, there were other issues that arose repeatedly, such as female modesty and the degree to which a caste should modernise its image. In short, I became interested in the whole field of clothing and identity, and in particular the question of how, within the often limited confines of village life, individuals and groups changed their clothes.

The fact that I was female, young and unmarried meant that villagers developed an extremely protective attitude towards me which was at once invaluable and constraining. In particular, I had considerably more limited access to men than to women. Furthermore, men's dress seemed a much less controversial issue than women's dress, for most young men were wearing Western-style trousers and shirts which were accepted in the village by almost every caste. Yet I was aware that many of the contemporary controversies over women's dress were in fact transformations of similar issues that had arisen over men's dress earlier in the twentieth century. And although these women's clothing disputes had no direct link with colonialism, they were none the less infused with certain issues which had emerged under British rule, if not before. In order to understand these links, I felt the need to delve deeper into the recent history of clothing disputes in India. I therefore left the village and spent five months in Delhi where I embarked on a different kind of fieldwork.

My fieldwork in Delhi took place largely in the Nehru Memorial Museum and Library (I call it fieldwork because it was a form of ethnographic research). My aim was to find firsthand accounts of the experience of the problem of what to wear as it was faced by Indian people in the late colonial period. For this purpose secondhand sources, which usually weeded out such details, were of little assistance. Diaries, autobiographies, newspapers and journals proved more rewarding. In particular the *Collected Works of Mahatma Gandhi*, volumes 1–90 (1958–84) proved an invaluable source of information. These impressive tomes contain not only Gandhi's speeches, correspondence and writing, but also newspaper reports and, more important, letters from the public to him. These gave insights into the problem of what to wear in a way that is rarely provided in history books.[19]

Having researched this issue, I returned to Saurashtra for a further two-month stay which enabled me to examine afresh the relationship between different levels of sartorial change. On leaving there, I spent a further month of fieldwork in a second village, this time in the capital itself. This 'urban village' was in the process of being converted into an 'ethnic' shopping centre, where clothes of the type worn in village Saurashtra were being converted into exclusive designer fashion garments. It was here, in the urban fashion village of Hauz Khas in South Delhi, that the links and disjunctions between the clothing dilemmas of colonialism, nationalism and village life finally became apparent.

The end-result of these various different methods of enquiry is not perhaps the standard anthropological work, but as a researcher I found a multidisciplinary approach rewarding. As Nita Kumar so rightly argues, the 'meanings' of a cultural tradition can be understood 'neither simply from their context, nor merely as intentionality', for they are also 'part of a larger system that goes beyond the actors' will, and indeed, consciousness' (N. Kumar 1988:5). As anthropologists, we must be willing to look beyond the

---

19 The articles by Cohn (1989) and Bean (1989), which do to some extent deal with this question, were published in the United States while I was in the field. At the time when I embarked on the subject it seemed an untouched territory, and it was therefore rewarding to read these publications after my return.

Introduction: The Problem of What to Wear

'field', even if it does mean stepping into the risky territory of other disciplines. History has recently benefited from redrawing its borders and incorporating subaltern perspectives within its vision (cf. Guha [ed.] 1982–9). Similarly the development of ethno-archaeology has enabled the archaeologist to use contemporary fieldwork experience as a key to understanding the past (cf. Hodder 1982, Miller 1985). My own approach is an endeavour to incorporate the historian's idea that the past makes sense of the present with the ethno-archaeologist's idea that the present throws light and understanding on the past.

The book is organised around the central theme of the problem of what to wear, with each chapter exploring this problem from a different angle and within a specific context. Many of the examples refer to the clothing dilemmas of Hindus in North India, and the book does not claim to be representative of Indian people as a whole. Chapters 2–4 focus mainly on questions of national identity through the clothing dilemmas of Indian men in the late nineteenth and early twentieth centuries. These are analysed within the context of British imperialism and the Indian struggle for independence. Chapters 5–8 concentrate mainly on women's clothing issues in a Gujarati village in the period from the attainment of independence (1947) to the late 1980s.[20] Here the clothing choices of individuals and groups are analysed in relation to such factors as caste, education, urbanisation and ideas of female modesty. Questions of local and national identity are brought together in the penultimate chapter which traces the development of contemporary 'ethnic' fashions in an urban village in Delhi, where in the late 1980s members of the educated élite were returning to the clothes that rural women were in the process of rejecting. Finally I seek to demonstrate how all these sartorial trends are part of a long-term cultural debate on Indian identity, which is played out at different levels of society from the village to the nation. By incorporating the attitudes of people both to their own clothing choices and to the choices made by others, I offer a dynamic model with which anthropologists can approach the complex and intriguing relationship between clothing and identity.

---

20 By discussing male clothing issues in a historical context and women's clothing issues in a contemporary context, I am not suggesting that women did not participate in history any more than that men do not participate in contemporary village life. My bias simply reflects that of both my fieldwork experience and of historical writings. While I had firsthand access to the perceptions of women in a contemporary village setting, I had very little access to their thoughts and opinions in the late colonial period, for few Indian women recorded their experiences and very few men (Indian or British) thought them worth recording. Conversely, while I had limited access to men's opinions in the village, I had easy access to the veritable plethora of literature written by Indian men during the struggle for independence.

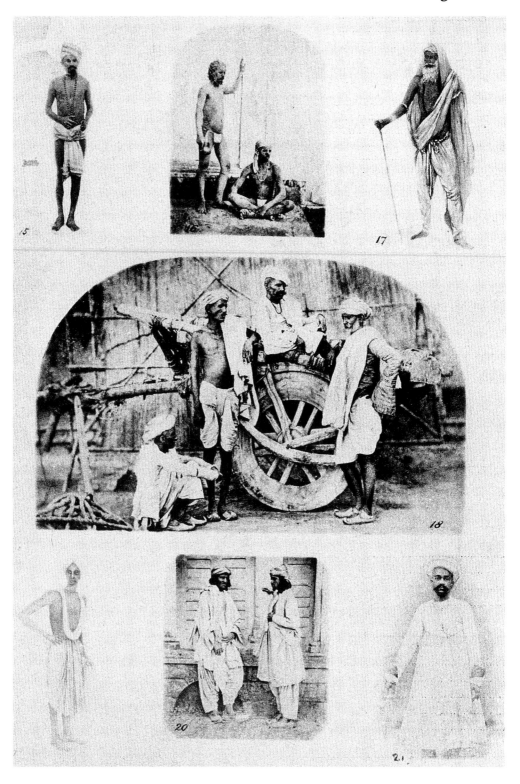

2 Searching for a Solution in the late Nineteenth Century

The nineteenth-century Bengali poet Michael Madhusudan Datta once shocked his friends and acquaintances by attending a Raja's party in full European dress. When the Raja asked him why he was not wearing the customary *dhoti* (waist-cloth) and *chadar* (shawl), the poet replied with a laugh: 'If I came wearing them I'd have to help carry pitchers and napkins; but these are the clothes of the Ruling Race; so there's no fear of that' (cited in Radice 1986: 203). On another occasion, Datta was seen emerging from a lake, this time dressed in a *dhoti*. When a friend taunted him, 'Where is your hat and coat now?', the poet replied, 'Man is many-formed: he takes on different forms according to the situation in which he finds himself' (*ibid.*: 203–4).

In the late nineteenth and early twentieth centuries, men like Madhusudan Datta were to find themselves in an increasing variety of sartorially perplexing situations. British imperial presence in India had introduced not only new forms of government, language, education and social etiquette, but also a new set of criteria of civilisation with a new set of clothes to go with it. Most British men and women took it for granted that their customs and lifestyle were part and proof of their superior place on the evolutionary ladder, and many members of the Indian intelligentsia were greatly impressed by the European perception of progress. But Indian responses to the British were never straightforward, either in dress or in other modes of behaviour. While many admired Europe's scientific discoveries and educational standards, they were often critical of other aspects of European culture and remained highly selective over which elements should be adopted or absorbed into Indian life. Clothes were among the many manifestations of British

Fig. 2.1 Different forms of cotton dress popular among Indian men in the mid- to late 19th century, published in J. Forbes Watson's *The Textile Manufactures and Costumes of the People of India*, 1866. The plate contains both Hindus and Muslims wearing both draped and stitched cloth. Watson describes the dress bottom right as a 'long Hindu Coat' and the dress bottom centre as a 'Mussulman coat'. Also depicted are the '*dhotee*' (*top left* and *middle centre*, worn by Hindus), the '*loongee*' (here translated as 'shoulder scarf') and '*paejama*' (*top right*, worn here by a *Brahman*). The central panel also contains a Hindu man wearing a long-sleeved quilted jacket. Watson's work was intended to demonstrate the clothes worn by Indians with a view to aiding the British to reproduce them and so gain a better hold of the Indian textiles market. Courtesy of SOAS.

culture which were carefully assessed and partly assimilated by a small but influential Indian élite.

Since clothing had always been an important sign of affiliation to different social and religious groups in India, few people were prepared to abandon their raiments of identity overnight. Indeed, a vast proportion of the rural population and almost all the female population continued to dress in predominantly Indian styles throughout the period of British rule. Yet for the small minority of Indian men who had been educated in the British manner, European clothes posed a significant problem. They were such an essential component of the European notion of civilisation that they could not simply be ignored by the educated Indian man. Yet to adopt them without hesitation seemed tantamount to a desertion of one's own people. The result was that individuals began to juggle their sartorial identities, sometimes awkwardly, sometimes with ease and sometimes, like Madhusudan Datta, with a good dose of self-conscious humour and provocation.

There was, of course, nothing new about such sartorial juggling. Throughout Indian history, traders, travellers, migrants and invaders had all contributed to the repertoire of clothing styles in India, thereby presenting new choices to the local population. Furthermore, during the Moghul period the ruling élite had actively insisted on the adoption of Moghul styles by all officials in government employment. This had forced many élite Indians into Moghul dress in the public sphere. As a strategy of resistance, most Hindus used to remove their foreign apparel before entering their own homes, thereby distinguishing their imposed identity from their chosen identity, which expressed itself in social, religious and domestic situations (cf. Watson 1866: 11). But unlike the Moghuls, the British did not try to force their own garb upon Indians. On the contrary, they actively sought to discourage what they called 'meaningless imitation'. This meant that when an Indian man adopted European dress he did so not because it was forcefully imposed on him but because, for one motivation or another, he actually chose to wear European clothes. This made his decision more controversial than that of the man who unwillingly compromised his sartorial identity for the sake of his employment under the Moghuls.

The arrival of European clothes was therefore met by a peculiarly complex variety of sartorial strategies which were soon further complicated by the ready availability of imported machine-woven cloth from abroad. While some Indian men wore a combination of Indian and Western[1] garments, others varied their clothes according to the situation, while yet others tried to combine both Indian and Western features within a single garment.

1 The term 'Western' refers here to garments originally popularised in Western countries.

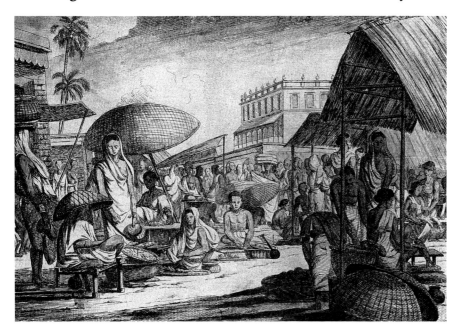

Fig. 2.2 A late 18th-century etching by Balt Solvyns entitled 'A Bazar, or Indian Market', illustrating both male and female draped dress. Note that the women do not wear blouses under their saris and that many of the men do not wear turbans. The architecture and dress suggest that the market is in Calcutta. Reproduced from Solvyns' *A Collection of two hundred and fifty coloured etchings descriptive of the Manners, Customs and Dresses of the Hindoos*, (1799). Courtesy of SOAS.

These different solutions to the problem of what to wear generated in turn a variety of responses from family, caste, friends, work and religious associates. They were also scrutinised by the British, who tried to control developments in Indian dress (cf. Cohn 1989, Chaudhuri 1976) and ridiculed what they considered 'inappropriate dressing'. Awareness of these potential responses from different audiences formed part of the framework in which the problem of what to wear had to be tackled.

This chapter seeks to explore the various factors that motivated Indian men to adopt European fashions or discouraged them from doing so. It begins with an introduction to different clothing types in India, emphasising both British and Indian attitudes to them. This provides a context for understanding why clothing choices posed a dilemma to certain members of the Indian intelligensia, and how different individuals and groups dealt with it.

SOME CLOTHING TYPES IN INDIA

For the purpose of clarity it is helpful to give a brief overview of certain basic clothing types in India, but it should be remembered that there is

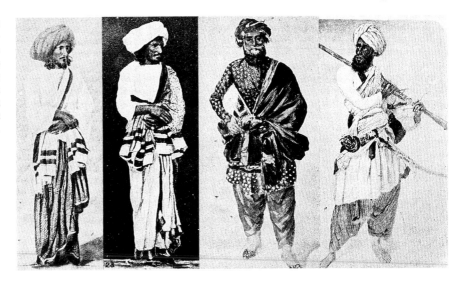

Fig. 2.3 Popular forms of cotton and silk men's attire in the mid-to late 19th century, published in Watson (op. cit.). Referring to the right-hand plates, Watson writes that the 'frock or coat reaching to the knee' is 'in common use amongst Mussulmans'. Courtesy of SOAS.

far greater variety than I can possibly record here. Furthermore, the act of labelling is artificial in many respects, not only because it crystallises forms which are in reality in a state of flux, but also because the terminology employed for different garments often varies not only according to language and region, but also sometimes according to author. For this reason I have tried merely to outline certain basic types of clothing in India rather than to enter the complex labyrinth of definitions of different garments and styles.[2]

Draped clothes

Probably the oldest and commonest form of dress in pre-colonial India consisted of various cloths draped around the body and held together by tucks and folds. Men's clothes were often white, and either plain or with simple borders. They were usually made from cotton, but were sometimes of silk. The poorest men wore little more than a basic loincloth (*langoti*), but the longer waist-cloth (*dhoti*), which could be wrapped and tucked in various ways, was more common. The upper body was either left uncovered or draped with a shawl (*chadar*), depending on the season and occasion. The head was wrapped by some form of turban (*pugri*) which could be tied in a number of different regional and specialised ways.[3] By the nineteenth century many men had added long tunics or shirts to their

2 Those wanting more detailed information should refer to the specialist works of the art historians G. S. Ghuyre (1951) and Moti Chandra (1973). More recently B. N. Goswamy has completed a superb volume, *Indian Costumes* (1993), in which he discusses the history of competing clothing terminologies and styles.
3 In some parts of Bengal and South India men did not wear turbans or hats (cf. Crill 1985).

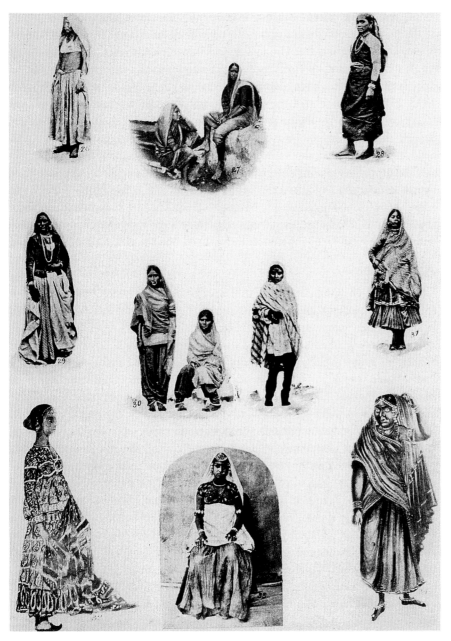

Fig. 2.4 Different forms of women's dress popular in the mid- to late 19th century, from Watson (op. cit.). The three women to the left wear skirts and bodices with head-scarves. Top centre and bottom right the women are dressed in saris, the former being 'women employed on the railway near Bombay'. In the centre are women wearing what Watson calls the 'Mahomedan Trowser' in its 'loose' and 'narrow' form. Courtesy of SOAS.

dhotis, and some were wearing whole outfits of stitched cloth.

Women's draped dress appears to have been undifferentiated from men's in early Vedic times, but the lower and upper cloths later gave way to the single length of draped cloth, nowadays known as the sari. This transformation is thought to have taken place by the late Vedic period (cf. Joshi 1993: 218). The sari, still the most popular form of women's dress in India today, was worn by being wrapped around the lower body with one end draped over the upper body. Later it was also manipulated to cover the head and sometimes the face. It was generally made from cotton or silk and decorated by dyeing, printing and/or embroidering. By the late nineteenth century many educated urban women and some rural women had added blouses and underskirts to their saris. The most striking feature of the *dhoti*, sari, *chadar* and *pugri* was that they were worn entirely by draping and tucking, and their manufacture required neither tailoring nor stitching.

Stitched clothes
Contrary to the popular belief that stitched clothes were first brought to India in the medieval period by Muslims, there is in fact evidence that some Indian women were wearing stitched skirts (*ghaghras*), bodices (*cholis*) and head-cloths (*odhnis*) even as early as the eleventh century BC (Joshi 1993: 219). Similarly, some Indian men, particularly in parts of northern and western India, were wearing stitched tunics and trousers many centuries before the Muslim conquest. The comparatively limited range of stitched clothes available in pre-medieval India was, however, greatly expanded during the Sultanate and Moghul periods when various types of trousers, robes and tunics gained in popularity (Chaudhuri 1976: 51). By the nineteenth century a long-sleeved outer robe (*jama*, *angarkha*) or tunic (*kurta*) worn with trousers (*pyjamas*) had become the acceptable outfit for an educated Indian man in public, if not in private. Muslim women generally wore a veil (*dupatta*), a long tunic (*kamiz*) with trousers (*shalwar*) or the wide flared skirt-like trouser (*gharara*). Following the Muslim conquest of northern India, many Hindu women gradually adopted such dress, eventually making it the regional style for parts of Northern India.[4]

The distinction between draped and stitched clothing has often been treated as if it were a distinction between 'Hindu' and 'Muslim' dress (cf. Bayly 1986, Cohn 1989). Certainly some Hindus, accustomed to wearing draped clothes, opposed the introduction of tailored garments on the grounds that they were ritually defiling (cf. Watson 1866: 11, Chaudhuri

4 The *shalwar kamiz* is often known by the name 'Punjabi dress'.

1976, Bayly 1986). Uncut, unstitched cloth was considered less permeable to pollution and was preferred for all ritual performances. Many of the Hindu men who wore stitched clothes to work during the Moghul period would change back into draped garments before re-entering the sacred space of their own homes (*ibid.*).

However, this practice does not confirm the notion that there were once clear-cut religious orders of clothing. There is no clear evidence of an ancient Hindu injunction against stitched clothes, and it therefore seems likely that certain Hindus used religious arguments as a means of preserving their favoured dress and preventing the widespread acceptance of stitched garments (Chaudhuri 1976: 52). Meanwhile certain Muslims used the plea of Islamic moral decency in their attempts to convert Hindus to stitched clothes. As we have seen, stitched garments were already worn in India before the Muslim invasions, when they were not regarded as 'Muslim dress', which suggests that their designation as 'Muslim' was indeed a later interpretation which Hindus used as a justification for sartorial resistance.[5] By the late nineteenth century many educated Hindu families regarded stitched clothes as superior to the comparatively scanty *dhoti*. While in religious contexts they saw them as defiling,[6] in secular contexts they saw them as proof of educational advancement and sophistication.

This association of tailored garments with advancement and sophistication was to gain further importance with the arrival of European styles introduced principally by European traders, missionaries and colonial administrators. European dress differed from most forms of Indian dress in the way it was cut, stitched and shaped to the contours of the body.[7] Gender differences were also strongly demarcated in European dress, with women's skirts and dresses giving them a distinctive and exaggeratedly curvaceous outline in relation to the more linear forms of men's dress.

In comparison to most Indian styles, European dress appeared physically

5 The arbitrary nature of 'religious' differentiation in dress is perhaps best demonstrated by the observation that in the plains Hindus used to fasten their outer robes to the right and Muslims to the left, whereas in North India the practice was generally reversed (Crooke 1906: 163). This suggests that the *fact* of differentiation was more important than the specific *form* these differences took. Furthermore, differentiation worked on a number of levels; hence poor Muslims wore *dhotis* like poor Hindus (Watson 1866: 21), whereas the male élite, both Hindu and Muslim, often shared the same or similar stitched styles.

6 Hinduism is not alone in advocating the use of draped clothing in ritual contexts. The Muslim pilgrim is forbidden to wear stitched clothes and dons two pieces of white cloth, known as *ihram* (holy, consecrated) dress for great and lesser pilgrimages (*Encyclopaedia of Islam* 1971, vol. 3: 1052–3).

7 For an analysis of the distinctive differences between European and other clothing traditions, see N. Tarrant, 1994.

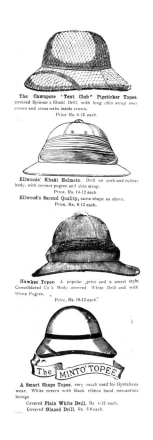

The Cawnpore "Tent Club" Pigsticker Topee. covered Spinner's Khaki Drill, with long chin strap over crown and cross webs inside crown.
Price Rs. 4-12 each.

Ellwoods' Khaki Helmets. Drill on cork and rubber body, with correct pugree and chin strap.
Price, Rs. 14-12 each.
Ellwood's Second Quality, same shape as above.
Price, Rs. 8-12 each.

Hawkes' Topee. A popular price and a smart style. Consolidated Co.'s Body, covered White Drill and with White Pugree.
Price, Rs. 15-12 each.

The MINTO TOPEE.

A Smart Shape Topee, very much used for Gymkhana wear. White covers with black ribbon band, non-actinic linings
Covered Plain White Drill, Rs. 4-12 each.
Covered Glazed Drill, Rs. 5-8 each.

Fig. 2.6 (*above and opposite*) Selection of *sola topis*, reproduced from *Whiteaway* 1911 (op. cit.). Such 'topees' were worn principally by British and Eurasian men and came to symbolise the authority of the British Raj.

TERMS CASH. "WHITEAWAYS, BOMBAY."

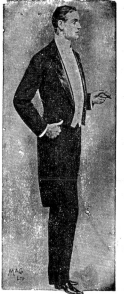

Dress Suit.

Dress Wear.

Exceptional light weight materials have been secured this season with just enough body to give the correct hang so desirable in Dinner or Full Dress Jackets. Every care is taken in the lowest as well as the first quality to see that only work of a

FIRST CLASS FINISH

is allowed to leave the premises. We specialize in

VICUNAS AND COATINGS

in tropical weights.

PRICES.

Semi Dress from Rs. 62 the suit.
Silk lining extra.

Dress Suit from Rs. 65-8.
Silk lining extra

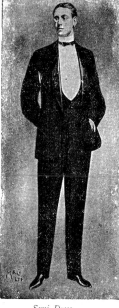

Semi Dress.

Mess Kit.

Sound value in Washing Whites, smartly cut from good wearing material is our aim in this section. That we have succeeded can be seen by the numerous clients we have all over India.

PRICES:

Mess Suits.

Rs. 10-8, 12-8, 14-8.

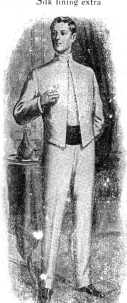

Light Weight Suits.

Pure Silk, Tussorette, or White Suits are a leading feature of our tailoring trade. The China Silks are wonderful, and cannot be equalled. Full range of samples, plainly marked, can be had at any time post free.

PRICES:

Silk Suits, Rs. 35-8 to Rs. 45-8.

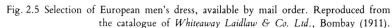
WHITEAWAY, LAIDLAW & CO. LD. POST BOX 220. BOMBAY.

Fig. 2.5 Selection of European men's dress, available by mail order. Reproduced from the catalogue of *Whiteaway Laidlaw & Co. Ltd.*, Bombay (1911).

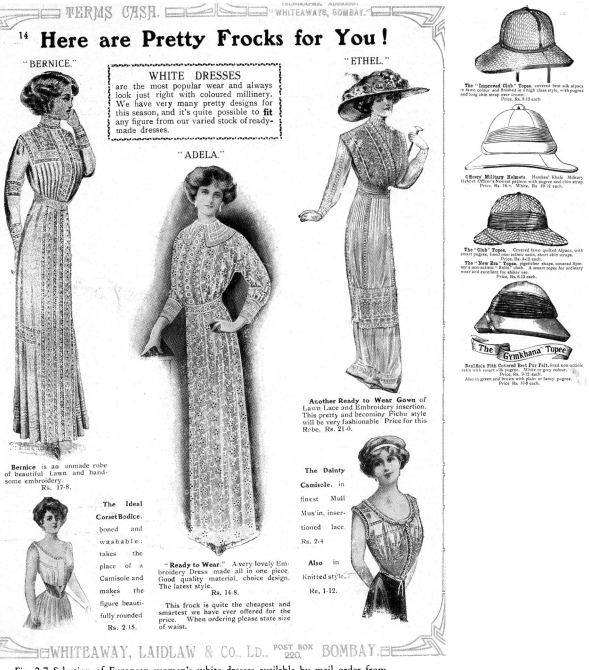

¹⁴ Here are Pretty Frocks for You !

"BERNICE."

WHITE DRESSES
are the most popular wear and always look just right with coloured millinery. We have very many pretty designs for this season, and it's quite possible to **fit** any figure from our varied stock of ready-made dresses.

"ETHEL."

"ADELA."

The "Improved Club" Topee, covered best silk alpaca in fawn colour and finished in a high class style, with pugree and long chin strap over crown. Price, Rs. 5-12 each.

Officers' Military Helmets. Hawkes' Khaki Military Helmet. Officer's Newest pattern with pugree and chin strap. Price, Rs. 18-8. White, Rs 18-12 each.

The "Club" Topee. Covered fawn quilted Alpaca, with smart pugree, lined non-actinic satin, short chin straps. Price, Rs. 3-12 each.
The "New Era" Topee, pigsticker shape, covered Spinner's non-actinic "Solio" cloth. A smart topee for ordinary wear and excellent for shikar use. Price, Rs. 6-12 each.

The "Gymkhana" Topee

Real Sola Pith Covered Best Fur Felt, lined non-actinic satin with smart silk pugree. White or grey colour. Price, Rs. 9-12 each. Also in green and brown with plain or fancy pugree. Price Rs. 10-8 each.

Another Ready to Wear Gown of Lawn Lace and Embroidery insertion. This pretty and becoming Fichu style will be very fashionable Price for this Robe, Rs. 21-0.

Bernice is an unmade robe of beautiful Lawn and handsome embroidery. Rs. 17-8.

The Dainty

Camisole, in

finest Mull

Muslin, insertioned lace.

Rs. 2-4

Also in

Knitted style."

Re. 1-12.

The Ideal

Corset Bodice,

boned and

washable ;

takes the

place of a

Camisole and

makes the

figure beautifully rounded

Rs. 2-15.

"**Ready to Wear.**" A very lovely Embroidery Dress made all in one piece. Good quality material, choice design. The latest style. Rs. 14-8.

This frock is quite the cheapest and smartest we have ever offered for the price. When ordering please state size of waist.

WHITEAWAY, LAIDLAW & CO., LD., POST BOX 220. BOMBAY.

Fig. 2.7 Selection of European women's white dresses available by mail order from Bombay in 1911. Virginal white was popular among British women but not with many Indian women, being associated with widowhood. From *Whiteaway* (op. cit.).

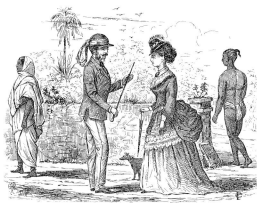

Fig. 2.8 New Arrivals
Mr Griffin: 'Well Miss Green, what are your impressions of the manners and customs of the natives?'
Miss Green: 'I have not been sufficiently long in the country to judge, but the costume is really charming, somewhat scanty perhaps: but so *picturesque*, so *graceful*, don't *you* think?'
Mr Griffin: 'Hem! It strikes me at times as being rather *dis*-graceful!'
N.B. Miss Green is looking *one* way, and Mr Griffin the *other!!!*
Reproduced from *The Indian Charivari*, 19 Sept. 1873. Courtesy of OIOC.

restrictive and was often ill-adapted to the Indian climate. This was particularly true of the types of dress worn in official circles on public occasions where practicality and comfort had to yield before the rigours of formality. None the less, some attempts were made by the British to adapt their daytime wardrobes to the Indian context while at the same time making sure that they did not lose their distinctively European style. The use of light-coloured linen suits for the summer and lightweight woollen fabrics in the winter were examples of such adaptations. More radical was the invention of a new form of hat, specially designed in the 1840s to protect imperial heads from the torturous rays of the tropical sun. Made from the pith of the sola plant, this light but bulbous hat was initially called a *sola topi* (pith helmet), but its function soon got confused with its fabric and it became known to many as the solar *topi* (cf. Cohn 1983a: 103). By the late nineteenth century it was worn fastidiously by European men in India and slightly less by the women and children, who often wore fancier versions. It was the distinctive nature of various forms of European headwear that inspired Indians to refer to Europeans as *topi walas* (hat-wearing people).

The problem of how to obtain and maintain a fashionable European wardrobe in India was one that caused the British some anxiety. They could consult catalogues and read books of advice before crossing the ocean, but they still had to face the problem of letting their clothes get into the hands of local washermen, with the latter's alien washing techniques. Not only did clothes have to be maintained but they also had to be transported, often in difficult circumstances where the officers concerned would not be able to obtain substitutes in case of a mishap. If necessary, Europeans could of course resort to local tailors, but it seems that, given the choice, they prefer-

Searching for a Solution in the late Nineteenth Century

red to order the genuine article from abroad. Authentic European men's clothes, owing partly no doubt to their rarity and partly to their associations with the ruling élite, fetched high prices when they entered local Indian markets as secondhand rejects. It is with an understanding of the distinctiveness and exclusivity of European styles that we can better understand not only how Indians reacted to European dress but also how the British reacted to Indian dress.

BRITISH ATTITUDES TO INDIAN AND EUROPEAN DRESS

B. Cohn has pointed out how Europeans, arriving in India for the first time, were invariably shocked by the 'nakedness' of the loinclothed Indian boatmen (Cohn 1990: 331). Fig. 2.8 portrays two stereotyped British reactions to Indian dress. The notion of the 'graceful' (or picturesque) and the 'disgraceful' (or indecent) were in fact frequently applied to both male and female attire. Where men's dress was concerned, the 'graceful' referred to the stitched robes worn by the Indian élite and the 'disgraceful' to the draped clothing popular among vast sections of the Indian population. In other words, subsumed within these two categories was a European assessment of most of the types of clothing worn by Indian men. We should therefore look briefly at just what such assessments implied.

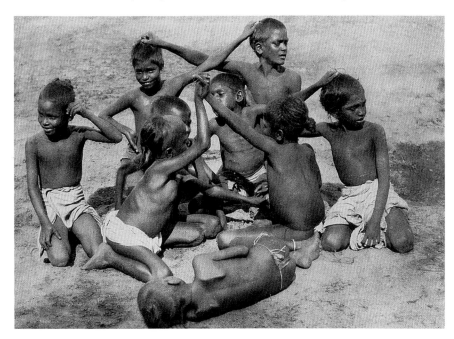

Fig. 2.9 Hindu children playing, revealing the nakedness that so shocked Europeans in India. Reproduced from H.V. Glasenapp's *Indien*, 1925. Courtesy of SOAS.

The 'disgraceful' sight of the loinclothed boatmen was not merely shocking to Europeans. It also confirmed their notion of the evolutionary inferiority of the Indian race – of its backwardness and barbarism. Furthermore, it revealed the blackness of the skin which was in itself regarded as a biological sign of racial inferiority. The effects of such a sight have been graphically described by Lieut.-Col. John Briggs in a letter to a young British man. Briggs's intention was to warn the novice about the strangeness of Indian customs which he defended on the grounds of cultural relativism and 'ignorance'. Describing the Madras boatmen, he wrote:

> To the European the sight is hardly human, to see a black animal kneeling on three bits of wood, connected only with the fibres of a coconut, paddling away alone several miles from land. . . .
>
> What then must be the feelings of a person, landing fresh from London, without having witnessed any intermediate state of society between the height of European civilization in the finest city in the universe, and that to which he is so suddenly brought! (Briggs 1828: 26–8).

The notion of the 'gracefulness' of Indian men's dress held more ambiguous connotations. On the one hand, the term 'graceful' was clearly a sign of appreciation and many British men and women were impressed by the flowing nature of Indian robes (cf. Crooke 1906: 163, E. F. Elwin 1907: 44). On the other hand, it implied unmanliness. As Briggs put it, the male Indian élite 'are habited in long flowing linen robes, giving them in our eyes, an air of effeminacy' (Briggs 1828: 28). The terms 'effeminate' and 'childlike' were frequently used by the British to describe the clothes of the Indian élite, particularly the elaborate and colourful combinations worn by the maharajahs (for an example see Steevens 1899: 121–3). Such designations were part of a more general process by which the politically dominant group tried to define the Indian male as powerless and subordinate in his own country. Ashis Nandy has highlighted the homology between political and sexual dominance which became increasingly important to the British as their power in India increased (cf. Nandy 1983: 4–11). When the British described Indian men's clothes as 'pretty' (Stuart 1809: 152), 'graceful' (Crooke 1906: 163, Elwin 1907: 44) and 'effeminate' (Briggs *loc. cit.*) they simultaneously denigrated Indian men to the unenviable status of their own women, whom they perceived as attractive, pretty, dignified even, but largely irrelevant to serious political concerns. British attitudes to Indian dress therefore revealed their attitudes towards Indians in general.

Since my intention is to demonstrate the heterogeneity of Indian responses to European dress, it is perhaps unfair that I should speak of British attitudes as though they formed a homogeneous view. Clearly, if I were to examine the full gamut of British responses to Indian dress in the nineteenth century, I would find some variety. There were some Britons who appreciated differences in dress without assuming the superiority of European styles (cf. Shore 1837, Billington 1973 [1895]). Others actively sought to revive Indian dress in an attempt to protect a threatened culture and aesthetic (cf. Birdwood 1880; repr. 1988: 244, Havell 1912: 21–4). But the aim here is to expose the characteristics of the dominant racist stereotype rather than the views of the sympathetic minority. Furthermore this stereotype was so widely expressed in British diaries, novels, newspapers and political cartoons that it came to represent something akin to a shared imperialist view. This was increasingly the case in the nineteenth century. Whereas in earlier times British travellers mingled to some extent with Indians, the men often settling with Indian women and adopting at least some Indian customs (Bayly 1990: 73), by the nineteenth century British civil servants were increasingly expected to conform to a well-defined set of social values and codes of conduct. What had been a scattered and heterogeneous group of European merchants and entrepreneurs leading individualistic lives gradually became a more structured body of British political authority, the credibility of which rested to some extent on its ability to present a cohesive official view. According to this view, the British were superior beings and Indians inferiors. Furthermore the British, through improving 'native' behaviour and customs, felt that they could enable Indians to better themselves. The 'graceful' and, more particularly, the 'disgraceful' nature of Indian clothes acted for the British not only as proof of Indian effeminacy and barbarism but also as a justification for their civilising presence in India.[8]

Like British attitudes and policies, British clothes became, over time, increasingly homogeneous. Early European travellers in India were, it seems, comparatively free to choose their own clothing styles, and often adapted or discarded their heavy European attire in quest of clothes more suitable to Indian customs and climate (Bayly 1990: 73, Dar 1969: 73). Woodruff for example describes seventeenth-century British traders in Surat as wearing 'fine white linen coats', girdles, scarves, turbans and 'moorman's

---

8   The desire to 'civilise' the native's dress was particularly apparent in missionary activities where the naked were often quite literally clothed (cf. Cohn 1983a: 78–87). Elwin, a Poona missionary, aware of the problems of imposing European dress, wrote that 'people have sometimes sarcastically spoken of the spread of Christianity amongst the heathen as being made a matter of trousers' (E. F. Elwin 1907: 43). Elwin himself felt that 'advancing refinement and civilization' was producing in Indians 'an instinctive desire to be more fully clothed' (ibid.: 43). Ultimately, however, he favoured the idea that Christian converts should be clearly distinguishable from Hindus. It was therefore 'advisable for them to adopt trousers' (ibid.: 44).

trousers' (cited in Dar 1969: 73). From paintings and descriptions it seems that most British men who chose to adopt Indian styles favoured loose stitched garments of cotton and silk to which they sometimes added European touches such as buttons and shoes.

As the British consolidated their political dominance in India in the early nineteenth century, the wearing of Indian styles became increasingly unacceptable. It was seen as a 'sign of eccentricity' and even a 'cause of discredit' (Bayly 1990: 110). In 1830 legislation was introduced banning employees of the East India Company from wearing Indian dress at public functions (Cohn 1989: 310). Even in private, the British adhered increasingly to the sartorial standards of Europe. Those who became 'de-Europeanised' through 'long residence among undomesticated natives' were referred to disparagingly by Lord Lytton as 'white baboos'[9] (Yule and Burnell 1903: 44).

The Europeanisation of British public and domestic life was part of the wider process through which the British came to distance themselves increasingly from their Indian subjects (cf. Cohn 1989, Nandy 1983). Maintenance of differences through dress and other social customs was important both for British self-esteem and as a means of demonstrating British superiority to an Indian audience. Briggs described its importance as follows:

... yet we should always preserve the European; for to adopt their [Indian] manners is a departure from the very principle on which every impression of our superiority, that rests upon good foundation, is founded.... The European officer who assumes native manners and usages may please a few individuals, who are flattered or profited by his departure from the habits of his country; but even with these, familiarity will not be found to increase respect, and the adoption of such a course will be sure to sink him in the estimation of the mass of the community, both European and native, among whom he resides (Briggs 1828: 201).

Thus, along with the positive – the sense of security gained by maintaining sartorial standards – went the negative: fear that failure to maintain those standards could result in a British man sinking or being morally weakened.

---

9 The Bengali term 'baboo' was originally used as a term of respect attached to a person's name. It was reserved for men of distinction, but by the late nineteenth century the British frequently used it on its own. Used thus, it took on a negative connotation with insulting implications. It referred to what the British described as the 'superficially cultivated', ambitious, semi-anglicised, educated and 'effeminate' Bengali man, and was often used to refer to those native clerks who wrote English (Yule and Burnell 1903: 44). When Lytton accused Indianised Europeans of being 'white baboos' he was referring to their hybrid nature, an unsatisfactory mixture of the negative aspects of both races.

Searching for a Solution in the late Nineteenth Century

It was essentially a fear that members of this small white minority might somehow be absorbed or at least tainted by the mass of Indians around them. Maintaining British standards of dress was a means of avoiding such deterioration. It became important for the Englishman in India to prove that he was as English as his fellows at home. If foreign influences were detected in his dress when he returned to England, they would be viewed critically. Woodruff tells how Hickey's 'gay coats caused so much talk when he first went home that he had to discard them' (cited in Dar 1969: 74).

This need to preserve impeccable British standards frequently featured in Anglo-Indian literature and journals. In 1873 the satirical journal *The Indian Charivari* published a column entitled 'Hints on Modern Etiquette'. In it, the fictional Lord Lushingslop warned his son of the sartorial perils of serving in India, 'a land so deplorably far from the centre of civilization'. He urged:

> Nothing can be worse taste than to adopt unhesitatingly the manners and customs of a strange country. An English gentleman should *always* be dressed, so that, were he suddenly dropped into Bond Street, he would pass *unnoticed* in the crowd (*The Indian Charivari* 27 June 1873).

While such extracts betray a certain humour concerning dress, other accounts reveal the essential seriousness with which the British in India regarded their clothes. Aldous Huxley, for example, noticed the British civil servant's obsession with sartorial rituals even as late as the 1930s when such customs were no longer considered so important in England. He observed:

> From the Viceroy to the young clerk who, at home, consumes high tea at sunset, every Englishman in India solemnly dresses. It is as though the integrity of the British Empire depended in some directly magical way upon the donning of black jackets and hard-boiled shirts (cited in Alexander 1987: 268).

Huxley astutely recognised the British psychological dependence on such rituals.[10] One civil servant, Kenneth Warren, posted to an isolated out-post in Upper Assam, has left a revealing account of just what they meant for him:

> If you lost your self-respect you were not looked upon in a respectful manner. So in order to maintain my self-respect I put on a dinner jacket and dressed for dinner and I said to my servants, who were quite likely to get a bit slack just looking after a man by himself in the middle of

---

10 I have recently come across Helen Callaway's article 'Dressing for Dinner in the Bush', which gives some excellent Indian and African examples of how the British depended on such rituals, and a fuller analysis than I have space for here (cf. Barnes and Eicher 1993).

the jungle, 'Now this is a dinner party and every night is a dinner party and you will serve dinner as though there are other people at the dinner table' (cited in Allen 1985: 62).

Naturally, retaining such levels of Britishness was a physical strain at times. In remote areas European clothes and the facilities for maintaining them were not easily available. Added to this was the inconvenience caused by their extreme unsuitability to the Indian climate. Not even children were exempt from wearing excessive layers of elaborate clothing in the afternoons (Allen 1985: 13). Women too complained of suffocating customs such as wearing kid or suede gloves at public functions in the heat of the mid-day sun (Barwell 1960: 109). Failure to abide by such rules could incur the risk of being asked to leave.

British obsession over dress related not only to social and psychological factors but also to their perceptions of the physical environment. The combination of alien customs and climate induced a fear of the unknown, and clothes provided an important means of physical as well as psychological protection. Cohn has written at some length about the development of British theories on the relationship between clothing and the prevention of tropical diseases (Cohn 1983a: 88–111). In particular Britons of both sexes were recommended to wear flannel underwear rather than linen since flannel, being a slow conductor of heat, was thought to guard the body against sudden changes in the atmosphere (*ibid.*: 1983a: 94). By the mid to late nineteenth century they were also recommended to wear their *sola topis* whenever they went out of doors.[11] The *topi* not only protected them from the much-feared sun, but it also provided a distinctive type of head-wear, which made them – men, women and children alike – immediately recognisable as European.

To understand the political dimension of British clothing habits, it is necessary to examine not only British clothes but also British policy more generally. Why should the British have chosen to emphasise their social distance from Indians at precisely the time when they were apparently lessening the gap between British and Indian customs through advocating European education in India? In order to appreciate the British need to develop sartorial distance, developments in Indian men's dress in the same period also need to be examined. Throughout the nineteenth century, while the British were intensifying their Britishness, members of the Indian élite were beginning to adopt various articles of European dress, and a few

11 If caught outside without their *topis*, BORs ('British Other Ranks') were confined to barracks for fourteen days (Allen 1985: 37).

adopted an entirely European image. The sartorial fastidiousness that developed among the British therefore coincided with, and was by no means unrelated to, the adoption of European dress by Indians. The fact that some Indian men were coming to look increasingly like Europeans actually had the effect of encouraging the British to make their own sense of sartorial correctness more rigid. In so doing they continually made their clothes and their accompanying rituals less accessible to the Indian élite. They were trying to escape 'imitation'.

The British desire to differentiate themselves from Indians was thus the opposite side of the coin from the Indian desire to integrate with the British. Similarly, the British fear of 'sinking' was inextricably linked to their fear of Indians 'rising'.

Civilisation by degrees: British attempts to control Indian dress
Indian dress posed not merely a clothing dilemma but also an ethical dilemma for the British. On the one hand they felt it their duty to civilise barbaric natives and rescue them from their own primitiveness. It was with such notions of 'improvement' in mind that Captain Johnstone clothed the 'naked savages' of the Juang hills (see Preface). But on the other hand the British did not want these natives to become *too* civilised. Captain Johnstone, for example, clothed them in Manchester saris, not European styles. If the British wanted to offer India the raiment of civilisation, it was civilisation with a cut-off point above which Indians were not supposed to climb.

The problem of how to clothe the Indian was further linked to the pro-

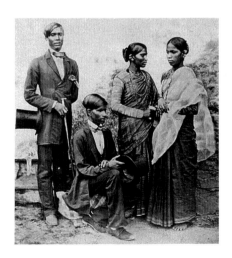

Fig. 2.10 'Goanese Christians' who have clearly experienced the 'civilizing' influence of Europeans. Note that the men wear full European dress while the women have retained Indian styles. European missionaries were mixed in their opinions as to whether or not Indian Christians should adopt European dress, an ambivalence reflected in the sarcastic saying that the spread of Christianity had become 'a matter of trousers' (Elwin 1907:43). Reproduced from W. Johnson's *The Oriental Races and Tribes, Residents and Visitors of Bombay*, vol. 2, (1866). Courtesy of Chris Pinney.

blem of the British economy. Although the British did not want Indians to adopt European styles, they did want them to buy and wear British manufactured textiles. By the late eighteenth century, Britain had developed sufficient technology in machine-spinning and weaving to produce large quantities of cheap cotton textiles for home use and for export. Previously, cotton textiles had been imported from India but from this time onwards Britain's need for Indian hand-woven textiles diminished. Its interests now lay in importing raw cotton which it could then export back to India in the form of cloth, spun and woven by machine in Britain.[12] But in order to produce textiles for the Indian market the British had to decide on the type of textiles they wished the Indian to wear. The choice was not entirely theirs, since the majority of rural Indians were conservative in their tastes.

British interests and intentions were carefully codified in John Forbes Watson's famous work *The Textile Manufactures and Costumes of the People of India* (1866). It was accompanied by eighteen volumes containing 700 'working specimens' of Indian textiles. These were to be regarded as 'Industrial museums' that would enable British manufacturers to study Indian tastes and imitate indigenous designs. Watson wrote: 'India is in a position to become a magnificent customer. . . . *What is wanted and what to be copied to meet that want*, is thus accessible for study in these museums' (Watson 1866: 2–3, his emphasis). He pointed out that most of the clothes worn by the poorer sections of Indian society consisted of unstitched pieces of cloth. It was these 'plainer cheaper stuffs' worn by the 'hundreds and millions of lower grades' that the British should imitate (*ibid.*: 7). The more complex and elaborate garments worn by wealthy Indians were not, however, worth imitating since they could not be produced cheaply in England.

The British were successful in capturing a large proportion of the Indian demand for cotton textiles.[13] Aided by Indian conservatism, they could supply clothes for the Indian 'lower grades', and in doing so they could simultaneously keep the Indian masses looking suitably Indian. But it was more difficult to control the clothes of the Indian élite. Furthermore it was this small educated minority, not the Indian masses, that posed a threat to the British since it consisted of the most anglicised Indians who came dangerously close to integrating themselves with the ruling British élite.

The British had of course invented their own problem. It was succinctly

---

12   For a concise account of the history of Indian and British textile relations, see Swallow 1982, Bean 1989. For detailed historical accounts see Irwin and Schwartz 1966, B. Chandra 1966.
13   Between 1849 and 1889 the value of British cotton cloth exports to India increased from just over £2m. a year to just under £27m. a year (Bean 1989: 362).

Searching for a Solution in the late Nineteenth Century

expressed in Macaulay's famous 'Minute on Education' (1835). Macaulay, who favoured the introduction of European education in India, argued the need for 'a class who may be interpreters between us and the millions whom we govern; a class of persons, Indian in blood and colour, but English in taste, in opinions, in morals and in intellect' (cited in Vittachi 1987: 36). The inevitable consequence of such a policy was the narrowing of the cultural divide between the British and the educated Indian élite. The British attempted to subdue this uncomfortable closeness not only by increasing the rigidity of their own dress codes, but also by trying to limit the Indian adoption of Western styles (Chaudhuri 1976: 58, Cohn 1989). The idea was to keep differences apparent. An incident in the life of Madhusudan Datta reveals this process of racial differentiation at work. Datta had been sent to Bishop's College in Calcutta, where he was given a Western education and developed the Western tastes that Macaulay so recommended. Yet he was discouraged from sharing the college uniform of his fellows. Krishnamohan Bandyopadhay recalls:

> The ecclesiastical authorities had an idea at the time that natives in India should not be encouraged to imitate the English dress – the tail coat and the beaver hat. It would have been infinitely better if they had not interfered with questions beyond their province – for it was this interference that goaded a fiery spirit like Datta's into an obstinate resistance. The collegiate costume was a black cassock and band and the square cap.... The authorities wished him to put on a white cassock instead of black. Datta said, *either collegiate costume or his own national dress* (cited in Radice 1986: 202).

Datta, playing the British at their own game, appeared in college dressed in an elaborate Indian outfit of white silk with a highly colourful turban and shawl. The authorities, who felt this was embarrassingly like 'fancy dress', were finally forced to allow him to wear the ordinary uniform (*ibid.*). But the fact that he had to fight for such a basic right highlights the peculiarly self-centred aspect of British policies for 'improving' the Indian. As Macaulay's speech made clear, the British needed educated anglicised Indians as 'interpreters'. They were therefore willing to share their education system, but not their physical identity, with the Indian. As Chaudhuri put it:

> The Englishman in India ... considered his way of life superior to every other ... but was wholly opposed to sharing its higher or more respec-table features with anybody who was not to the manner born.... They were violently repelled by English in our mouths, and even more violently by English clothes on our backs (Chaudhuri 1976: 57–8).

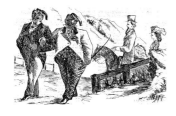

Fig. 2.11 Our 'Wallahs'.
1st Wallah 'Who's that old
bloke?' *2nd Wallah* 'Oh, he's
only the fellow that educated
me. He's devilish low, but I'm
obliged to notice him. Though
between ourselves, if it wasn't for
his daughters, I'd be inclined to
snub the old fool.' Reproduced
from *The Indian Charivari*, 18
Aug. 1876. Courtesy of OIOC.

Underlying this control of dress was a fear that the Indian male might be a little too successful in his 'imitation', and even rise above the very people who had enabled him to rise in the first place (fig. 2.11).

British attempts to control Indian dress were by no means limited to the sphere of education. Cohn has illustrated how the British chose to orientalise the uniform of the army and the official dress of the Maharajas (cf. Cohn 1989). They also laid down regulations concerning what Indians should wear for official and ceremonial occasions (see fig. 2.12, also Chaudhuri 1976: 58). Such legislative demands caused considerable tensions which often became manifest over the controversial issues of headwear and footwear (cf. Cohn 1989).

To summarise, the British authorities disliked Indian men wearing European dress, but regarded Indian dress as primitive. They wanted Indians to progress from barbarism, but not to the full heights of European civilisation. These preoccupations are perhaps best summarised in fig. 2.13. Not even the improved and educated Indian male is portrayed in full European dress. It is a blatantly racist portrait of how far the British were prepared to let the Indian 'advance'. But there were some Indians who were not prepared to accept the somewhat grudging offer of partial civilisation. It is to their divergent opinions and imaginative outfits that we now turn.

INDIAN ATTITUDES TO EUROPEAN DRESS

It is impossible to define an 'Indian view' of Western clothes. Indian reactions to 'the other' were neither as rigid nor as stereotyped as British ones. This is hardly surprising since the Indians who came into contact with or simply saw the peculiar white man with his strange apparel were from a variety of different religious, educational and regional backgrounds. The British and their clothes were seen variously as peculiar, exotic, ugly, smart,

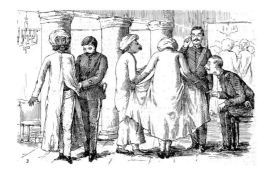

Fig. 2.12 Madras fashions
'We imagine something like the above will be necessary in the anti-chamber of Government House Madras, vide, the following notice, dated March 1876. "Hindu and Mahomedan gentlemen . . . are requested to observe the following instructions with regard to dress:- The head dress should consist of a turban. The external dress should be a long robe; a waist-band or girdle should be worn under or over the robe; and the lower limbs should be carefully covered . . ." '
Reproduced from *The Indian Charivari*, 14 April 1876. Courtesy of OIOC.

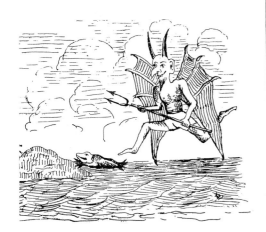

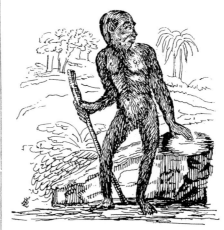

1st Geological Period.

First Protoplasm, shapeless thing,
From which all Human kind did spring;
A spirit, jealous at the sight,
Gave it a kick, just out of spite, *

* Note.—See introduction to Moore's "Lalla Rookh."

2nd Period.

Now Protoplasm lives on dry land,
"Baboon" he's called, with club in hand;
Baboons, however, talking shirk,
For fear they might be made to work!

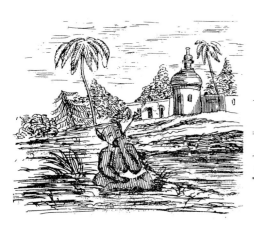

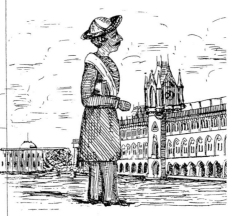

3rd Period.

Immense improvement now he shows,
He takes on human shape, and woes;
He drops the "n," and tail at once,
And calls himself "Baboo the dunce."

4th, or Modern Period.

The scanty dress he used to use,
He now casts off for pants and shoes;
From "dunce" to scholar, man of parts,
He's changed, and "Master" is of "Arts."
This, and more titles all combined,
In Baboos of our day you'll find.

Fig. 2.13 'Origin of Species' or Improvement by 'Natural Selection' after Darwin. Reproduced from *The Indian Charivari*, 9 Jan. 1874. Courtesy of OIOC.

funny, sacrilegious and unclean. Many saw them as civilised but rarely, it would appear, did they find them beautiful. The fascination with European garments was related more to what they represented than to either their practicality or their aesthetic appeal.

People's attitudes to European styles varied to some extent according to the closeness of their contact with Europeans. In areas with a strong missionary influence such as parts of South India, or with a strong British presence such as Calcutta, Western clothes were more available and were more rapidly adopted than in other parts of India. In many rural areas the inhabitants had little contact either with Europeans or with their dress. Where such contact was minimal, European clothes were seldom adopted, although European manufactured cloth was often worn in Indian styles.

There were plenty of reasons why Indians might not have wanted to adopt European dress. It was heavy, restrictive, unsuitable to India's climate, expensive by comparison to Indian dress and comparatively difficult to obtain. Furthermore, Western clothes did not fit into the existing classifications of appropriate caste, regional or religious styles. A number of Hindus felt that dressing in European clothes, like eating foreign food or travelling abroad, was a violation of caste. Those who succumbed to such foreign influences risked being excommunicated. Certainly many of the first Indians who crossed the seas to Europe and returned with the unclean foreigner's customs and dress were regarded as a category apart from other Hindus. They became known as the 'England-returneds', a sort of ritually impure group with a peculiarly high status in secular terms.

There were other risks in adopting European dress. It not only made an Indian man look different from his fellows, but meant that he also behaved differently. With the clothes of the European came a whole new etiquette which often conflicted with accepted Indian ideas of respectable behaviour. This was particularly clear with rituals surrounding head- and footwear (cf. Cohn 1989). Whereas Indians normally removed their shoes on entering a building, the British kept theirs on. They thought naked feet disgusting while Indians thought shoes inside the house polluting. Similarly, the Indian idea that the head should be covered as a sign of respect[14] conflicted with the British idea that a man should uncover his head for the

14 Cohn discusses these differences in terms of a clash of cosmologies. He shows how the functionalist British failed to recognise the symbolic importance of the head and feet in Hindu thought. He suggests that the head, as the seat of pure substance and knowledge, and the feet as the seat of pollution, required covering in Hinduism (Cohn 1989: 346). This is undoubtedly so, although it should also be noted that the British too perceived the head as the locus of knowledge and viewed their own headwear in more than functional terms.

same reason. The adoption of European dress was not therefore merely a sartorial concern, but involved changes in lifestyle and values. A man in a suit would not for example sit on the floor Indian-fashion or eat with his hands. He would expect his house or at least his quarters of the house to be equipped with the appropriate furniture to suit his clothes. But the adoption of all these foreign customs risked alienating a man from his own people and often invited criticism from them. It also widened the social distance of men from women, who generally retained Indian customs and manners even when their husbands adopted European modes.

The decision to adopt European dress was therefore a risky one, implying a change of identity and lifestyle. Yet the emergence of Western clothes in India could not be ignored by educated Indians any more than that of the British themselves, since British dress represented all the values which the British boasted: superiority, progress, decency, refinement, masculinity and civilisation. These values came to be shared by some men of the Indian élite, particularly those educated in the Western fashion. If they wanted to be modern and participate in this civilisation, wearing the correct clothes was surely one means of doing so.

Hence, the problem of whether or not to adopt Western clothes revolved around the conflict between two sets of values, an Indian set[15] and a European set, which seemed incompatible and irreconcilable. What was honourable and polite in one set was often dishonourable and impolite in the other. But for many there was no clear-cut boundary between Indian and Western dress. Rather, there was a gradual incorporation of Western elements. The problem of what to wear for élite Indian men in the nineteenth century can perhaps best be defined as the problem of how much foreignness to allow into one's clothes.

Some Indian solutions to the problem of what to wear

Foreign fabrics in Indian styles. The simplest and least controversial way to resolve the difficulty of how to modernise one's dress without appearing to desert one's 'traditional' identity was to adopt European fabrics but retain Indian styles. This option was common in towns and cities and to some extent in villages where cloth was hawked by itinerant traders. The British, as we have seen, had taken care to reproduce cloth of the Indian type in order

15 In speaking of an Indian set of values, the intention is not to imply that these values were in any way cohesive, or that they were necessarily perceived as 'Indian' by the people who held them. Within the Indian set of values were numerous smaller sets of values which could be more or less in conflict with each other. Yet in relation to the British, these other sets may be regarded as Indian.

to capture the popular market. By producing cheap machine-made versions of the finely textured fabrics previously worn only by the higher echelons of Indian society, they attracted enthusiastic customers (cf. Bayly 1986).

Although British cloth was made in the land of the 'unclean' foreigner, it does not appear to have been too tainted with the negative aspect of foreignness. Silberrad wrote of the United Provinces in 1898: 'There is hardly a trace of preference for hand-woven over machine-woven articles on caste or sentimental grounds' (Bayly 1986: 308). Quite the contrary, many were attracted to the new variety that foreign cloth offered. The aniline dyes used in Europe introduced a whole new range of colours which had an exotic appeal in India. According to Mary Frances Billington, it was sheer brightness that attracted buyers: 'It is the gaudiness of rose-pink, of emerald green, of royal blue, or amber-yellow which constitutes a leading attraction of our European piece-goods, and commends them to native purchasers when they are displayed in native bazaars' (Billington 1973 [1895]: 185–6).

For some, it was the very 'foreignness' of European cloth that made it appealing. The Ceylonese writer J. Vijayatunga has described his local people's excitement when European goods were hawked in his village by itinerant traders at the turn of the century. Their merchandise varied from cloth to safety pins to Pears soap. All of them had a special value because foreignness was itself a value: 'Among us anything that is better, or considered better, has the adjective *Rata* (signifying abroad) fixed to its name. ... The merchandise of Europe is definitely *Rata Badu* (abroad goods) and that is why they are better than good' (Vijayatunga 1970 [1935]: 38).

The decision to adopt European fabrics while retaining Indian styles was a particular favourite with Indian women, both rural and urban. Those women whose husbands adopted European dress rarely followed suit by adopting European women's styles, for these contravened ideas of female modesty and respect too grossly.[16] At most, Indian women added accessories such as shoes, blouses, petticoats and jackets to their Indian dress.[17] But while they retained the distinctive sari, they simultaneously followed European fashions in fabrics, colours and designs, thereby incorporating the latest trends from Europe and giving them a new Indian form. Documentation of this process may be found in the *Indian Ladies Magazine* (published in Madras), one of the first English-language journals for women in India. In the 1920s and 1930s it ran a weekly editorial in which contemporary

16 For the relationship between women's dress and notions of female modesty, see chapter 5.
17 The widespread adoption of the blouse was probably the most noticeable effect of British influences on Indian women's dress.

fashions were discussed and suitable clothes recommended to women readers. Sometimes Indian women were accused of imitating the West, thereby detracting 'from the grace of Indian dress and even looking ridiculous' (*ILM* 1934, VII, 1: 77). At other times they were encouraged to observe and incorporate Western trends within their saris (*ILM* 1930, III, 8: 380). Whether these women were thought to be too fashionable or insufficiently fashionable is less significant than the fact that the 'fashion' was always defined in Western terms. Through constant comparisons and suggestions, the *Indian Ladies Magazine* processed the latest ideas from Europe into a new Indian form, providing continual reassurance that the Indian woman could be fashionable without sacrificing her traditionalism.[18]

There were many men who followed a similarly safe solution to the problem of what to wear, not only adopting Western fabrics but also tailoring various Indian garments until they took on a European veneer. The historian Abdul Halim Sharar has provided a detailed account of the gradual incorporation of European elements into men's dress in northern India. He shows how the Persian cape (*balaba* or *chapkan*) was gradually given a more Indian form (*angarkha*), and finally developed into the *sherwani* which had buttons down the front, following the European fashion. In their early stages wealthy men's robes were made from the luxury fabrics of muslin and silk and often embroidered. But as they became more Europeanised, they became increasingly like the Englishman's frock coat, made from heavy dull material with less ornamentation and given tight sleeves (Sharar 1975: 169–70). Some men added a white shirt collar to the *sherwani* to complete the look (*ibid.*).

The Westernisation of Indian garments was a gradual and subtle process, far less controversial than the actual adoption of European garments themselves. It was, in a sense, a safe compromise. For Indian men it was a means of looking respectable without having to desert one's Indian identity. Furthermore, by eliminating the more elaborate aspects of their former attire,

---

18 Indian women's reluctance to adopt European styles was indicated in a debate that arose in the 1930s concerning what Indian women should wear for tennis. It was recognised that the sari was cumbersome and restricted movement, but the European woman's tennis frock was not thought decent for the Indian woman. Finally it was suggested that the Indian woman could wear 'a blouse and a fairly thick white skirt . . ., reaching about half way between ankles and knees, and a thin half-sari on top, held in place at the waist with a gold belt'. This, it was thought, would indicate 'the modesty of the sari' while at the same time allowing scope for movement (*ILM*: 1933, VI, 3: 146). Rather than reject suitable Indian styles, Indian women found means of adapting their habitual clothes to suit the occasion.

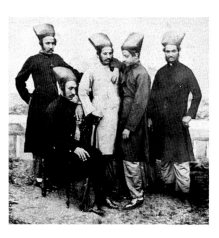

Fig. 2.14 Parsis in Bombay, wearing their distinctive headwear (*phenta*) with tailored collarless coats, baggy trousers and European-style boots. Reproduced from W. Johnson's *The Oriental Races and Tribes, Residents and Visitors of Bombay*, vol. 1, 1863. Courtesy of Chris Pinney.

Fig. 2.15 Village headmen from Ceylon (now Sri Lanka), wearing a mixture of Ceylonese and European garments. *Below*: Reproduced from W. Urwicks's *Indian Pictures drawn with Pen and Pencil*, 1891. *Opposite*: Reproduced from E. Schlaginweit's *Indien in Wort und Bild*, vol. 1, 1880. Courtesy of SOAS.

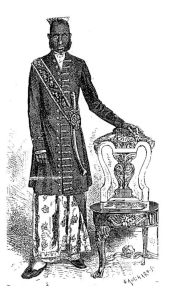

they could escape the accusation that they looked effeminate. Slim and tailored Indian garments were then a popular solution particularly among professional Indians who worked in the law courts in the mid to late nineteenth century. Such outfits were worn with the type of headwear (turban, *phenta*, cap) considered appropriate to an individual's social and religious standing. The British, as we have seen, admired this type of Indian professional dress since it was smart and decent without being too close to their own dress.

Mixing Indian and European garments. There were many Indians who wanted more than a European version of Indian dress. They wanted rather to adopt European garments themselves, not least because these appeared part and parcel of European civilisation. Some such men did not go the whole way but wore a mixture of both Indian and European garments simultaneously. In Bombay the wealthy Parsis (fig. 2.14) were probably the first men to adopt European shoes and trousers, which they wore with their own style of coat and distinctive Parsi hat (*phenta*). Umbrellas and watches also became important adjuncts to the outfit of the smart educated man.

In India's towns and occasionally the villages Maharajas and local élites also began to invent new combination outfits consisting of both Indian and European garments. The latter were not always easy to get hold of and this, combined with their expense, made them good status symbols that marked out a man's superiority and progressiveness to the local community (fig. 2.15). The status attached to such clothes in a small village has been humorously described in the following extract from Vijayatunga's essay 'White Man Passes Through' (first published in 1935):

It must not be supposed for a moment that we in our village are by

Searching for a Solution in the late Nineteenth Century

any means out of touch with Civilisation. Civilisation passes our way quite often, only it does not stop and stay with us. Nevertheless, we give Civilisation a very good scrutiny each time it passes us. . . .

Now and then the White Man himself flits past our village. Some half mile away beyond the bend of our road we hear the approach of his motorcycle. Then spluttering formidably, a cloud of dust in its trail, appears the Wondrous Machine and sitting astride it a figure whose head and face are hidden beneath a 'pig-sticker' topee. We are all eyes on the phenomenon. . . . we marvel at him and the Civilisation of which he is so marvellous a specimen.

The White Man then . . . is our standard. Once the standard is recognised and accepted, it is easy to emulate. . . .

. . . the President of the Village Tribunal . . . wears a white cotton suit of the so called European cut and wraps over his trousers a white cloth Sarong fashion in the native style, but leaving a good twelve inches of the trouser ends to be seen. Whether this is an additional respect for the European trousers or the covering up of a shameful lapse I have never fathomed, but all Gansabhava [village tribunal] Presidents, . . . in fact all the aristocrats and those who wish to pass as such . . . they all sport the mystic masonic all-round apron over their trousers.

Much as we appreciate the tranquility of our village, and its claims to distinction, we are even more thrilled by the knowledge that we are in touch with the secrets of Civilisation, that it flows past us and that we are not wholly isolated or ignored (Vijayatunga 1970: 32–4).

To the local élite of Vijayatunga's region, European dress was clearly a status symbol enabling them to distinguish themselves from the common people and participate in the mysteries of 'civilisation'. By wrapping a white *sarong* (wrap) over their trousers they were chosing what might be considered a diplomatic solution to the problem of what to wear, for they were able to express their acknowledgement and knowledge of both European and Ceylonese customs simultaneously. They could be modern without appearing to desert local tradition. Furthermore they did not have to worry about British reactions to their dress because their contact with the British was so minimal. Their reputation depended more on the opinions of members of the local community. If Vijayanutga's opinion is at all representative, the local community was impressed.

The adoption of a mixture of European and Indian clothes was extremely popular in India's cities, where European garments were readily available for purchasing or for copying. In particular Calcutta, the heart of British

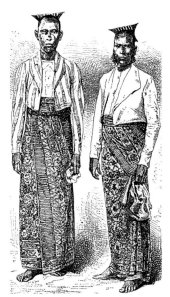

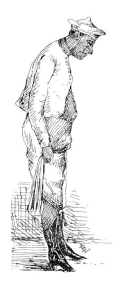

administration and home of many British residents, became the centre for these composite fashions. The various forms that such outfits took at the turn of the century have been described by Nirad Chaudhuri:

> In my boyhood the European dress-shirt in its stiff version was by itself a recognised formal wear for men. Wealthy people went to visit and even to parties in these shirts, looking very imposing with their starched fronts, gold diamond studs and links, sometimes a gold chain, and a very fine crinkled dhoti as diaphanous as the finest muslin, and also patent leather pumps with bows (Chaudhuri 1976: 6).

Other popular combinations described by Chaudhuri were the European coat worn over a *dhoti* with no shirt, and the European shirt worn without a collar or tie but with an embroidered shawl draped over the top (*ibid.*: 6–7). In other words, Bengali men invented their own new fashion which retained what they liked of Indian garments while adding what they admired from Europe. This enabled a man to be 'in fashion' without having to Westernise his appearance completely. Furthermore, it was an excellent solution for those Indians who could not afford full European dress. But one disadvantage of wearing such composite fashions was that they incited the disdain and ridicule of more conservative Bengalis and of the British. By the late nineteenth century, men who wore such hybrid outfits were often dismissed as 'baboos', their dress and language a constant source of ridicule in literature and the press (fig. 2.16).[19] One aspect of this British loathing of the 'baboo' was that he transgressed the boundary separating the British from the Indian — which, as we have seen, the British increasingly wished to maintain. Fears of the chaos that might ensue from the rise of unchecked baboodom are expressed in fig. 2.17, which portrays a reversal of Anglo-Indian societal norms when King Baboo takes the British throne.

The extent to which Indians were aware of British disdain and, for that matter, cared about it must have varied from individual to individual. But British mockery was difficult to ignore in a place like Calcutta where many Indians were actually employed as officials, clerks and bankers under the British. The fact that Indians later struggled to stamp out the use of the word 'baboo' suggests that many did care. The decision to wear a mixture of Indian and European dress was not then without its consequences.

Fig. 2.16 From *The Indian Charivari*, 23 Jan. 1874 (*above*) and 3 Oct. 1873 (*below*). Courtesy of OIOC.

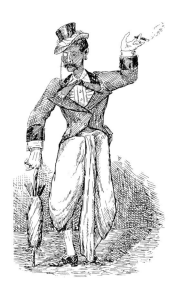

19 That the 'baboo' was a powerful source of criticism and amusement within Bengali society itself is evident from his frequent appearance in satirical literature, political cartoons and popular art forms such as the Kalighat paintings and Bat-tala wood engravings.

Fig. 2.17 Reproduced from *The Indian Charivari*, 7 March 1873. Courtesy of OIOC.

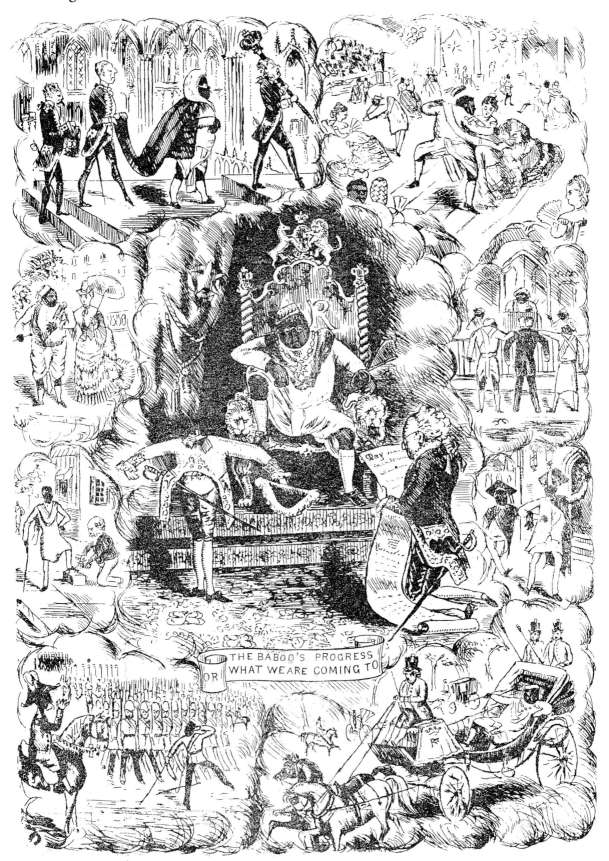

Though largely accepted and welcomed as fashion by many Indians, it was treated with contempt not only by the British but also by those sections of the Indian population who either totally accepted or totally rejected European styles. Many self-aware Indian men who wished to be respected by both their own people and the British took care to avoid such combinations. But there were other possible solutions to the problem of how to retain Indian garments while at the same time adopting European ones.

Changing clothes: a solution to cultural dualism? Changing one's clothes to suit the occasion allowed an Indian man to maintain, if necessary, two distinct sartorial identities, an Indian one and a European one. The advantage of this approach was that it enabled a person to dress according to two different and often incompatible standards of cultural correctness. Rather than incurring the ridicule of the British by wearing hybrid combinations, a man could wear full British dress when acting in an official capacity and full Indian dress in the presence of his family and Indian friends. By changing back into Indian clothes before entering his own home, he could express his ultimate loyalty to his own people. In the same way that Hindus had protected the sanctity of their houses from the threatening and polluting 'Muslim dress', so they began to protect their homes from the clothes of the European:

> So, when the wealthy and conservative Hindus of Calcutta put on European clothing either for business or fashion, they were very scrupulous in putting them off before going into the inner courtyard, all of which were under the jurisdiction of the family deities and the women (Chaudhuri 1976: 57).

The advantage of this solution was that a man could be suitably dressed wherever he went. But he had to decide where to draw the line between his European appearance and his Indian appearance, a decision that was not always simple. The threshold of the house was, as we have seen, a popular transformation point, but even here there was the problem of what to wear when people one normally mixed with outside the home came inside it. This was a problem experienced by the wealthy and fashionable lawyer Motilal Nehru, who found himself having to remain in European dress for a solid week because he had a British guest and journalist staying in his house (M. Nehru 1982, vol. 1: 136). Presumably he felt he would not be taken seriously enough in Indian apparel. There were, then, times when the private self had to be sacrificed to the public image even in the private space of one's own home.

Searching for a Solution in the late Nineteenth Century

Some men confined their European image to a work context only and continued to wear Indian dress in private and in other public contexts not related to work. To them the office or the workplace was the boundary line between an Indian and a European image. Some would change their clothes while still at home. Others would perform the act in public. Elwin describes how Poona policemen, going off duty, would actually take their trousers off in the street and walk home in 'just tunic and undergarments fluttering in the wind' (E. F. Elwin 1907: 45). More recently, a Nayar man informed the anthropologist Kathleen Gough: 'When I put on my shirt to go to the office, I take off my caste, and when I come home and take off my shirt, I put on my caste' (cited in Srinivas 1968: 123).

Sometimes the sartorial border was drawn in wider geographical terms. A man employed in an urban setting would often wear European dress in the city, but revert to Indian clothes when returning to his natal village, a custom not uncommon even today. He could choose whether to draw the boundary line at the entrance to the village or the entrance to his state or anywhere in between, but failure to draw it at all could cause considerable offence. Ramanujan writes:

> My father, on his annual trips to his home state of Kerala, in the 1940s, felt compelled to remove his Western suit at the border town of Alwaye. On one occasion he forgot to take off his suit and ran into ridicule everywhere he stopped. People who waited on him made it clear that they found his suit an affront (Ramanujan 1984: 32).

Drawing the boundary wider still, many Indians maintained distinctive European and Indian sartorial identities according to the country they were in. For most Indians, visiting Europe involved wearing European dress and for some returning to India involved returning to Indian dress. Dadabhai Naoroji, otherwise known as the Grand Old Man of India, wore immaculate European clothes throughout his time in London in the 1880s, but when he returned to India in 1893 he stepped from the boat in Bombay harbour 'dressed in the Parsi style, in black coat and turban and red silk trousers' (R. Masani 1960: 122). But even the solution of changing one's clothes according to the country was not without its complications. A man travelling to Europe had to decide at which point to change his clothes. Should he, like the young M. K. Gandhi, buy his European apparel in India and wear it throughout the voyage, or should he, like Mahendra Pratap, buy his new clothes on reaching England, thereby travelling in Indian dress? In his autobiography Pratap describes the self-conscious sartorial anxiety he felt on his trip to England in 1911: 'I started on this trip in

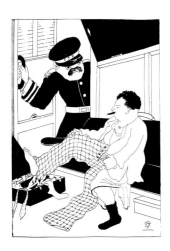

Fig. 2.18 'Don't disturb me now.
I'm about to become a sahib.'
Drawing by Gogonendranath
Tagore, reproduced from G.
Tagore's *Virup Vaira*, 1917.
Courtesy of OIOC.

pure Indian costume' and 'though the eyes kept gazing on my Indian uniform I managed to pass through in full dress to London via Paris. In London, however, I made a sudden change to European dress. I bought everything ready made all in a hurry' (cited in Walsh 1983: 35–6). Pratap's solution was perhaps more advisable than Gandhi's. The latter had the appropriate European clothes without the knowledge of when to wear them. His friends had rallied around in Bombay, equipping him with suitable outfits before his departure from India in 1888. Recalling his somewhat embarrassing arrival in England, Gandhi writes:

> On the boat I had worn a black suit, the white flannel one, which my friends had got me, having been kept especially for wearing when I landed. I had thought that white clothes would suit me better when I stepped ashore, and therefore I did so in white flannels. Those were the last days of September, and I found I was the only person wearing such clothes (Gandhi 1989: 38).

One of the major problems with changing one's clothes to suit the context was that one had to decide where one context ended and another began. This involved some kind of prior knowledge of the contexts in which one was going to move, but even if this knowledge was readily available, there was still the problem of the awkward moment of transformation itself. Where and how should a man actually perform the act of changing his clothes and how could he avoid being caught embarrassingly in the middle of the act? This problem has been pinpointed by the Bengali artist and satirist Gogonendranath Tagore in a satirical drawing of a man caught in the very act of transforming himself into an English gentleman (fig. 2.18). The cartoon was probably a jibe at the fact that Indians were sometimes forbidden to enter first-class railway carriages if they were not dressed in civilised European attire, but it also highlights the peculiarly schizophrenic existence of those people who were constantly switching identities so as to be appropriately dressed on each occasion.

Despite the inconvenience and discomfort of European dress, there were a number of reasons why Indian men might have wanted to wear it, even if it was only a temporary adoption. Being dressed in European clothes was not only a means of self-presentation, it was also a means by which one was judged by others. There were undoubtedly privileges in being dressed like the proverbial English gentleman. Even if the British did not actually want Indians to wear European dress, they none the less treated them with greater respect if they did. This was revealed by an incident in 1917 when the Maharaja of Bikaner returned to Bombay from Europe and was immediately ordered to show his passport. It had not been demanded when he left Bombay, so he wanted to know why it should be demanded on his return. The police officer on duty apparently explained that the Maharaja had been in 'European garb' when he left the country but was now dressed in 'native costume' (*Hindi Punch* 22 July 1917).

To many Britons Indian clothes, whatever their form, clearly remained a mark of inferior status. Chaudhuri demonstrates this with reference to the rhetoric of lavatory signs in Calcutta where the local corporation replaced blatant racial discrimination with the more subtle discrimination by clothes:

> When I was young the public conveniences of Calcutta were always segregated: there used to be, on one side, a set of them meant for us, the natives of the country, and, on the other, another set for 'Europeans'. When the Corporation of Calcutta became completely Indianized at the end of 1924, the signboard 'Europeans Only' was changed to 'Gentlemen in European Dress', to avoid giving offence to racial sensitiveness (Chaudhuri 1976: 88).

But Indian men were not always the victims of these prejudices. At times they used them to their advantage. In the same way that young boys deliberately dressed to look impoverished and so dupe the local memsahib into giving them clothes (see Chapter 1:7–8), so some men adopted Western dress as a strategic move. Elwin tells how a young boy at the mission school successfully disguised his humble background by learning good English, wearing European dress, *sola topi* and all, and adopting an Indian name. He got immediate admission into Government Office and advanced rapidly (E. F. Elwin 1907: 49). By contrast a boy in a *dhoti* who turned up at the railway office for an interview was curtly ordered outside (*ibid.*).

The British were not alone in their discriminatory judgements. Members of the Indian élite who had adopted Western dress were often equally prejudiced against their own people, whom they now considered insufficiently dressed. Rabindranath Tagore suffered in his youth when he went on holiday near the Ganges but was not allowed to accompany the elders into a nearby village on account of his 'indecent' dress. He recalls:

> My feet were bare, I had no scarf or upper robe over my tunic, I was not dressed fit to come out; as if it was my fault! I never owned any socks or superfluous apparel, so not only went back disappointed for that morning, but had no chance of repairing my shortcomings and being allowed to come out any other day (R. Tagore 1917: 48).

By the early twentieth century an increasing number of Indian men had travelled to England, attended British universities (usually Oxford or Cambridge) and become accustomed to a British standard of living. As these 'England-returneds' took up important professional posts and became reincorporated into the Indian élite (who had at first shunned them), they set new standards for the anglicised Indian male. Instead of changing back into Indian apparel for domestic life, some began to retain Western standards even within their own homes. Among such men Indian clothes were kept largely for ceremonial use on religious occasions; they no longer felt the need to wear their Indian identity on their sleeves. While their wives maintained an Indian appearance, they succumbed to a full European look. But the number of men who adopted full European dress was surprisingly small.

Full European dress. It was perhaps a combination of British prejudice against Indian dress and an Indian desire to be taken seriously and participate in 'civilisation' that motivated some Indians from the educated élite classes to adopt full European dress. Madhusudan Datta is said to have been the first Indian to wear a complete European outfit in the high court in Calcutta. The year was 1866, when other professional 'England-returned' Bengalis were wearing *chapkan* and cap (Radice 1986: 202–3). Not only did Datta flout this convention, but he also 'let it be known that England-returned Bengalis would not be welcome at his house unless they dressed similarly' (*ibid.*: 203). This upset some of his more orthodox contemporaries. The Bengali writer Bhudev Mukhopadhay, for example, frequently lamented what he called 'Madhu's despicable inclination to imitate' (Raychaudhuri 1988: 30) which manifested itself in his dress, his lifestyle and his later conversion to Christianity.

Datta's behaviour was judged particularly harshly by his fellows because he was among the first to break the unspoken code that an Indian man must look Indian within his own home and with his fellows. For second- and third-generation 'England-returneds' it became easier to break the rule. It also became increasingly common for Indians to wear European dress at social functions, even when there were no Europeans present. But the desire to wear full European dress was by no means shared by all educated Indians. There were always some who maintained a critical distance. Gogonendranath Tagore was not alone in fearing that too much Westernisation would result in a complete loss of Indian identity (see fig. 2.19).

Surprisingly few Indian men did in fact adopt the Western look on a full-time basis. Many continued to change their clothes on entering their homes. Comfort may have been a consideration here as much as culture,

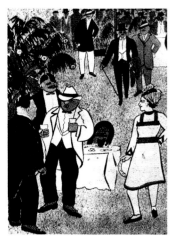

Fig. 2.19 'Party at an Indian House. Find the Indian? A Puzzle for the Younger Generation.' Reproduced from O.C. Gangoly's *The Humorous Art of Gogonendranath Tagore* (n.d.). Courtesy of OIOC.

for European clothes were hot and heavy for the Indian climate and were unsuited to conventional Indian modes of sitting. But there was also the implication of cultural loyalty that was rarely abandoned. This was most often expressed in a man's headwear. Many Indian men who wore European dress maintained some form of Indian turban or cap. Not only was the head regarded as the centre of purity in Indian culture, but a man's head-dress was also his most distinctive badge of affiliation to different caste or religious groups (cf. Cohn 1989, Crill 1985). The fact that many Indians continued to sport their own headwear implied a desire both to protect themselves from whole-hearted identification with the British, and to retain their own sense of religious, regional or caste identity while wearing the otherwise secularising European dress. Throughout the difficult relationship between Indian and European dress, the head usually emerged as the most sensitive of all sartorial issues: those Indians who adopted European hats were often accused of taking on superior British airs. Most, though by no means all, took care to avoid wearing the *sola topi* which almost amounted to the British equivalent of caste dress.

Loyalty to one's culture was by no means the only reason why 'England-returneds' rarely adhered to full European dress. They were probably also motivated by an increasing awareness that, however like the proverbial English gentleman they looked, Indians would never quite be accepted in British society. European dress may have been a passport to respectability, but it was not a passport to full integration. An Indian could only *look* the English gentleman; he could not expect to be treated as such. The colour of his skin remained the last but vital stamp of Indian identity, acting for the British both as a cause and as a justification for racial prejudice.[20]

The reality of British attitudes to Indian skin, and hence to Indians, was brought home to many by an incident in the life of Dadabhai Naoroji. In 1886 this much-respected Parsi was the first Indian ever to stand as a candidate for the British parliament. To the shock of Indians at home and abroad, his failure to get elected was publicly justified in a speech by the

20 This was particularly clear in British attitudes to Eurasians (those born of a European father and Indian mother). If their skin was pale enough and if they dressed in suitable European clothes, they could 'pass' as Italians, Greeks or Spaniards and thus gain access to the exclusive British social milieu with its European-only clubs (Younger 1983). Here, looking convincingly European was not merely a matter of 'imitation', it was a matter of cultural and social integration. But if a Eurasian's ancestry was known, then, despite pale skin, he or she was no longer accepted in British society. Eurasians were notorious for dressing in European styles and for wearing the *sola topi*, even after the British departed from India. Even today Eurasian men and women cling to European styles as a means of demonstrating their difference from Indians (cf. Gaikwad 1967).

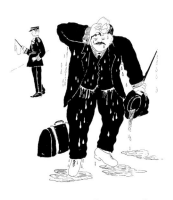

Fig. 2.20 'By the sweat of my brow I tried to be mistaken for a *Shaheb* but still that man calls me Baboo.' Drawing by Gogonandranath Tagore. Reproduced from G. Tagore (op. cit.). Courtesy of OIOC.

British prime minister, Lord Salisbury, on the grounds that Naoroji was a 'black man'. Those two words 'black man' kicked him into fame (R. Masani 1960: 100–6) and heightened Indian awareness of the extent of British prejudice. Many, like Naoroji, had received personal insults from the British, despite their dress. It was the realisation of the fact that racial prejudice went beyond clothes that led to a turning-point in their clothing habits. Gogonendranath Tagore, always critical of the Westernised Indian, has portrayed this painful moment of realisation (fig. 2.20). He demonstrates the futility of Indian attempts to 'pass' as English.

But if an Indian man wanted to avoid wearing Western dress, this still did not solve the problem of what he should wear. There were many types of Indian clothes from which he could choose, and furthermore many of these options were now considered old-fashioned by educated Indians themselves, who were not used to wearing them and sometimes thought them indecent. That there had never been a uniform 'Indian dress' but rather an immense variety of different types of clothing seemed to emphasise India's cultural diversity more than its homogeneity. Thus, the desire to avoid wearing European dress was linked to the further problem of how to define Indian dress. While some tried to invent new pan-Indian styles, others tried to revive existing forms. The central problem was to find a form of Indian dress that could be respectable without being European at a time when respectability was defined in European terms.

Redefining Indian dress
Some of the earliest attempts to redefine Indian dress emerged in Calcutta – not only the seat of British authority but also the most fertile territory for emerging nationalist sentiment. In particular the Tagore family were prominent in the search for both a new Indian aesthetic and a new Indian dress. As early as the 1870s, Jyotirindranath Tagore, brother of the poet Rabindranath, instigated one of the most valiant attempts to unite the Indian with the European without privileging one type of dress over another. Not content with the solution of wearing European garments in combination with Indian ones, or the solution of opting for either European or Indian dress, he tried to invent a national dress which combined both Indian and European features within a single garment.

Always an innovator, Jyotirindranath Tagore had started up a political association in the mid-1870s and felt that a change of clothes could be a starting-point for political change. His brother Rabindranath, who was only fourteen at the time, later recalled these sartorial experiments:

Searching for a Solution in the late Nineteenth Century

> My brother Jyotirindra began to busy himself with a national costume
> for all India, and submitted various designs to the association. The dhoti
> was not deemed business-like; trousers were too foreign; so he hit upon
> a compromise which considerably detracted from the dhoti while failing
> to improve the trousers. That is to say, the trousers were decorated with
> the addition of a false dhoti-fold in front and behind. The fearsome thing
> that resulted from combining a turban with a topee our most enthusiastic
> member would not have had the temerity to call ornamental. No person
> of ordinary courage would have dared it, but my brother wore the com-
> plete suit in broad daylight, passing through the house of an afternoon
> to the carriage waiting outside, indifferent alike to the stare of relation
> or friend, doorkeeper or coachman. There may be many a brave Indian
> ready to die for his country, but there are but few, I am sure, who even
> for the good of the nation, would face the public streets in such pan-
> Indian garb (R. Tagore 1917: 143–4).

Jyotirindra's invention seems not to have been a great success. Though
ideologically sound, it failed dismally to fulfil either Indian or British
notions of aesthetics. Unable to convince even members of his own political
association to wear these composite garments, he certainly could not persuade the nation to adopt them. But Jyotirindranath was ahead of his time
in realising the importance of dress, and was one of the first Indians to
suggest that a redefinition of Indian dress could bring about a sense of
political unity. He was also one of the first to link his own personal problem
of what to wear to the national problem of Indian identity.

His brother Rabindranath later took up the challenge. He found a very
different solution to the problem of defining national dress. He felt that
members of the Indian élite had isolated themselves by deserting their own
people but at the same time failing to become integrated with the European
community: 'The mischief with us is that we have lost what we had, but
have not the means of building afresh on the European standard, with the
result that our home-life has become joyless' (R. Tagore 1917: 124) He
criticised the British for their insularity as much as the Indians for emulating
the British, who he felt had remained aloof from Indian culture and, unlike
the Moghuls, had contributed little to it. Because of this, there was no reason
to include them in the Indian definition of national dress. Therefore, rather
than seeking an Indo-European solution to the problem, he sought what he
called a Hindu-Muslim combination which excluded any British component
whatever. His aim was not so much to invent a new Hindu-Muslim style
but rather to prove that the *chapkan*, often regarded as Muslim dress, was

Clothing Matters

in fact a Hindu-Muslim combination and was suitable as Indian dress:

> The chapkan is the dress of Hindus and Muslims combined. Hindus and Muslims have both contributed to all the changes it has gone through to make up its present form. And still in Western India, in various princely states, one can see a lot of variety in the capkan. And in this variety one does not only see Muslim inventiveness but also the creativity and freedom of the Hindus. ... If a race is forming that can be called an Indian race, then by no means can the Muslim aspect of that race be omitted. ... So the dress that will be our national dress will be a Hindu-Muslim dress (R. Tagore 1960: 227–8).[21]

Tagore expressed these thoughts early in 1905. At that time it seemed unlikely that Indian men would revert to the Indian *dhoti*, and he even suggested that it was unsuitable for office work or the courts. It was no doubt also unsuitable for combining Hindu and Muslim elements since it was associated primarily with Hindus. Yet only a few months later, *dhotis* were re-emerging on the streets of Calcutta with a vengeance. Sparked off by Lord Curzon's announcement of the partition of Bengal, they became for about five years the ultimate symbol of *swadeshi*[22] (home industry) and of the Bengali man's opposition to British policies.

Of course *swadeshi* was not a new idea when it emerged in Bengal in 1905, but the expression of a rumbling dissatisfaction with British economic policies, particularly those connected with the decline of the Indian textile industry. As early as 1872 Justice Ranade had delivered a series of lectures popularising 'the idea of swadeshi, of preferring the goods produced in one's own country even though they may prove to be dearer or less satisfactory than finer cotton products' (Chandra, cited in Bean 1989). Some members of his audiences had vowed to wear Indian-made textiles. In particular Ganesh Vasudeao Joshi began to spin yarn daily for his own *dhoti*, shirt and turban (*ibid.*). For him the *dhoti*, despite its backward associations among both the British and élite Indians, was a suitable means of expressing patriotic sentiment.

When the *dhoti* re-emerged in Bengal in 1905, it was as a sign of protest over British policies. Those who adopted *dhotis* expressed the incompatibility of mixing Indian and Western styles which were as incompatible as Indian and British interests in India's future. True allegiance to the Indian people was expressed in the boycott of foreign cloth and the burning of European clothes (Bayly 1986: 313). Hindu protesters organised mass processions which ended with cleansing dips in the Ganges from which people emerged

---

21 I am grateful to William Radice for translating this passage from Bengali.
22 The word *swadeshi*, from *swa* (own) and *desh* (country), refers to home industry, i.e. all things produced in India.

in the pure, preferably hand-woven cloth of the Indian peasant (*ibid.*). The British may have had little respect for these 'indecent' *dhotis* but, as Motilal Nehru pointed out in a letter to his son, they had no choice but to accept the Bengali *despite* his *dhoti*. Motilal writes with his characteristic enthusiasm:

> The Bengali reigns supreme throughout Bengal. He goes to office bare-footed in his dhoti and chaddar and refuses to use anything of English manufacture at the risk of losing his employment. His employees cannot do without him and give him free admittance. Bengali High Court judges, barristers, solicitors, noblemen, merchants, have all discarded English costume. Thousands of indigenous industries have sprung up. We are passing through the most critical period of British Indian history (letter 16 Nov. 1905. in M. Nehru vol. 1, 1982: 91)

By 1910 the presence of the *dhoti* was subsiding again in the streets of Calcutta, and many wealthy Indians returned to a European or semi-European look. For the next fifteen years most respectable educated and professional Indian men wore European dress or extreme forms of Euro-peanised Indian dress in their public life.[23] But the seeds of a search for a national dress had been planted.

The clothing dilemmas of the Indian élite in the late nineteenth and early twentieth centuries were but one expression of a more general growing discomfort with colonialism. They revealed the impossibility of respectability or neutrality in an environment in which all sartorial options were loaded with negative implications of one kind or another. How significant a role this sartorial dissatisfaction played in the development of an early critique of British rule it is difficult to assess. For many the problem of what to wear remained largely personal and was not generally discussed in the public sphere. The pain, humour and confusion it caused were recorded mainly in private letters, autobiographies and journals rather than in speeches and at political meetings. And although clothing came briefly to the political forefront with the *swadeshi* movement in Bengal, this was largely a regional struggle and failed to have any major effect on the clothing choices of the nation at large. From this we may conclude that while clothes were recognised as a medium through which dissatisfaction with the British could be expressed, they were not central to public political debate in this period. This was soon to change with the emergence on the political scene of M. K. Gandhi.

---

23   There were of course always a few prominent Indian patriots who never converted to European dress, such as B. G. Tilak.

3 Gandhi and the Recreation of Indian Dress

> Only their insularity and unimaginativeness have made the English retain the English style [of dress] in India, even though they admit that it is most uncomfortable for this Indian climate. I venture to think that thoughtless imitation is no sign of progress. Nor is every reversion to old habits tantamount to accepting back the hand of time. Retracing a hasty erroneous step is surely a sign of progress (Gandhi, *Young India* 22 June 1921, CWMG, vol. 20: 251).

No Indian leader took the problem of what to wear more seriously than Mohandas Karamchand Gandhi and probably no other leader changed his clothes so dramatically. The story of his rejection of the European suit in favour of a simple loincloth has attained almost folkloric proportions.[1] Yet the image of Gandhi in his loincloth is so reassuringly familiar that its significance is rarely analysed systematically. It is somehow assumed that we all understand what Gandhi meant by his loincloth. It is one of the facts of history that by its very familiarity remains unexplored.

There has of course been wide recognition that clothes were significant to Gandhi (cf. Brown 1990: 161, Kumar 1984). As early as 1949, Millie Graham Polak, who had spent some years with him in South Africa, commented: 'What different phases in Mr Gandhi's mental career had been proclaimed by the clothes he wore! Each costume, I think, denoted an attitude of mind' (M. G. Polak 1950: 142). More recently Susan Bean has provided the first thorough analysis of the role of clothes in the struggle for Indian independence (cf. Bean 1989). She portrays Gandhi as a 'semiotician', who experimented with clothes until he 'achieved an understanding of the role of cloth in Indian life' (*ibid.*). She concludes that by finally adopting the loincloth he was able to communicate all his most important messages through the medium of dress, while by encouraging hand-spinning, weaving and the wearing of Indian *khadi* (hand-spun, hand-woven cloth),[2] he was

---

1 In India the image of Gandhi as the thin loinclothed saint who threw aside European dress in favour of the clothes of Indian poverty and simplicity is kept alive in popular representations on calendars and religious posters. In the West, Richard Attenborough's film *Gandhi* (1981) rekindled that image.

2 The term *khadi* refers to handwoven cloth. By 1920 Gandhi used it in the stricter sense to refer to cloth that had been handwoven from handspun yarn.

able to raise the issue of cloth to primary economic and political importance.

Bean's work has provided valuable documentation and analysis both of Gandhi's clothes and of his economic policy. Bayly meanwhile has highlighted the symbolically charged moral language that Gandhi employed when speaking of *khadi*. Bayly suggests that in using such language, he was reviving the semi-dormant 'magical' and 'moral' beliefs that had always been attributed to cloth in Indian society (Bayly 1986). Yet, despite these valuable contributions to understanding the role of clothes in the rise of Indian nationalism, a number of questions remain unanswered. Did Gandhi really rediscover the significance of cloth in Indian life, as Bean and Bayly suggest, or did he rather create his own symbolism and theory of cloth and clothes? And if clothes were symbolic to Gandhi, what exactly did they represent? Was he able to fix their meaning and did he even try to do so? Furthermore, if he hoped to use clothes as a means of communication, how great was his success in actually achieving this communication through his dress?

Much of the confusion revolves around the question of whether, in order to understand Gandhi's clothes, we should interpret their visual effect, or whether instead we should try to interpret his written and spoken 'intention'. Bean begins by tracing the clothing changes and interpreting them according to what he wrote about them in his autobiography.[3] But by the time he adopted the loincloth, which is little mentioned in the autobiography, Bean favours her own interpretation of what she thinks Gandhi meant by his clothes. She concludes:

> He used his appearance to communicate his most important messages in a form comprehensible to all Indians. Engaged in the simple labor of spinning, dressed as one of the poor in a loincloth and chadar, this important and powerful man communicated the dignity of poverty, the dignity of labour, the equality of all Indians, the greatness of Indian civilisation, as well as his own saintliness. The communicative power of costume transcended the limitations of language in multilingual and illiterate India. The image transcended cultural barriers as well. His impact on the West was enhanced by his resemblance, in his simplicity of dress and his saintly manner, to Christ on the Cross (Bean 1989: 368).

Here, the meaning of the loincloth appears clear and easy for Indians and

---

3 Gandhi's autobiography, otherwise known as *The Story of my Experiments with Truth*, was first published in 1927. It contains a number of personal details concerning its author's clothes. But it has to be remembered that it was written retrospectively with the self-consciousness of one who recreates his own history. In this it differs from his speeches and letters concerning his clothing changes, which were written without hindsight and do not reveal the same overall sense of consistency or certainty (cf. CWMG, vols 1–90).

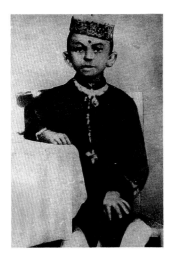

Fig. 3.1 Gandhi, aged seven, wearing a *dhoti*, long coat and woollen cap of the type commonly worn in North India. Courtesy of NGM.

Westerners alike to interpret. But if we examine the way it was interpreted by his contemporaries, it is evident that the meaning was far from clear and that interpretations were varied and confused. Was Gandhi a saint, a lunatic, a pauper or a fraud? All of these were common explanations. And if we turn to his own speeches about his dress, we find that what he wrote and said about the loincloth was invariably different from all the above interpretations. It is precisely this discrepancy between intention and interpretation that made clothes a highly problematic issue throughout Gandhi's life. For however much he tried to control the way his dress was understood, he invariably found that people favoured their own explanations.

Gandhi was highly aware of this discrepancy between intention and interpretation and therefore considered all his clothing changes with 'deep deliberation' (CWMG, vol. 21: 225) before putting them into practice. It was also his awareness of the possibility of 'misinterpretation' that led him to proclaim the meaning of his dress in speeches and letters to the press. If dress was truly capable of communicating his message clearly, there would have been little need for such explicit verbal explanations. But, as Gandhi well knew, dress, like other symbolic phenomena, was capable of signifying a variety of different things simultaneously.

This chapter explores the development of Gandhi's very particular theory of clothes and examines his attempts to persuade the Indian nation to understand and share his sartorial beliefs. It begins with a brief overview of his most significant clothing changes, concentrating in particular on his loincloth, the garment he wore for the last twenty-seven years of his life. Emphasis is placed on the ambiguity of the symbolism of Gandhi's dress. This same question of the multiple meanings of clothes is then considered in relation to his attempts to control the clothing of the nation through encouraging all Indians to wear *khadi* and all Indian men to wear the so-called 'Gandhi cap'.

GANDHI AND HIS CLOTHES: A BRIEF HISTORY[4]

From Kathiawadi boy to English gentleman
Unlike many Indian men who adopted European dress in the late nineteenth century, Gandhi was not from a particularly élite family, nor was he brought up in an environment with a strong British presence. Born in 1869

---

4 Many readers will be familiar with at least some of Gandhi's clothing changes from reading his autobiography or Bean's article (1989), but a brief summary of these changes is necessary here in order to include missing details and provide a context for the ensuing analysis.

Gandhi and the Recreation of Indian Dress

into a respectable middle-caste *Baniya*[5] family, he was raised in the towns of Kathiawad (now Saurashtra), a region slow to realise the impact of British influences. Like many educated urban boys, he often wore a shirt and sometimes a coat with his *dhoti*, and favoured the use of the fashionable Ahmedabad mill-cloth known as 'Rifle brand' (Pyarelal 1965: 196). But he was disparaging of those local Indians who had succumbed to full European dress, an act he associated with conversion to Christianity (cf. Gandhi 1989 [1927]: 29). None the less when the young Gandhi heard that he was going to London to study law, he immediately equipped himself with the appropriate garb, despite finding the short jacket 'immodest' (*ibid.*: 35). He was anxious not to look out of place. For him London was 'the very centre of civilization' (CWMG vol. 1: 54) and he was willing to compromise any external signs of his Indianness in order to fit in. He even removed his *shika* (tuft of uncut hair worn by Hindus) on the eve of his departure for fear it would expose him to ridicule and make him look a 'barbarian in the eyes of the Englishmen' (Gandhi 1989 [1927]: 327).

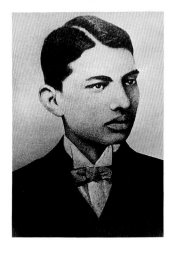

Fig. 3.2 Gandhi as a law student in London. Courtesy of NGM.

Although the nineteen-year-old Gandhi was inexperienced in European customs and shy of Europeans on board the ship, he clearly felt that he had mastered sartorial matters and even lent his black coat to a fellow Indian passenger who seemed less well equipped than himself (CWMG vol. 1: 12). It was therefore a considerable shock and embarrassment when he stepped ashore at Southampton to find he was the only person in white flannels. His intention to blend into the English scene had been sorely frustrated; he looked precisely the inexperienced young Indian student that he was.[6] And his embarrassment was by no means over. On his first evening he was visited by Dr P. J. Mehta, an Indian experienced in British lifestyle and etiquette, and fascinated by the smoothness of Dr Mehta's top hat, he picked it up and stroked it, only to be angrily rebuked for bad manners. Gandhi recalls: 'The incident was a warning for the future. This was my first lesson in European etiquette' (Gandhi 1989 [1927]: 38). The psychological impact of these incidents may be measured by the fact that he bothered to record them nearly forty years later. They were perhaps his first experience of the unfortunate disparity between how he thought he looked and how he actually looked in the eyes of other people.

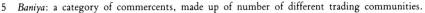

5 *Baniya*: a category of commercents, made up of number of different trading communities.
6 This did not stop him commenting rather snobbishly on the clothes of one of his fellow-passengers with whom he arrived at a hotel. He recorded in his diary: 'Mr Abdul Majid thought very highly of himself, but let me write here that the dress which he had put on was perhaps worse than that of the porter' (CWMG vol. 1: 20).

ing his three-year stay in London (1888–91). His initial attempt to 'become' an English gentleman, not only through elaborate dressing but also through learning French, elocution, how to play the violin and how to dance, soon proved futile even to him. The vows of vegetarianism he had taken under the influence of his mother seemed to haunt him with a sense of his own Indianness.[7] The dancing, French and violin-playing lasted only a few months, but it was years before he cast off his Western appearance. For although he had lost faith in the ability of European clothes to transform him into an English gentleman, he still felt they were more 'civilised' than Indian dress and firmly believed in the value of Westernisation (Bean 1989: 356–9). Furthermore, part of his original desire to become 'polished' was that it might compensate for his vegetarianism (Gandhi 1989 [1927]: 43). A Western exterior was becoming a suitable mask for an increasingly Indian interior, which he first became aware of when he stepped outside his local Kathiawad and into a very foreign Western world.[8]

Gandhi not only preserved his civilised Westernised exterior when he returned to India in 1891, but also encouraged his family in Rajkot to adopt European dress (*ibid.*: 77). However, like many Western educated Indians he appears to have favoured Indian rather than European headwear while living in India. For when we next read of Gandhi's dress, he was wearing a turban with his European suit (*ibid.*: 88).

South Africa: from sophistication to simplification
If the self-conscious young Gandhi was embarrassed by the inadequacy of his British image when he first arrived in England in 1888, he was also embarrassed by the efficiency of his British image when he first arrived in

---

7 Gandhi's mother, who opposed his visit to England, had persuaded him to take a vow not to touch wine, women or meat (Gandhi 1989: 33). Vegetarianism was at first an embarrassment to Gandhi, but later in England he came to see it as a moral and religious virtue. Throughout his stay, however, it singled him out from mainstream meat-eating British culture.
8 Sachchiddananda Sinha's enthusiastic description of Gandhi walking down Piccadilly in 1890 suggests that this shy Indian student was highly successful in covering up his peculiarities with a good set of European clothes: 'He was wearing a silk top hat, burnished and bright, a Gladstonian collar, stiff and starched; a rather flashy tie displaying almost all the colours of the rainbow, under which there was a fine, striped silk shirt. He wore as his outer clothes a morning coat, a double-breasted vest, and dark striped trousers to match and not only patent leather boots but spats over them. He carried leather gloves and a silver mounted stick, but wore no spectacles. He was, to use the contemporary slang, a nut, a masher, a blood – a student more interested in fashion and frivolities than in his studies' (cited in Nanda 1989: 24).

66

Gandhi and the Recreation of Indian Dress

1893 in South Africa, where he had been offered a post as a barrister representing Indian rights (*ibid.*). Other expatriate Indians were dressed either in long robes or in *dhotis*, and Gandhi's immaculate frock coat and expensive Western appearance were, he felt, an instant disappointment to the Muslim merchant who greeted him at the port. The only Indian feature of his attire was an imitation Bengali turban and this soon proved an equal embarrassment when he was asked to remove it by a magistrate in the Durban court. Removing headwear was a gesture of humiliation in India, and being ordered to remove it was an insult (Bayly 1986: 292). Gandhi reacted by leaving the court with his turban on but intent on wearing a British hat in future to avoid 'unpleasant controversies' (Gandhi 1989: 90). Only the patriotic persuasions of the Muslim merchant convinced him that the incident was worth highlighting (*ibid.*: 90–1). Gandhi therefore wrote to the press, exposing the matter.

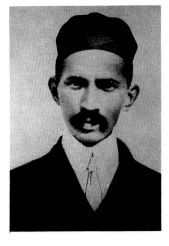

Fig. 3.3 Gandhi in 1900 during the early years of his legal practice in Johannesburg. He has replaced his 'Bengali turban' with a small black skull cap. Courtesy of NGM.

This incident marked a turning-point in Gandhi's attitude to dress as it was 'much discussed in the papers' and gave him 'an unexpected advertisement' in the first week after his arrival (*ibid.*: 91). From this period onwards, instead of wearing only what was socially acceptable and obligatory, he began to adopt clothes which he knew to be socially unacceptable and provocative. It marked the beginning of a period of sartorial experimentation (cf. Bean 1989) when Gandhi began to convert his own embarrassment at being wrongly dressed into a strategy for exposing injustice and embarrassing others. This technique was probably first employed when he was imprisoned in Johannesburg in 1908 for failing to register under the Asiatic Law Amendment Act. Along with other Indians, he was stripped naked, then given a prison uniform, stamped with the letter N for 'Native'. After initial horror at being classified with the 'natives', Gandhi soon decided to accept voluntarily those rules for natives from which Indians were exempt. 'It was my intention', he writes, 'to go through all the experiences of a prisoner. I therefore asked the chief warder to have my hair cropped and my moustache shaved off' (*ibid.*: 141). This the Governor had strictly forbidden, presumably because he did not wish it to appear as if the authorities were maltreating their non-violent Indian prisoners. But, much to the embarrassment of the authorities, Gandhi insisted on removing his own hair and even spent two hours cropping the hair of fellow Indian inmates. The incident was the first of a number of occasions in which Gandhi chose to adopt visual signs of public humiliation.

Throughout his time in South Africa (1893–1914), Gandhi's dress became increasingly humble, if not eccentric. By 1910 he had replaced his smart business suit, stiff collar and tie with a ready-made 'rather sloppy' lounge

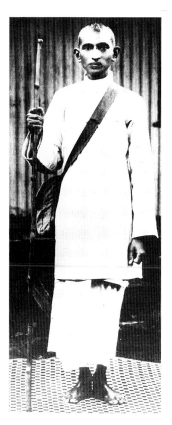

Fig. 3.4 Gandhi dressed for the *Satyagraha* struggle (1914). This was the dress he first adopted at a mass meeting in Durban in 1913 when he referred to his clothes as a sign of mourning. Courtesy of NGM.

suit and 'clumsy' shoes. This in turn gave way to trousers, a loose cotton shirt and sandals (M. G. Polak 1950: 142–3). At times he was even seen wearing 'shorts and shirts made from Australian flour-sacks' (cited in Rai 1945: 50), but he continued to wear European styles throughout most of his stay (Nanda 1989: 74–5). His adoption of an increasingly simple lifestyle, in which he washed his own clothes, cut his own hair and experimented with food, was greatly influenced by Ruskin's book, *Unto This Last*, which Gandhi read in 1904. He was impressed by Ruskin's condemnation of industrialisation and his praise of the simple life. He wrote his own critique of Western civilisation some five years later, called *Hind Swaraj* (Indian self-rule), in which he expressed disdain for a society based on the fulfilment of bodily rather than spiritual satisfaction, and he criticised the idea that European dress could have a civilising effect on the Indian people (CWMG vol. 10: 19). He accused Manchester of causing India's impoverishment and approved of the *swadeshi* movement in Bengal where Indian men were parading in public in Indian rather than European dress (*ibid.*: 57).

As early as 1911 Gandhi was recommending that 'every intelligent person' should learn weaving (CWMG vol. 10: 398–9), but he continued to dress in European rather than Indian styles. However, it was not India's economic distress but rather the shooting of Indian coalminers by the South African authorities that finally prompted him to make his first public appearance in Indian dress in 1913. The occasion was a meeting in Durban of between 6,000 and 7,000 people, including a number of prominent Europeans. Gandhi appeared with his head shaven, and dressed in a *lungi*[9] and *kurta* (fig. 3.4); this was a gesture of sorrow. Realising that people might be confused by his appearance, he immediately explained his dress in a speech to the crowd which was reported in the *Natal Mercury* the following day:

> They [the audience] would notice he had changed his dress from that he had formerly adopted for the last 20 years, and he had decided on the change when he heard of the shooting of his fellow countrymen.... He felt that he should go into mourning at least for a period, which should be co-extensive with the end of the struggle, and that he should accept some mourning not only inwardly, but outwardly as well, as a humble example to his fellow countrymen.... He was not prepared himself to accept the European mourning dress for this purpose and, with some modification in deference to the feelings of his European friends,

9 *Lungi*: stitched waistcloth, often worn by Muslims.

Gandhi and the Recreation of Indian Dress

he adopted the dress similar to that of an indentured labourer.[10] He asked his fellow countrymen to adopt some sign of mourning to show to the world that they were mourning, and further to adopt some inward observance also. And perhaps he might tell them what his inward observance was – to restrict himself to one meal a day (CWMG vol. 12: 274–5).

This was the first of a number of speeches in which Gandhi advocated the reduction of dress as an outward sign of inner grief. He called on all present to participate in this visual display of sorrow, urging harmony between a person's innermost feeling and exterior appearance. For him it was the visual equivalent of a reduction of food. He believed that through suffering, self-sacrifice and renunciation of physical comfort wrongs could be purged. These ideas were to become central to his perception of the significance of dress.

Returning to India: symbolic dismissal of Western civilisation
When Gandhi finally left South Africa, with the success of his *satyagraha*[11] campaign murmuring if not resounding back in his homeland, he chose to make his Indian return conspicuous by dressing as a Kathiawadi peasant (fig. 3.5 right). Having first arrived inappropriately dressed both in England (1888) and in South Africa (1893), he knew the level of attention that unexpected clothing could attract. Now, in Bombay in 1915, he tried to turn this public attention to his advantage by revealing his decision to favour the clothes of the Indian peasantry above those of Europeans. He must have ordered his peasant outfit while still in South Africa or in England, where he spent four months[12] before arriving in Bombay. His decision to identify with the Kathiawadi peasantry was a highly self-conscious and somewhat strange choice, particularly since he had spent so little of his adult life in Kathiawad and was not even from a peasant family. But how did people react to his choice of clothes, and did they understand what he was trying to convey by them? Some Indians were clearly impressed. The young Jamnadas Dwarkadas, for example, wrote: '... there was something

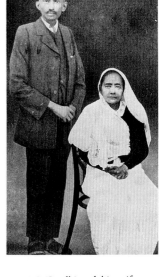

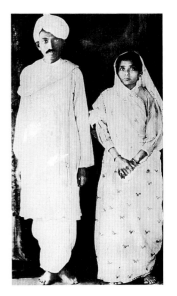

Fig. 3.5 Gandhi and his wife, Kasturba. *Above*: Photographed in 1914 shortly before leaving South Africa. *Below*: Photographed on their arrival in Bombay (Jan. 1915). Gandhi has replaced his suit with the dress of a Kathiawadi peasant. Courtesy of NGM.

10 'Indentured labourers' were Indians who came to South Africa under an agreement to serve there for five years. Many remained there as labourers for the rest of their lives. They usually dressed in *lungis* or *dhotis*. When Gandhi claimed that he had modified his dress in deference to Europeans, he was probably referring to the fact that he was wearing a *kurta*. Many labourers would have gone bare-chested.

11 *Satyagraha*, literally 'truth force': Gandhi's name for non-violent resistance which he saw as superior to aggressive revolution. His last *satyagraha* campaign in South Africa had involved organising a strike of Indian miners and leading them illegally across the border into the Transvaal in 1913.

12 During this time Gandhi worked in the Indian Ambulance Corps, and helped to nurse soldiers wounded in the war. For this he did wear a regulation uniform.

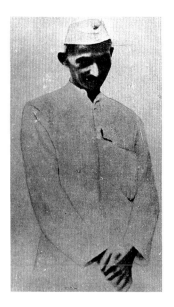

Fig. 3.6 Gandhi in 1920, dressed in a *khadi* kurta and the famous 'Gandhi cap' which he invented. Courtesy of NGM.

extraordinarily simple and unique in Gandhiji's mode of dressing, which made a very deep impression on me and a vast number of young people in the country' (Dwarkadas 1969: 3). But there were many, like J. B. Kripalani and Gaganvihari Mehta, who found him more òdd than inspiring: the latter, on meeting him in Shantiniketan in 1915, described him as a 'crank' (G. Mehta 1949: 180), while the former recalled: 'He was only Mr Gandhi then, and rather an eccentric specimen of an England-returned-educated-Indian. Everything about him appeared queer and even quixotic' (Kripalani 1949: 118). Sometimes his rustic appearance failed to have the desired effect simply because it was altogether too convincing. At the National Congress meeting in Lucknow (1916), two grandly dressed landlords actually mistook him for a stray village peasant (Lal 1969: 52).

Clearly appreciation of Gandhi's dress depended to some extent on people's prior knowledge of who he was. There was a profound difference between the man who chose to reject alternatives in favour of peasant dress and the peasant who wore the same dress without premeditation simply because he was a peasant. Therefore, if Gandhi was to communicate effectively through his dress, he had simultaneously to explain what it meant. He alternated between publicly explaining his clothes and enjoying the anonymity of being mistaken for any old pauper or a religious ascetic in his private life (Gandhi 1989: 335).

During the first few years after his return to India, Gandhi frequently experimented with his clothes (cf. Bean 1989: 366–7). Sometimes he wore a *dhoti* with a decorative border, sometimes *pyjamas* and a loose shirt, and sometimes a simple plain *dhoti* with a shawl (M. G. Polak 1950: 142–3). He frequently alternated between his large Kathiawadi turban and a small cheap Kashmiri cap. For a brief period in 1917, when he was collecting recruits for the British war effort, he even adopted a *sola topi* (Dwarkadas 1969: 240). At this time, he received abusive mail including one letter addressed to 'Traitor Gandhi' (*ibid.*). To have worn a *sola topi*, that potent symbol of British imperialism, cannot have added to his popularity,[13] however much he appreciated it on practical grounds (CWMG vol. 41: 25). However, the objections of his fellow-Indians were yet another indication to Gandhi of the symbolic importance of headwear in India. Two years later he was to exploit this symbolism by inventing his own personalised form of headwear – a white folding *khadi* version of the Kashmiri cap – which later became known as the 'Gandhi cap'. Gandhi wore it for less than two years (see fig. 3.6), but it became one of the key popular symbols of the nationalist struggle.

13 It is interesting that in his autobiography Gandhi does not mention wearing the *sola topi*, especially since he mentions a variety of other headwear: the top hat, the Bengali turban and various caps.

Gandhi and the Recreation of Indian Dress

Of course, Gandhi's experiments with clothes were not merely concerned with visual effects. They were also intrinsically linked to his desire to restore the Indian hand-weaving and hand-spinning industries (cf. Bean 1989, Cohn 1989: 343). In 1915 he established the Sabarmati ashram in Ahmedabad and immediately began to experiment with weaving and later spinning. He wanted Indians to boycott foreign goods and to wear *khadi* cloth made from yarn they had spun themselves by hand. He 'grew impatient' to adopt pure *khadi* in his own dress (Gandhi 1989: 411) which, up till this point, was hand-woven from machine-spun yarn. Only with great difficulty did the ashramites finally locate some people who still knew the art of hand-spinning, then almost in total decline. From them they purchased hand-spun yarn and began to weave it, initially into strips of cloth only 30 inches wide. Gandhi threatened one woman that if she could not weave a 45-inch strip within a month, he would make do with a short *dhoti*. She fulfilled his demand and relieved him from what he claims would have been 'a very difficult situation' (*ibid.*). He later embraced that 'difficult situation' when, in 1921, he adopted a short *khadi* loincloth. What encouraged him to take this final step?

The loincloth[14]
Gandhi first mentioned the idea of wearing loincloths in April 1919, when he looked forward to the time when men would say 'We shall confine ourselves to pure *swadeshi* cloth, even though we may have to remain satisfied with a mere loincloth' (CWMG vol 15: 199), a comment addressed to those who argued that they could not afford to discard their foreign cloth in favour of the more expensive Indian *khadi*.[15] Gandhi himself still dressed at this time in the comparatively respectable *dhoti* and did not express any intention to adopt a loincloth himself. During the Khulna famine, however, he was criticised for encouraging people to burn foreign cloth while others were dying from starvation and nakedness. Moved by the accusation, he contemplated sending his shirt and *dhoti* to relief workers and contenting himself with a 'mere loincloth'. But he seems to have mistrusted his motives: 'I restrained my emotion. It was tinged with egotism. I knew the taunt was groundless' (*The Hindu* 15 Oct. 1921, CWMG vol. 21: 225). Gandhi next contemplated the gesture after witnessing the arrest of his Muslim co-worker Maulana Mahomed Ali in mid-September 1921. He later

14 Gandhi's waistcloth was usually referred to either as a *langoti* or a loincloth. It was in fact much longer than either term suggests and could more accurately be called a short *dhoti*.
15 Cost was always one of the major problems with *khadi*. It was considerably more expensive to buy than mill-cloth because of the time needed to produce it by hand. Many economists have argued that this was the main factor which prevented a more substantial *khadi* revival.

recalled: 'I addressed a meeting soon after his arrest. I thought of dispensing with my cap and shirt that moment, but then I restrained myself fearing that I might create a scene' (CWMG vol. 21: 225).

Why was Gandhi so hesitant? Clearly he was attracted to the idea but could not anticipate how people would react. What finally precipitated him into action was his realisation in Madras of the failure of his *khadi* programme. In September 1920 he had launched the non-cooperation programme, aimed at attaining *swaraj* (home rule) in one year. He had hoped that by the end of September 1921 every Indian would be wearing *khadi* and that there would be a complete boycott of foreign cloth, but instead the year was nearly up and he was disturbed to find that there was not even enough *khadi* available and that many poor Madrassi labourers could not afford it:

> The plea of the poor overpowered me. . . . I began telling people in my speeches: 'If you don't get khadi, you will do with a mere loincloth but discard foreign cloth.' I know that I was hesitating whilst I uttered those words. They lacked the necessary force, as long as I had my dhoti and shirt on (*ibid.*: 225–6).

But Gandhi was not prepared to set the drastic example of wearing a loincloth until he had discussed it at length with some of his closest followers. He knew that it could be misinterpreted, and was aware of the connotations of indecency and primitiveness that it would imply. Maulana Azad Sobhani was sympathetic to the idea but Krishnadas and other friends were sceptical and viewed the prospect with 'a feeling of indefinite fear' (Krishnadas 1928: 203). Gandhi recalls: 'They felt that such a radical change might make people uneasy, some might not understand it; some might take me to be a lunatic, and that all would find it difficult, if not impossible to follow my example' (CWMG vol. 21: 225). Some of Gandhi's associates also feared that he might be beginning the life of a Hindu ascetic and would renounce everything (Krishnadas 1928: 203).

Despite the laborious attempts of his friends to dissuade him from such a step, Gandhi finally decided to take the risk and on 22 September 1921 wrote a declaration of his intention, which was published the next day in *The Hindu*. In it he proposed to wear a loincloth for a period of just over five weeks, until the allotted deadline for *swaraj*:

> I propose to discard at least up to the 31st of October my topi and vest and to content myself with only a loincloth and a chaddar whenever necessary for protection of the body. I adopt the change because I have always hesitated to advise anything I may not be prepared to follow. . . .

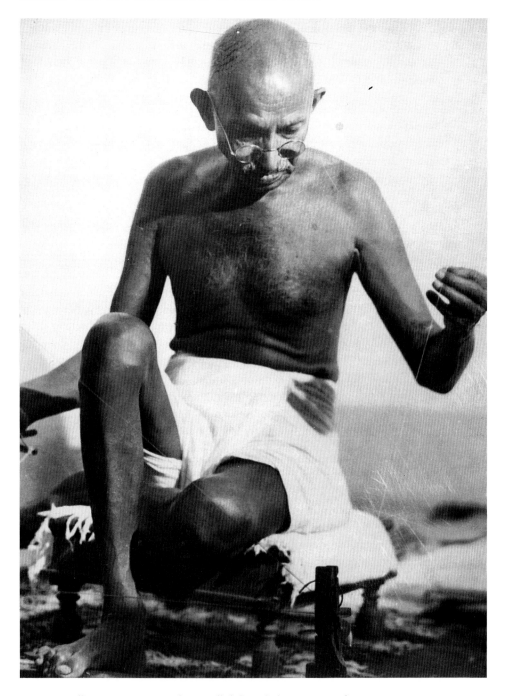

Fig. 3.7 Gandhi spinning, wearing his so called 'loin cloth'. Courtesy of NGM.

I consider the renunciation to be also necessary for me as a sign of mourning. . . . That we are in mourning is more and more being brought home to me as the end of the year is approaching and we are still without swaraj. . . . (CWMG vol. 21: 181).

At 10 o'clock that evening a barber shaved his head, after which he spent a restless and contemplative night. He was particularly anxious about the reaction of his fellow Gujaratis who would find his loincloth a 'sore trial' (Krishnadas 1928: 204). More generally he worried that people might think it indecent (CWMG vol. 24: 456). He none the less set out the next morning, dressed in his scanty attire, to deliver a speech to some Madura weavers. On his third day of wearing the loincloth, Gandhi was still plainly a little apprehensive about people's reactions. He wrote in *The Hindu*:

The masses in Madras watch me with bewilderment. . . . But if India calls me a lunatic, what then? If the co-workers do not copy my example, what then? Of course this is not meant to be copied by co-workers. It is meant simply to hearten the people and to make my way clear. Unless I went about with a loincloth, how might I advise others to do likewise? What should I do where millions have to go naked? At any rate why not try the experiment for a month and a quarter? Why not satisfy myself that I left no stone unturned? . . .

I want the reader to measure from this the agony of my soul. . . . I do wish they may understand that swadeshi means everything (*The Hindu*, 15 Oct. 1921; CWMG vol. 21: 226).

It is clear from Gandhi's speeches that when he first adopted the loincloth he was not intending to wear it all his life as a definitive statement of his beliefs. It was another of his 'experiments' and an expression of his innermost grief and 'mourning'. It was intended to enable the poor to discard their foreign cloth more easily without feeling ashamed of their nakedness, and to provoke people into spinning more yarn. It was probably never intended to communicate the 'dignity of poverty' or the 'greatness of Indian civilization' (cited in Bean 1989: 368). Gandhi never confused the positive benefits of his own 'voluntary poverty' with the crushing effects of the enforced poverty of the 'Indian masses'. If a 'mere loincloth' was the habitual dress of his countrymen, this was more a cause of pain to Gandhi than of pride. Back in 1919, he had told a crowd in Baroda: 'If we go naked in these days, it is for want of cloth' (CWMG vol. 16: 225). The loincloth was the dress of necessity not desire, and Gandhi claimed he was ready to revert to his 'normal dress' if only people would adopt full *swadeshi*

Gandhi and the Recreation of Indian Dress

(CWMG vol. 21: 277). To a Muslim who wrote to him in 1924, accusing him of indecency, he replied:

> It [the loincloth] will go when men and women of India help me to discard it. . . . I wish to be in tune with the poorest of the poor among Indians. . . . How can these poor people afford a long shirt with a collar? Who will give them a cap? If we wear so many garments, we cannot clothe the poor, but it is our duty to dress them first and then ourselves, to feed them first and then ourselves. . . . When Hindu and Muslim sisters have adopted the spinning-wheel and come to look upon khadi as their adornment, I shall feel that I have got all I wanted. I shall then certainly please my correspondent by wearing a dhoti and a long shirt and collar (CWMG vol. 24: 456).

In Gandhi's own perception, the loincloth was a sign of India's dire poverty and of the need to improve its wealth through *swadeshi* and through a wholesale rejection of European civilisation.[16] It was a rejection not only of the material products of Europe, but also of the European value system with its criteria of decency. It was better for the poor to wear scanty loincloths than to clothe themselves in garments from abroad. But while the loincloth was indeed a full-scale promotion of Indianness, it was not a glorification of poverty. Rather, through his nakedness, Gandhi hoped visually to expose Indian poverty while simultaneously suggesting its resolution through hand-spinning, weaving, and freedom from British rule. When in 1931 he insisted on wearing his loincloth to London where he had been invited to participate in the Round Table Conference, he argued that it was because of his duty to the poor that he refused to wear more clothes.[17] He was the representative of 'Daridranarayana, the semi starved almost naked villager' (CWMG vol. 47: 119). Defending his loincloth in an article he wrote for the *Daily Herald* while in England, Gandhi declared:

> My dress, which is described in the newspapers as a loincloth, is criticized, made fun of. I am asked why I wear it. Some seem to resent me wearing it. . . . But I am here on a great and special mission and my

---

16   It is important to make the distinction here between European civilisation and Europeans, a distinction which Gandhi always kept very firmly. It was not Europeans themselves he opposed, but rather their civilisation with its emphasis on materialism and egoism (CWMG vol. 10: 174).

17   It is interesting that in 1922 Gandhi had argued that if he went abroad he would discard his loincloth out of respect for foreign notions of decency. He claimed that to wear it was tantamount to lack of consideration for others and would be 'a form of violence' (CWMG vol. 23: 40).

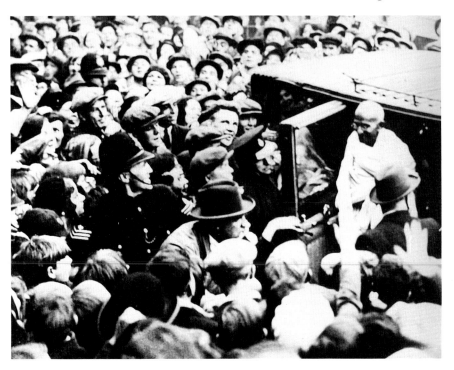

Fig. 3.8 Gandhi in England, 1931. *Right*: leaving a taxi on his way to meet Charlie Chaplin in London. *Opposite*: with Lancashire mill workers. Miraben (*far right*) recalls the moment when the photograph was taken: 'Bapu said a few words, then two women workers hooked him by the arms, one on each side, and throwing up their unengaged arms shouted, 'Three cheers for Mr. Ganddye, hip, hip-' (cited in Hunt 1978:290). Courtesy of NGM.

loincloth . . . is the dress of my principals, the people of India. Into my keeping a sacred trust has been put. . . . I must therefore wear the symbol of my mission (*Daily Herald* 28 Sept. 1931; CWMG vol. 48: 79–80).

Gandhi stubbornly wore his loincloth throughout his stay in Britain, refusing to compromise his dress, even in front of King George V at Buckingham Palace. In fact, he wore it for the rest of his life[18] because his 'mission' was never completed. He never obtained his objective of clothing the entire Indian nation in *khadi* and re-establishing a self-sufficient craft-based society. So even after the attainment of independence, he had no reason to return to his 'normal dress'.

From an outsider's point of view Gandhi's loincloth may be considered one of the most successful and ingenious attempts symbolically to oppose British rule. Yet if we try to evaluate its success in Gandhi's own terms, it is clear that it failed to provoke the realisation of his political dream. It was adopted in 1921 as a desperate measure because *swaraj* was still far off and the Indian people were still dressed in foreign cloth. It was a temporary 'sign of mourning', intended to provoke people into spinning, weav-

18   Gandhi was assassinated in 1948.

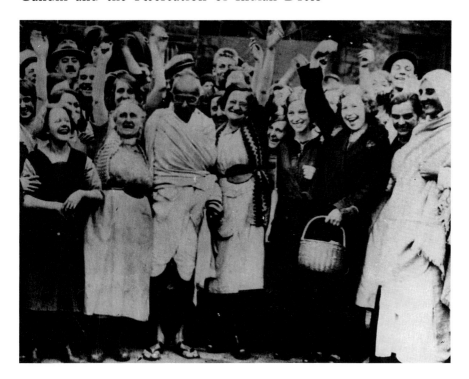

ing and clothing the poor. The fact that Gandhi still wore the loincloth when he died was a sign that the Indian people had rejected his version of progress and national development. To him it was a cause of great sorrow that after independence those who had once adopted *khadi* were now returning to foreign cloth (CWMG vol. 90: 206). His loincloth had been unable to effect the national sartorial changes he had hoped for.

Of course, one can never fully know Gandhi's 'intention' in wearing a loincloth, for what he actually wrote and declared in his speeches may have differed to some extent from his personal reflections. Yet through analysing the content of his expressed intention, one can gain considerable insight into how he tried to construct the meaning of his loincloth publicly. It is suggested here that Gandhi wrote and spoke so much about his dress because he wanted people to understand it and because he realised that it could easily be misinterpreted.[19] Misinterpreted it was, but this does not mean that the misinterpretations were necessarily detrimental to Gandhi, or that Gandhi did not to some extent enjoy the ambiguity of his own sartorial gesture.

19 Misinterpretation, in this case, is any interpretation at variance with Gandhi's proposed intention. For detailed analysis of the potential of clothes to miscommunicate information about their wearers, see Lurie 1992.

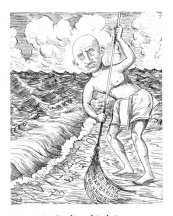

Fig. 3.9 'Girding his loins to mop sea civilization'. Reproduced from the *Hindi Punch*, Bombay (original included Gujarati inscription), 2 Oct. 1921. Courtesy of OIOC.

Some misinterpretations of the loincloth

When Gandhi first announced his intention to shed his *dhoti* and cap, a cartoon appeared in the *Hindi Punch* showing him sweeping back the tide of civilisation with the broom of 'old time barbarism' (fig. 3.9). To many Britons and educated Indians alike, his loincloth was a backward step, a return to the nakedness of the 'primitive' and 'barbaric'. Even his closest followers were concerned, as we have seen, to dissuade him from taking such a drastic measure. Some feared that they too might be expected to shed their clothes. Since Gandhi discussed his decision with them at length, they became the people closest to understanding his proposed intention. Maulana Azad Sobhani immediately reacted by reducing his own dress, replacing his pantaloons with a *lungi* and his shirt with a waistcoat, and removing his cap which, from then on, he wore only for prayer (Krishnadas 1928: 210). Krishnadas, after agonising reflection, finally decided to discard his vest but not to adopt the more drastic and 'humiliating' loincloth (*ibid.*: 207).[20]

First reactions to Gandhi's change of dress from those outside his immediate circle varied from puzzlement to fear and misapprehension. Some, like the ex-chief justice of Baroda, Abbas Tyabji, laughed.[21] Others, like the Muslim Maulana Abdul Bari, feared that Gandhi's loincloth violated Islamic codes of decency.[22] But whatever the reaction, it certainly attracted attention and drew the crowds (*ibid.*: 245). As it became a well-known feature of his identity, people came to interpret it increasingly as a sign of Gandhi's saintliness since he looked like a religious ascetic. He had already been labelled *Mahatma* (Great Soul) some years before he adopted the loincloth and by 1921 he was frequently perceived as a saint (Amin 1984). But somehow his new loincloth garb seemed like the confirmation of his sainthood (Jog 1945: 125, Dey 1948: Preface). People came from miles around to get Gandhi's *darshan* (holy sight) (Bean 1989, Krishnadas 1928). The loinclothed ascetic was an image they could relate to and admire. Even today it is the image of Gandhi that is most preserved in popular posters and calendars.

But there were two major problems with people interpreting the loin-

20 Krishnadas felt that Gandhi had adopted the loincloth as a sign of the intensity of his own inner pain at the sight of the naked masses. For others to do likewise, without the same intensity of feeling, would therefore be 'mere blind imitation or affection, and nothing else'. None the less Krishnadas felt guilty witnessing Gandhi's suffering without sharing it. He claims to have 'suffered a good deal under the stress of these conflicting emotions' concerning whether or not to adopt a loincloth himself (Krishnadas 1928: 206–7).

21 Tyabji's words at the time were: 'See, Mahatmaji has turned mad, but not merely that; he has devised a new way of making others mad also' (Krishnadas 1928: 253).

22 His words were: 'We have all come to see you, but it is against our scripture to keep the knees bare in this fashion' (Krishnadas 1928: 252).

Gandhi and the Recreation of Indian Dress

cloth as confirmation of Gandhi's sainthood. The first was that Gandhi himself hotly denied being a saint on many occasions and cursed what he called his 'mahatmaship'.[23] And the second was that by seeing Gandhi's dress as the clothes of a Hindu ascetic, people 'naturalised' his loincloth and accepted his poverty. It was after all what you would expect of a holy man. If these interpretations are judged according to Gandhi's proclamations about the meaning of the loincloth, they are clearly wrong. For he did not want people to accept his nakedness passively as if it were a purely religious act or a sign of asceticism. He wanted them to 'measure the agony of his soul' (CWMG vol. 21: 226) and to spin in order that he and the poor whom he represented might be clothed. In fact, Gandhi was so vehemently opposed to the notion of 'saintly garbs' that he even refused to grant Ashram membership to the well-known *sanyasi*, Swami Satyadev, on the grounds that the latter would not replace his ochre robes with plain white *khadi* (cf. Kalelkar 1950: 32). The *sanyasi*'s robes were, he felt, inappropriate to the task of serving the nation, for they invited the adoration of the people and distracted both the wearer and his followers from their path of duty.

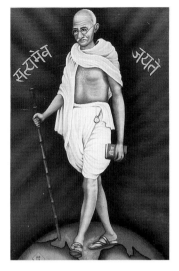

Fig. 3.10 'The way of truth triumphs'. Contemporary oleograph of Gandhi as saint. Courtesy of Chris Pinney.

To reduce Gandhi's own clothes to a mere symbol of sainthood was clearly to undermine most of what he had to say about them. But the situation was, of course, ambiguous for although religious interpretations deconstructed Gandhi's message, they simultaneously brought the crowds to him and actively increased his popularity 'as a saint'. Furthermore much of Gandhi's behaviour, including his adoption of 'voluntary poverty', was typically characteristic of Indian saints, if not saints in general. This ambiquity was further exploited by Gandhi himself, who frequently used highly emotive religious terminology when speaking of *khadi* (cf. Bayly 1986).

Another common interpretation of Gandhi's loincloth was that it was purely strategic. Most famous was Winston Churchill's description of Gandhi as 'a seditious Middle Temple lawyer' now 'posing as a half-naked fakir'[24] (cited in Templewood 1954: 54). More extreme still was Beverly Nichols's assertion that Gandhi was really a fascist and that *khadi* was the equivalent of the Nazi shirt and swastika (Nichols 1944: 164–5). Fig. 3.11 plays on this idea that Gandhi, like other world leaders, had created his own uniform which was all the more distinctive for being shirtless. Some were even

23 See his declaration in the British press in 1931: 'Some call me a saint. Others call me a rogue. I am neither one nor the other' (CWMG vol. 48: 79). See also his speech in Sholapur in 1927: 'I assure you the words darshan and Mahatma stink in my nostrils' (CWMG vol. 33: 101).
24 Following this statement the journalist and Liberal MP Robert Bernays published a book about Gandhi entitled *Naked Fakir* (1931). Churchill's phrase gained legendary fame and is quoted in most biographies of Gandhi.

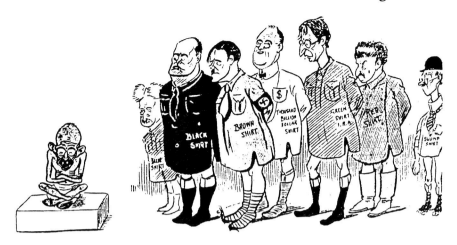

Fig. 3.11 'And he ain't wearing any blooming shirt at all!' Cartoon by J. C. Hill, published in the *Auckland Star*, 1931. Courtesy of the *Auckland Star*.

suspicious of this very shirtlessness. One communist group, on hearing of his imminent arrival in Britain, issued a statement warning that 'the dramatic tactics of his not putting on a shirt and living on vegetables and goat's milk should not mislead the working class. Such tactics are adopted to serve the ends of capitalist interests in the East' (cited in Lester 1932: 35).

Clearly people were capable of reading all manner of things into Gandhi's loincloth regardless of what he himself said about it. It was partly because of this ambiguity that so many of his followers tried to persuade him to reclothe himself when visiting Britain in 1931. Apart from anything else, they worried that he would not be taken seriously (S. Bose 1964: 137) and that 'he may become a music hall joke' (Bernays 1931: 300). Even before his arrival, there was much talk of Gandhi's appearance in letters and in the British press. Sometimes he was described as 'Christlike'. On one occasion he was dismissed as a 'naked nigger' (cited in Lester 1932: 36). But to the British authorities he was largely an embarrassment, particularly when it came to the question of whether he should be invited to afternoon tea at Buckingham Palace. King George V had intended to welcome all the Indian delegates from the Round Table Conference but he was reluctant to invite 'the little man' with 'no proper clothes on, and bare knees' (Templewood 1954: 59). The situation was awkward since his dress was a blatant breach of court etiquette, but Gandhi had already announced in a speech that even if he met the King he would not reclothe while the Indian poor were still naked at Britain's expense (CWMG vol. 48: 72–3). Finally the King relented and Gandhi appeared in his habitual loincloth and a large white shawl which he turned inside out since he had not had time to wash it (Slade 1984: 138). The event was much enjoyed by journalists and cartoonists, and Gandhi himself participated in the general air of sartorial amusement. Asked if he had been wearing enough clothes for his meeting with the King, Gandhi is said to have replied: 'The King had enough on for both of us' (Lal 1969: 20).

While remaining naked and thereby exposing Indian poverty was a vital priority to Gandhi, it was not always easy to sustain, for there were often a number of well-wishers anxious to reclothe him. This was true not only of children,[25] but also of some of his closest followers. Gandhi's frustration at their lack of understanding was revealed in an incident on the ship bound for England in 1931. Unknown to Gandhi, many of his supporters, anxious that he might be cold or uncomfortable, had offered him gifts of stockings, shawls, mufflers, bags, wallets and even an American-made folding camp-bed (Slade 1984: 129). These had been packed on board the ship by Gandhi's closest associates who were accompanying him to Britain. Gandhi was furious when he discovered them, remonstrating that he was a representative of a poor country and could not possibly arrive in England with a collection of 'swanky suitcases'. It was an embarrassing situation which was finally resolved by posting all the most expensive-looking luggage back to Bombay from Aden so that he could still arrive in Britain looking the poor man.

Not only was Gandhi's nakedness physically difficult to maintain but it also became problematic in the metaphorical sense, particularly among some of his Western admirers. Out of their immense respect, they could not resist reclothing him in their minds, thereby making him more decent in Western terms. Bernays, for example, preferred to describe Gandhi as 'not half naked, but three quarters naked' (Bernays 1931: 299). And the American Haynes Holmes talked of his 'royal air', saying he looked and spoke 'like a king' (Haynes Holmes 1945: 101). It is difficult to imagine any description of him that is further away from what Gandhi was trying to portray: the poverty and needs of his naked, illiterate countrymen. Yet, like the religious interpretations of his dress, these interpretations were well meant, even though they entirely deconstructed most of what he was trying to communicate. The ambiguity of his symbolic dressing did not necessarily harm his reputation. On the contrary, the fact that he looked like a Hindu

---

25 Children both in England and in India seemed to have an instinctive desire to give Gandhi clothes. To a young Indian boy who wanted to ask his mother to make Gandhi a shirt, Gandhi replied that he would only accept it if she could provide shirts for every poor man in India (Kalarthi 1960: 14).

ascetic or Christ or even a 'king' actually served to increase his popularity. Furthermore his nakedness and simplicity remained a powerful contrast to the pedantically clad European image. And even if he did not recommend nakedness as an ideal, he none the less advocated a complete rejection of the previously idealised European look.[26]

Examination of Gandhi's speeches and writings concerning dress reveals that he developed a personal theory of clothes. For him they were an outward expression of the moral integrity of the wearer – an expression of truth. He first voiced these ideas in South Africa, but later came to concretise them after his return to India. They became a consistent theme and in later life he usually described his own dress in these terms. But if one examines his attempts to encourage the Indian nation to adopt *khadi* and the Gandhi cap, one finds him utilising a number of different and often contradictory arguments about the meaning of clothes. The final section of this chapter explores Gandhi's elaborate rhetoric as he tried to fulfil his ambition: 'The whole country will be clothed in khadi. That is my dream. This is a fight to finish' (cited in Bakshi 1987b: 173).

THE MAHATMA AS CLOTHING MANAGER OF THE NATION

Designing the Gandhi cap

In a little-known conversation with his friend Kakasahib, Gandhi explained how he came to choose the form of the Gandhi cap:[27]

> I considered carefully all the caps and head-coverings which obtain in the various parts of Bharat [India]. I bore in mind that it is a hot country, and therefore, our heads need to be kept covered. The Bengalis and some South Bharati Brahmins go bare-headed of course, but, as a rule, Bharatis [Indians] always wear something or other on their heads. The Punjabi phenta [turban] looks fine, but it takes up too much cloth. The pugree is a dirty thing. It goes on absorbing perspiration, but does not show

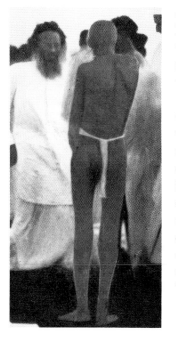

Fig. 3.12 Gandhi at his most naked, pictured after bathing in the sea at Nandi in 1930.

26   The rejection of the European look was part of a more general rejection of a European way of life. Gandhi wanted people to change not only their appearances but also their very physical composition and lifestyle. His advocacy of an extreme form of strict vegetarianism, of fasting and celibacy were all part of an attempt to decolonise the body and to re-Indianise it. They were also part of the 'purification' process. Gandhi felt that 'self-purification' and 'penance' were essential to India's wellbeing. In 1927 he argued: 'I must go on purifying myself and hoping that only thereby would I react on my surroundings' (CWMG vol. 33: 100)

27   Lack of information has hitherto led to a number of speculative guesses about the origins of the Gandhi cap. Ashe thought it derived from Gandhi's prison uniform in South Africa (in Bean 1989: 367), while Bean has suggested it was linked to his interest in Hindu-Muslim unity (*ibid.*).

it, and so seldom gets washed. Our Gujarati conical Bangalore caps look hideous to me. The Maharashtran Hungarian caps are a little better, but they are made of felt. As for the U.P. [Uttar Pradesh] and Bihari caps, they are so thin and useless that they can hardly be considered caps at all! They are not even becoming. So, thinking over all these various types of headgear, I came to the conclusion that the Kashmiri cap was the best. It is light as well as elegant; it is easy to make; it can be folded, which makes it easily portable. One can put it in one's pocket, or pack it comfortably in one's trunk. The Kashmiri cap is made from wool. I thought it should be made of cotton cloth. Having thus chosen the form, I then began to consider the colour. Which colour would be most suitable for the cap? Not a single colour appealed to me. So I fixed upon white. White shows up dirt and grease, so white caps would have to be frequently washed (a great recommendation!). Also, white cloth is easily washable. The cap being of the folding sort, it would be quite easy to press after washing, and iron out into a fresh, clean, smooth, white cap! What could be better or more becoming? So, having thought this out, I made this cap. As a matter of fact, the climatic conditions of our country render the sola topee the most suitable headgear for Bharatis. It affords perfect protection for the head, eyes, and back of the neck from the burning sun, and, being made of pith, is delightfully light and cool. It lets in a little air, too. The only reason why I do not advocate the sola topee is that it does not harmonize at all with our Bharati dress. Moreover, people these days dislike anything that has a European flavour. If our craftsmen would evolve a head-gear which combined all the qualities of the sola hat with a Bharati shape, they would be doing a great service to the whole country. It only needs a bit of thought. I am sure they would not find it difficult (Kalelkar 1950: 97–8).

Although it is clear that Gandhi was deliberately searching for a suitable national cap, the fact that he wished to combine aspects of the *sola topi* with an Indian form[28] suggests he was not fully aware of how important a symbol of opposition to the British his invention would become. His primary motive was to invent a form of pan-Indian headwear which anyone could afford and wear. As we have seen, a man's headwear was important for revealing his social and religious identity. By promoting this small *khadi* cap, Gandhi hoped to attain a level of visual uniformity which had never existed in Indian headwear. Such uniformity was very important to Gandhi, who argued:

28 This is, of course, precisely what Jyotirindranath Tagore had invented when he combined the *sola topi* with the Indian turban with somewhat unsuccessful results (see previous chapter).

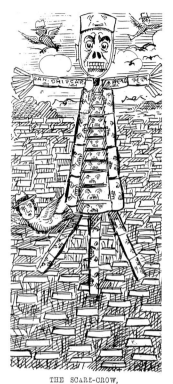

THE SCARE-CROW,
that frightens some white birds!

Fig. 3.13 Reproduced from *Hindi Punch*, Bombay 21 Aug. 1921. Courtesy of OIOC.

One who is eager to dress himself in khadi from head to foot should begin with the head straight away. The khadi cap can be used by all, the rich and the poor.... the idea that all should have the same kind of cap on their heads is well worth considering (CWMG vol. 20: 386).

When coloured imitations of the cap were sold in Bombay, Gandhi reiterated the importance of keeping all hats identical: 'A swadeshi cap should be one that can be identified even by children' (CWMG vol. 20: 385).

Gandhi himself was wearing the cap by 1919, by which time he was already vigorously promoting *khadi*, hand-spinning and the burning of foreign cloth. The cap spread quickly among his supporters and he made it an obligatory part of the Congress uniform (Cohn 1989: 344). During the non-cooperation movement, it was sold at all major political meetings and on street corners. By 1920 substantial numbers of the Indian male population were wearing it. The British authorities were unhappy at this sudden mushrooming of white caps on Indian heads: as we have seen, they had long been trying to control Indian headwear and they now began to clamp down on Gandhi cap-wearers by dismissing them from government jobs, fining them and at times physically beating them. Fig. 3.13, drawn in response to the British decision to ban government servants from wearing Gandhi caps in the Central Provinces, criticises the British for their cowardice. The cartoonist recognised that the significance of the cap was created as much by British responses to it as by Gandhi's personal attempts to promote it.

Once the cap had gained symbolic importance from a combination of Indian and British uses and abuses, Gandhi himself took up the symbolic challenge. What is interesting is the language he employed in defending and promoting the cap: aware that his invention could be interpreted as anything from an innocent piece of headwear to a potent symbol of subversion, he made substantial use of this ambiguity, emphasising different aspects of the cap's significance according to the situation and event. His rhetoric shows a certain mastery in exploiting the ambiguity of symbolic phenomena.

At times the arguments Gandhi employed were in tune with his own personal belief in the moral, political and economic importance of dress. He described the Gandhi cap as a garment of 'truth' and argued that if everyone followed the truth, the government would be forced either to respect public opinion, to put everyone in jail, or to leave the country (CWMG vol. 19: 482). When the chief justice of the high court at Ratnagari declared in 1922 that 'any pleader wearing a Gandhi cap in court' would be considered 'guilty of disrespect to the Judge', Gandhi responded by highlighting the cap's vital symbolic value:

... the principle underlying this war against khadi caps is of the highest importance. It shows how innocent but moral and economic movements are attempted to be killed by their adversaries. ... Nor do pleaders who adopt the national cap do so out of any disrespect for the court, but they do it out of respect for themselves and the nation to which they belong. They do it because they do not wish to conceal their religion or their politics, whichever way one regards the adoption of the khadi cap (CWMG vol. 22: 16).

But while Gandhi considered his new cap so important that he hoped that 'thousands will be prepared to die for the khadi cap which is fast becoming a visible mark of swadeshi and swaraj' (CWMG vol. 21: 507), he claimed at other times that it was really nothing more than a 'beautiful, light, inoffensive' garment, valued for its practicality more than its political significance (CWMG vol. 20: 105). This was a vital part of Gandhi's political technique.[29] By emphasising the apparent innocence of the cap, he was able to make government suppression of the garment appear both unnecessary and unreasonable. He even went so far as to suggest that the symbolic significance of the Gandhi cap was less his own doing than a product of the government's overcharged imagination. In response to a cap prohibition introduced by an officer of the Gwalior state, who saw the cap as a symbol of non-cooperation, Gandhi wrote:

I am sorry for this unnecessary prejudice against a harmless and cheap cap. I venture to inform the Gwalior authorities that, whilst it is true that many non-co-operators wear what are known as 'Gandhi caps', there are thousands who wear them simply for convenience and cheapness, but who are no more non-co-operators than the Peshi Officer himself (*Young India*, 9 March 1922, CWMG vol. 23: 35).

But although Gandhi sometimes argued the political neutrality of the cap when it came under persecution, it is clear that he himself saw cap-wearing as an important statement of a person's political belief. This was poignantly revealed when, journeying to Calcutta in April 1925, he was disappointed

---

29 Gandhi invariably chose apparently innocent objects (spinning-wheel, *khadi*, the Gandhi cap and so on) as political symbols. This enabled him to make British repression appear more unreasonable. This was clearly illustrated in his choice of the salt law as a symbol of government repression. The salt tax was one of the least draining taxes on the Indian economy. But by encouraging people to ignore the British monopoly and to make their own salt, Gandhi chose an action which appeared thoroughly reasonable but which was politically and symbolically subversive. Clothes and salt were also basic human rights, necessary to all, which made them accessible symbols to which the Indian masses could relate.

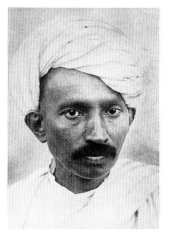

to see from his train window not 'a forest of white khaddar caps', but 'provoking black foreign caps on almost every head' (CWMG vol. 26: 574). When a black-capped crowd struggled to get a glimpse of his holy sight on the platform at Nagpur, he recoiled at the hypocrisy: 'My name on their lips and black caps on their heads, – what a terrible contrast! What a lie! I could not fight the battle of Swaraj with that crowd.... I was in agony' (*ibid.*: 575). He demanded their foreign caps, but no more than a hundred were thrown and four of these were not thrown by their owners. This was yet another cause of remorse for Gandhi, for he wanted *swadeshi* to be peaceful and not coercive. But there were those who interpreted his symbols of 'truth force' as symbols of aggression and an excuse for violence. Such incidents revealed yet again that Gandhi, master of symbolism though he was, could not persuade others to adopt his own belief in the meaning of dress. This was further revealed in his attempts to persuade all Indians into *khadi* clothes.

Converting the nation to khadi

Fig. 3.14 The evolution of Gandhi's headwear (1915–21). *Above*: Gandhi with a turban (1915). *Below*: With an embroidered Kashmiri cap (1915). *Opposite top*: Wearing the Gandhi cap (1920). *Opposite bottom*: Pictured the night before he adopted the loincloth, having just removed his cap and had his head shaved by a barber (1921).

Gandhi's main personal emphasis was, as we have seen, on the moral significance of clothes. He hoped to convey this significance to the entire Indian nation, changing people's attitudes to their dress. As with many of his theories, he used the Sabarmati ashram as the laboratory for his experiments. As early as May 1915, soon after his return from South Africa, he had written a draft version of the ashram constitution which included a 'vow of *swadeshi*' to be taken by all ashram members.[30] Place of origin and means of production were to be the key factors determining a garment's moral worth. All machine-made cloth, even if it was produced in India, violated Gandhi's concept of truth, non-violence, non-stealing, non-possession and celibate living. Once he had revived the hand-spinning industry, making

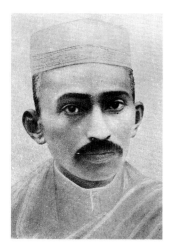

30   The full vow went as follows: 'The person who has taken the vow of Swadeshi will never use articles which conceivably involve violation of truth in their manufacture or on the part of their manufacturers. It follows, for instance, that a votary of truth will not use articles manufactured in the mills of Manchester, Germany or India, for he cannot be sure that they have involved no such violation of truth. Moreover, labourers suffer much in the mills. The generation of tremendous heat causes enormous destruction of life. Besides, the loss of workers' lives in the manufacture of machines and of other creatures through excessive heat is something impossible to describe. Foreign cloth and cloth made by machinery are, therefore, tabooed to a votary of non-violence as they involve triple violence. Further reflection will show that the use of foreign cloth can be held to involve a breach of the vows of non-stealing and non-possession. We follow custom, and for better appearance, wear foreign cloth in preference to the cloth made on our own handlooms with so little effort. Artificial beautifying of the body is a hindrance to a *brahmachari* [celibate] and so, even from the point of view of that vow, machine-made cloth is taboo. Therefore the vow of Swadeshi requires the use of simple clothing made on simple handlooms and stitched in simple style, foreign buttons, cuts, etc., being avoided. The same line of reasoning may be applied to all other articles' (CWMG vol. 13: 93).

Gandhi and the Recreation of Indian Dress

the spinning-wheel (*charkha*) a national symbol, he added another criterion to his *swadeshi* vow: that the cloth should be woven from hand-spun yarn. This was a *swadeshi* far stricter than that practised a decade earlier by the Bengali nationalists, who had used the country of origin and not the means of production as their criterion for determining the morality of cloth.

By 1919 Gandhi was appealing to all Indian men and women to adopt *khadi* and take a vow of *swadeshi*.[31] Added to the moral value of *khadi* were the social, political and economic benefits of making and wearing *swadeshi* cloth. By the end of his life Gandhi had woven almost all his beliefs into the concept of *swadeshi*. In brief, he felt that through stimulating the production and use of indigenous cloth he could provide supplementary employment to the masses, remove untouchability, promote the self-sufficiency of India's villages, weld together people of all religions and castes, drive out British rule by non-violent means and introduce an improved standard of morality and sense of national unity. *Khadi* and spinning were to become not only the unifying national cause in the peaceful struggle for freedom but also the basis of a new non-industrial, craft-based economic structure in independent India. As Gandhi himself admitted, *khadi* to him was something of an obsession: 'Of all my foibles, of all my weaknesses and fanaticisms or whatever you like to call them, *khadi* is my pet one. . . . This is sacred cloth' (CWMG vol. 23: 106).

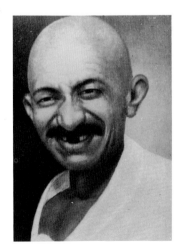

Gandhi set about converting the nation to *khadi* in a systematic and structured manner. He established numerous organisations and associations for its promotion, as well as training centres for spinning and weaving. He also persuaded the Congress Party to give *khadi* an important place at the centre of its policies. By 1920 the non-cooperation movement included a boycott on imported textiles and the organisation of pickets at the entrance to foreign cloth shops. Furthermore, all Congress politicians were expected to wear white *khadi* (loose shirts with *dhoti* or *pyjama*), and were later requested to spin for a minimum of half an hour a day. And while Congress was to set the example, all Indian men and women were called on to burn their foreign cloth as part of their acceptance of the *swadeshi* vow. Volunteers hawked *khadi* through the streets, providing door-to-door collections of foreign cloth for burning or distribution to the destitute. Meanwhile, substantial efforts were made to stimulate the production and wearing of *khadi* through constructive education schemes, exhibitions, shops and national schools.

31 The precise wording of these vows varied considerably from speech to speech.

So fastidious was Gandhi over the necessity of wearing *khadi* that he even objected to an actor wearing foreign cloth in a national school production of Shakespeare's *Hamlet* (CWMG vol. 29: 319–20). He criticised priests for dressing images of the gods in machine-made foreign cloth (CWMG vol. 16: 188). And he attempted to replace the use of flower garlands, traditionally distributed to honoured guests on auspicious occasions, by 'yarn garlands' made from hand-spun cotton thread which could be collected and later used to provide cheap clothing for the poor (CWMG vol. 26: 74). He also sought to revolutionise women's clothing by trying to persuade women to hand over their jewellery for use in public works (Gandhi 1946: 195) and adopt plain undecorated *khadi* saris, preferably white. *Khadi* and its counterpart, hand-spinning, were a potential solution to all India's problems. For Gandhi they were an act of faith.

In view of Gandhi's personal belief in the moral importance of *khadi*, it is interesting to follow his various arguments as he tried to define and redefine the meaning of clothing for the Indian nation, for it is here that we encounter the many conflicts and ambiguities of his sartorial teachings. Because of his belief in unity of thought and action, he chose *khadi* as the fabric of truth *par excellence*, the ultimate expression of moral duty and personal belief. Yet at the same time, he was forced to acknowledge that it was economically and politically expedient for all to wear *khadi*, regardless of their beliefs, since this saved it from becoming the freakish garb of a small religious minority. Taking the examples of foreign cloth and *khadi*, it is possible to untangle some of the inescapable ambiguities of Gandhi's theory of dress as his idea of clothing as truth (an end in itself) was forced to make concessions to a more practical idea of clothing as strategy (a means to an end).

Khadi versus foreign cloth: battle of morality and tactics

There were numerous reasons why it was difficult to persuade people to adopt *khadi*. Many had internalised the belief that foreign cloth meant civilisation and that a return to *khadi* was a return to 'savage days' (CWMG vol. 26: 258). Furthermore, fine cloth had always been favoured in India above thick coarse *khadi*, even before the invention of mill-cloth. Gandhi was aware of *khadi*'s limitations. In 1920, he admitted

> ... that all khadi is not equally good quality; that it easily crumples and coat and trousers do not remain stiff; it shrinks so much that the sleeve recedes from the wrist to the elbow; it looks like a sieve so much that moong grains can easily pass through it: people perhaps have had experience of one or the other or all of these things.... (CWMG vol. 17: 16).

Gandhi and the Recreation of Indian Dress

In economic terms, *khadi's* position was equally tenuous for it represented poorer quality at higher prices. This inevitably deterred many from buying it and led Gandhi to propound an alternative economic theory[32] in which national wellbeing was the new criterion of value:

> Life is more than money. It is cheaper to kill our aged parents who can do no work and who are a drag on our slender resources. It is also cheaper to kill our children whom we do not need for our material comfort and whom we have to maintain without getting anything in return. But we kill neither our parents nor our children, but consider it a privilege to maintain them no matter what their maintenance costs us. Even so must we maintain khadi to the exclusion of all other cloth. . . . When we have studied them [*khadi* economics] from the point of view of national well-being, we shall find that khadi is never dear (*Harijan* 10 Dec. 1938 in Gandhi 1959: 70).

Khadi-wearing was to become a moral duty both to the nation and to the wearer, who should recognise the full implications of the 'khadi spirit': 'illimitable faith', 'illimitable patience', 'self-sacrifice', 'purity of life' and 'fellow feeling with every human being on earth' (Gandhi 1959: 104–5). In short, it was a matter of *dharma* (religious duty). In order to wear *khadi* a person should therefore maintain a lifestyle worthy of it, for 'the outward appearance must be fit with the expression within' (CWMG vol. 19: 345). It was not enough for people to don *khadi* simply because it was coming into vogue. For Gandhi a change of clothes was like a change of religion; it was a question of morality and belief (CWMG vol. 27: 334). Without this latter aspect, a sartorial conversion was worthless. In 1921, he wrote in Navajivan:

> Anyone who wears khadi out of ignorance, by way of imitating others or out of hypocrisy, will not be regarded as having taken the vow of khadi, despite the fact that he wears it. Such fashionable khadi wearers could not be regarded as advancing the sentiment of khadi (Gandhi in Bakshi 1987b: 89).

Directly opposed to *khadi* was foreign cloth which, with its superficial glamour and artifice, lured innocent people away from the path of truth and virtue. The battle between *khadi* and foreign cloth was therefore a symbolic encounter between good and evil. The very act of wearing or buying

---

32 Gandhi altered the emphasis of his economic arguments in later years when he tried to get villagers to spin, not for sale but for their own use. He wished to decentralise the *khadi* movement and make it an important part of his scheme for village uplift.

PUBLIC MEETING

AND

BONFIRE OF FOREIGN CLOTHES

Will take place at the Maidan near Elphinstone Mills
. . . Opp. Elphinstone Road Station . . .

On SUNDAY the 9th Inst. at 6-30 P. M.

When the Resolution of the Karachi Khilafat Conference and another Congratulating Ali Brothers and others will be passed.

All are requested to attend in Swadeshi Clothes of Khadi. Those who have not yet given away their Foreign Clothes are requested to send them to their respective Ward Congress Committees for inclusion in the

GREAT BONFIRE.

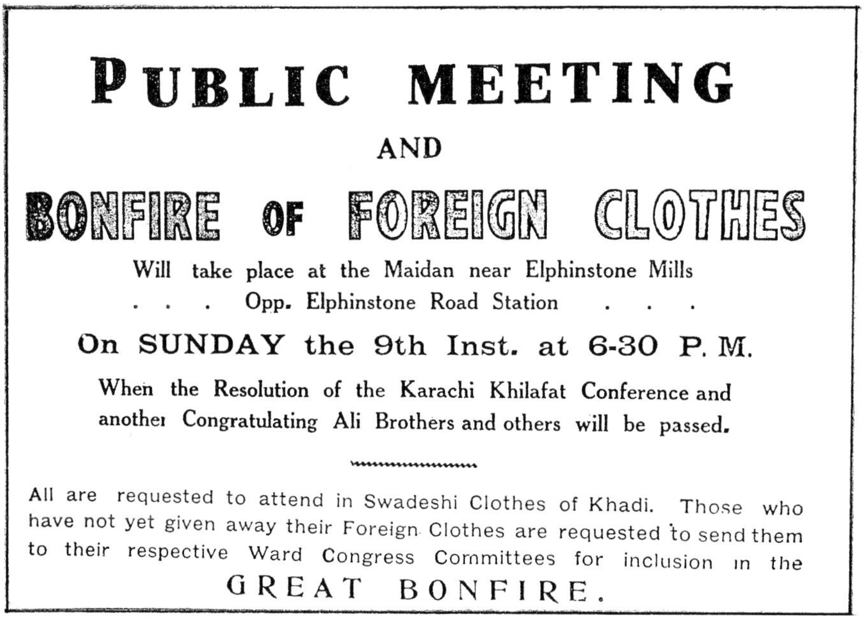

Fig. 3.15 Poster brought out during the non-cooperation movement. Courtesy of the Press Information Bureau, Government of India.

imported machine-manufactured textiles represented a fall to temptation. Rephrasing one of his favourite passages from the Sermon on the Mount, Gandhi preached: 'It is as sinful to cast covetous glances at imported cloth as it is for a man to cast lustful glances at another's wife' (CWMG vol. 18: 409). Gandhi therefore called on mill-owners to stop putting 'temptation' in the way of men and women 'in the shape of flimsy Japanese dhotis or saris or starchy calico'. Rather, they should seek to cultivate new consumer tastes, where art would be recognised in *khadi* itself (cited in Bakshi 1987b: 18). He even argued that the person who wears foreign cloth is no longer Indian 'since by his dress he has become a foreigner' (*ibid.*: 23). And just as nationality and religion were more or less permanent features of a person's identity, so the choice of *khadi* over foreign cloth was to represent a permanent and lifelong conversion. When people were tempted to give up *khadi* and spinning after independence, Gandhi remonstrated that it represented a way of life based on non-violence and that people had misunderstood him if they thought it was merely a strategy for attaining *swaraj* (CWMG vol. 90: 229).

Such remonstrations reveal that, at the ideal level, Gandhi hoped that people's clothing would match and indeed express their internal moral state. But at the pragmatic level he was faced with a number of difficulties. First, there was the fear that through over-emphasising the moral requirements of *khadi*, he might lose support from people who dared not wear *khadi* for fear that they were morally inadequate to do so. This would prevent it from becoming the national cloth it was intended to be. And secondly there was the problem that *khadi* was only powerful in the political and economic sense if sufficient numbers wore it on the streets. In other words, *sheer numbers* were essential to its success. So too was the idea that rich and poor, high caste and low, Hindu, Muslim, Sikh, Christian, Parsi and Jew should be indistinguishable from the fabric of their dress. These factors forced Gandhi to reject at times his original interpretation of the relationship between *khadi* and morality. In reply to a letter from someone who feared wearing *khadi* because he lacked the necessary qualities of 'sincerity, purity and self conquest', Gandhi wrote:

> Its one great merit is that it solves, as nothing else can, the economic problem of India and removes starvation. We want all, irrespective of character, to wear khaddar. Scoundrels, drunkards, the very scum of the land, must clothe and feed themselves. I would not hesitate to urge them to wear khaddar even though I cannot induce them to change their mode of inner life. We must cease to attribute to khaddar virtues which it cannot carry (CWMG vol. 23: 458–9).

In other words, he was calling now for all people to wear *khadi*, whatever their beliefs, a plea which directly contradicted his earlier cry for the integrity of the *khadi*-wearer. And although clothing was supposed to represent each person's spiritual and mental choice, he introduced a series of psychological pressures and regulatory measures to ensure that as many people as possible were persuaded to adopt *khadi* regardless of their faith in the '*khadi* spirit'.

Gandhi's most controversial tool of persuasion was his insistence on the 'transformative' qualities of cloth (Bayly 1986: 314). He shifted his original thesis that people must be worthy of *khadi* to a new one that through wearing it people could actually *become* more worthy. In other words the mere act of wearing *khadi* was so virtuous in itself that it could purify the wearer, whereas foreign cloth was so intrinsically vile that contact with it was physically and mentally defiling. The striking feature of this argument was that Gandhi was utilising the very concept of untouchability which in other contexts he abhorred.[33]

Gandhi's terminology was highly emotive, arousing mass hysteria from

---

33 Take, for example, his damning response when asked if it was wrong for menstruating women to touch books and paper and things connected with learning: 'Such a question can only be asked in a wretched country like India which is disgraced by foolish notions about touching and not touching things' (CWMG vol. 31: 89).

the crowds and stirring episodes where people stripped themselves of foreign garments and tossed them on to communal fires.[34] He referred to foreign cloth as 'filthy', 'defiling', 'untouchable' and 'our greatest outward pollution', and called on people to 'cleanse' themselves by assigning their garments to the 'sacrificial flames'. Foreign cloth, he argued, revived 'such black memories' and was such a mark of 'shame and degradation' that it was not even fit to give to the starving poor, for to wear it was to violate *dharma* (CWMG vol. 20: 433).[35] Those who refused to burn their clothes should send them abroad or confine their use to lavatory wearing only, since they were too defiling for any other purpose (CWMG vol. 20: 342). Gandhi's attitude disturbed the Indian intelligentsia, not least Rabindranath Tagore, who was vehemently opposed to persuasion by crowd psychology and who feared the consequences of the notion of 'untouchability', previously confined to the social sphere, spreading to infect economics and politics (Ahluwalia and Ahluwalia 1981: 99). *Khadi*, by contrast, was 'sacred cloth' (CWMG vol. 23: 106): its radiance influenced other aspects of living and its 'fragrance' made public life 'clean and wholesome' (CWMG vol. 22: 151). Gandhi even suggested that people should seek *darshan* not from himself but from *khadi* (CWMG vol. 33: 101).

The apparent inconsistencies of Gandhi's arguments were to some extent a product of the varied nature of his audiences. Unlike other politicians of his day, he chose to aim his teachings primarily at the masses, but relied on maintaining some credibility with the intellectual élite who held all the major political posts. Of all his policies, it was his obsession with *khadi* and spinning which the Indian intelligentsia found most difficult to stomach, and he was forced to modify his arguments when it appeared that he might lose their support. While he continued to fill his public speeches with passionate and emotional pleas for *khadi*, his language in press interviews and personal discussions was often considerably more restrained. To a perturbed C. F. Andrews[36] he said that although foreign cloth was itself

34 Krishnadas captured the atmosphere of hysteria and excitement that accompanied these fires when he described one lit by Gandhi in Assam: '. . . he set fire to a huge collection of foreign clothes lying in front of the platform. At that time a sort of frenzy seized the whole crowd, and from all sides foreign clothes rained in heaps upon the burning pile. In the crowd, some there were who were seen to cover their nakedness with their towels or their chuddars, consigning their dhoties to the flames. My pen fails to portray the fit of divine enthusiasm that had seized the audience. In such large quantities were clothes offered to the sacrificial fire that it kept on burning till the whole of the succeeding morning' (Krishnadas 1928: 66).

35 After being accused many times of confusing his priorities, Gandhi conceded finally that foreign cloth could be sent to the starving in Malabar, since one could not afford to be fastidious when clothing the naked (CWMG vol. 25: 2–3).

36 An Anglican clergyman who sympathised with a number of Indian causes.

impure, this did not make the wearer of foreign cloth an impure being. Neither did the wearer of *khadi* become a pure being simply through changing his clothes to pure *khadi* (CWMG vol. 25: 236). At times, the entire transformative argument was excluded altogether and replaced by the idea of economic welfare or national solidarity and duty. Thus in Kolupur in 1927 the virtues of the khaddarite were explained as follows: 'The khadi-wearer has distinctly something to his credit inasmuch as he serves both the poor and his country. Khadi immediately takes him up from a lower level and makes him the friend of the poor' (CWMG vol. 33: 194). Gandhi's many and varied explanations of the meaning of *khadi* reveal not the insincerity of his beliefs but rather the extraordinary strength of his conviction that in *khadi* lay the foundations of free India. With the zeal of an evangelist he therefore sought to convert all Indians to *khadi*, at least physically if not mentally. For ultimately he was forced to accept that the fact of people wearing *khadi* was more important than people's individual motives for doing so. Gandhi hoped that *khadi* dress could act as a blanket, covering internal differences with a façade of apparent sameness, implying national unity whether or not such unity actually existed.

By suggesting that all Indians should entirely reject foreign cloth and revert to *khadi* permanently, Gandhi was offering a resolution to the problem of the divided self that threatened Indian identity under British rule. But although he tried to reduce the problem of what to wear to the simple choice between foreign cloth (sin) and *khadi* (morality), for many the options were never that clear-cut.

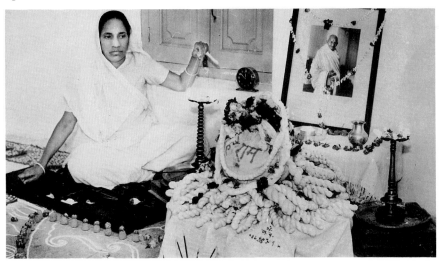

Fig. 3.16 Gandhi's shrine, covered in skeins of hand-spun cotton yarn (1948). Courtesy of NGM.

4   Is *Khadi* the Solution?

> I have done my packing racked with conflicts as to what to take and what not to take with me – whether to wear khaddar dress there while addressing the audience or swadeshi silk, the point of which will not be so well understood ... whether to be smart and fashionable as of old or to be simple and common only. I have at last chosen to be the latter. But it is taking time and trouble to assimilate the new method (Sarladevi Chaudhurani, 3 May 1920, letter to Gandhi, CWMG vol. 17:429).

Sarladevi Chaudhurani[1] was preparing for a conference in May 1920 when she experienced this sartorial anxiety. Her letter to Gandhi reveals that the problem of what to wear was still a thriving issue in India despite Gandhi's attempts to resolve it. But the problem had taken a new form. Rather than worrying about the extent to which they should Westernise their dress, the Indian élite were now worrying about the extent to which they should simplify and re-Indianise it. Far from effacing the problem of what to wear, Gandhi had in fact raised it to unprecedented heights for he had drawn it out of the political closet. It was no longer relegated to private journals, but was now a much-discussed public issue. Furthermore Gandhi's particular emphasis on the morality of *khadi* gave the problem a new flavour. Whereas in the past it was considered morally and culturally acceptable to alter one's dress to suit the occasion or to wear a combination of Indian and European dress, it was now, according to him, immoral to wear anything but *khadi* on a permanent and daily basis. Any hope of finding a neutral solution to the problem of what to wear seemed now to have been completely eradicated since Gandhi actively encouraged people to interpret one another's clothes as signs of personal and political belief. The result was that people became increasingly self-conscious about their public image and found their clothing choices the subject of more rigorous criticism and public scrutiny than ever before.

---

1   Sarladevi Chaudhurani was the wife of Pandit Rambhoj Dhutt Chaudhurani, a nationalist leader in the Punjab, and the niece of Rabindranath Tagore. In 1920 she became the first élite woman to adopt *khadi* and was exceptional for wearing it in coarse plain white undecorated form.

Is *Khadi* the Solution?

Khadi obligations

There were numerous pressures encouraging people to adopt *khadi* – not only from Gandhi's constant speeches but also, as we have seen, from a vast network of people and institutions spread from towns to villages, dedicated to the propagation of *khadi*, both the textile and the ideology surrounding it. As the ideology spread, it took on a variety of forms as different individuals chose to emphasise certain aspects, and to ignore and invent others.

Propaganda from *khadi* extremists ranged from the humorous to the physically threatening. At Jabalpur in Central India, the local Congress committee organised a parade of 111 washermen's donkeys dressed in English coats, trousers, waistcoats, hats and scarlet neckties, each donkey representing a different Indian who had been favoured or knighted by the 'satanic' government. The intention behind the demonstration was to encourage all Indians to return British honours and decorations, and adopt instead humble, simple Indian *khadi* (*The Times* 7 May 1930). Public ridicule of those still wearing foreign cloth did not always take such an elaborate form, but it acted as a constant reminder to wear *khadi*, especially when ridicule sometimes turned from mild intimidation to physical violence. *Khadi*-clad pickets not only prevented those wearing foreign cloth from entering foreign cloth shops but at times even barred them from entering Hindu temples (OIOC: L/1/2/14).

In their attempts to persuade the nation into *khadi*, those with 'khadi faith' resorted to arguments far removed from Gandhi's. In April 1930 one of his so-called 'lieutenants' made a speech in Gujarat, telling people not to touch foreign cloth since cows' fat was used in its manufacture.[2] By June the rumour had spread and leaflets were printed in Bombay explaining that in Manchester, 300 pounds of cow and pig blood were used in the production of every 1,000 pounds of coloured foreign cloth (*ibid.*). The mention of cows' blood was designed to upset Hindus for whom the cow is sacred, while that of pigs' blood would disgust Muslims for whom the pig is unclean. If such rumours had ever gained wide circulation they could have provided a powerful resistance to foreign cloth and incentive to adopt *khadi*.[3]

Apart from anti-foreign cloth propaganda and the emotional pressure of public scrutiny, there were, as we have seen, actual rules and regulations

---

2 This was of course a reworking of the famous old rumour that cows' fat was used to grease the sepoys' cartridges, which is thought to have sparked off the Indian rebellion of 1857.

3 These rumours were not entirely without basis. Animal fat was used in Manchester in the sizing process, but it was cheap mutton fat, not pig or cow fat. Colours were fixed using egg albumen, not blood (OIOC: L/1/2/14).

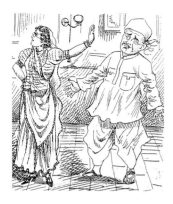

ALO, a briefless but hitherto fashionable lawyer, now courting Swadeshi clients,

to

ALI, his still fashionable wife :—

"*Be plain in dress, and sober in your diet,*

In short, my deary, kiss me, and be quiet ! "

Fig. 4.1 Reproduced from *Hindi Punch*, Bombay, 6 Nov. 1921. Courtesy of OIOC.

which constrained people's choices of what to wear. This applied especially to Congress politicians and all those attending national schools who were, according to membership regulations, obliged to wear *khadi* permanently. For women the pressure was less institutionalised but came instead from the authority structure of the family (see fig. 4.1). The degree to which women participated in the nationalist movement often depended on the degree to which the men of their family were involved (Kishwar 1985: 1698); a woman married to a *khadi*-wearing husband would generally be obliged to wear *khadi* herself. Such a situation has been sensitively described by the writer Kamala Das, whose mother was forced into *khadi* by her husband:

> My father, soon after the betrothal, stipulated firmly that his wife was not to wear anything but *khaddar* and preferably white or off-white. . . .
>
> After the wedding he made her remove all her gold ornaments from her person, all except the *mangalsutra*.[4] To her it must have seemed like taking on widow's weeds, but she did not protest. She was mortally afraid of the dark stranger who came forward to take her out of the village and its security (K. Das 1976: 4).

The success of clothing as a political symbol lay in the fact that, except for certain religious ascetics and poor beggars, every man and woman in India wore clothing of some sort and so was drawn automatically into this national debate. Once dress had attained such elaborate symbolic importance, there was no escape from participation in the battle of clothes, no matter whether a person actually wished to participate in it or not.[5] As always, headwear was a central issue.

Gandhi cap games continued
One of Gandhi's objectives in designing the Gandhi cap was, as we have seen, that all Indians should share the same form of headwear, thereby creating the effect of visual uniformity. What is interesting is the way in which this one material symbol, despite its visual consistency, was used by different groups to represent their own interests. For as the cap emerged on an increasing number of heads, so it was subject to an increasingly wide range of symbolic interpretations. Ultimately it participated not merely in British-Indian power struggles (cf. Cohn 1989) but also in inter-Indian struggles where it became the material focus of widespread communal ten-

---

4 *Mangalsutra*: type of necklace worn only by married women.
5 Lurie ends her book *The Language of Clothes* with the reminder: 'We can lie in the language of dress, or try to tell the truth; but unless we are naked and bald it is impossible to be silent' (Lurie 1992: 261).

Is *Khadi* the Solution?

sion. Even in England it became a provocative issue, used to define alternative attitudes to British administrative policy in India. Central to this
symbolic warfare was the technique of capping the capless and de-capping
the capped, a game played out at levels varying from verbal persuasion to
physical force. Most of these cap incidents took place during the Non
Cooperation Movement (1920–1) and the Civil Disobedience Movement
(1930–1), although isolated incidents were not uncommon.

Just as forceful as British attempts to curb the wearing of the cap through
prohibition, imprisonment and sometimes the violent assault of Gandhi cap-
wearers were the attempts made by cap-wearing Indians to remove foreign
headwear from non-Gandhians and to force them to wear the Gandhi cap.
Occasionally this took the simple form of a regulation, such as the rule
in Lahore insisting that all cab-drivers and similar municipal employees wear
khadi caps (CWMG vol. 20: 488). More often, however, the obligation to
wear them took a more imperative form. In August 1921 there were reports
of gangs of *khadi*-capped Gandhians rampaging on Chowpatty seafront in
Bombay, insulting and at times physically attacking anyone not wearing
a Gandhi cap (*Statesman* 5 Aug. 1921). Under such pressure, people were
more or less forced to buy and wear caps which were sold at high prices
and some of which, though looking like Gandhi caps, were not in fact made
from *khadi* (*ibid.*). That same month, Madan Mohan Malaviya was delayed
in addressing a meeting on *swadeshi* in Poona, owing to the uproar caused
by Gandhians at the sight of a finely woven turban on the head of one
of the local landlords in the audience. Attempts were made to seize the
turban, which was made from foreign cloth, and burn it. Malaviya refused
to speak until the crowds reluctantly agreed to allow the would-be victim
of this violence to remain in the audience with his turban still firmly in
place on his head (*Statesman* 11 Aug. 1921). Many accounts of the bonfires
of foreign cloth also report the forcible seizure and burning of foreign
headwear by Gandhi cap-wearers. Under the powerful intimidation of Congress volunteers, people would often hand over their foreign headwear out
of 'a sense of shame' (Krishnadas 1928: 116).

Both internal and external cap conflicts came to a head in Bombay in
November 1921 during the official visit of the Prince of Wales. As part
of non-cooperation policy, Congress was encouraging a boycott of all
official events linked to the Prince's arrival. After a peaceful mass meeting
of largely *khadi*-clad protesters at Elphinstone Mills, where Gandhi spoke
and lit a pile of foreign cloth, violence broke out among members of the
vast crowd returning to the city centre. People determined one another's
loyalties through the type of cap or turban they wore; clothes, and

especially headwear, soon became the central focus of this serious outbreak of communal violence, commonly known as the Bombay riots.

According to Gandhi's bitter report of the events (cf. CWMG vol. 21: 462–5), fighting started when a 'swelling mob' of *khadi*-capped aggressors began 'molesting peaceful passengers in tramcars ... forcibly depriving those who were wearing foreign caps of their head-dresses and pelting inoffensive Europeans'. The primary targets of these attacks were Parsis and Eurasians, most of whom had attended the Prince's reception and were sporting foreign cloth, often in European styles. In Bhindi Bazaar the angry mob started beating up all who refused to surrender their foreign headgear and at least one old Parsi was seriously maltreated for holding on to his turban which was made from foreign cloth. Yet even as these atrocities proceeded, reports were emerging of counter-attacks in Anglo-Indian quarters of the city where those wearing Gandhi caps were forced to uncover their heads and beaten if they refused to do so (*ibid.*). It was essentially a battle between bands of white-capped khaddarites (mainly Hindu and Muslim) and opposition forces (mainly Christians and Parsis), beturbaned and behatted in foreign cloth of varying colours and styles. The two sides subjected each other to humiliation through seizing items of opposition headwear which had become so imbued with symbolic potency that the mere sight of them could incense people to the point of murder (cf. Krishnadas 1928: 406–21). Gandhi, realising the extremities that clothing conflicts had reached, was full of self-reproach for not having curbed cap violence earlier, since he had often witnessed over-zealous supporters casting other people's headwear into his sacrificial fires. From this time on, he always condemned the forcible seizing of headwear, even if it was foreign. Such acts conflicted with his notion of non-violent action (*ahimsa*).

By 1930 the Congress call to civil disobedience brought the cap back into public focus. There were reports in May of British soldiers in Sholapur parading the streets armed with hooked sticks which they used to whip the caps off passers-by (OIOC: L/1/2/14). Later that year a series of incidents in the Kaira district of Gujarat resulted in an investigative inquiry by Lord Brailsford. He claimed that local police and revenue officials were not only using the Gandhi cap as an excuse for indiscriminate beatings, but were also encouraging social divisions in the area by inciting landless labourers to attack the wealthier *khadi*-capped peasantry of the region (OIOC: L/P&J/7/27). Many wealthy peasant landowners in Kaira supported the civil disobedience movement, including the non-payment of taxes and the wearing of *khadi* (Hardiman 1981: 125–8, Brailsford 1943:

Is *Khadi* the Solution?

191–6). It was Gandhi cap-wearers in particular who were singled out for abuse by frustrated revenue officials and police who confiscated land and offered it for sale at absurdly low prices to those prepared to refrain from civil disobedience. In the Borsad region the local subcollector not only tried to encourage poor labourers of the *Baraiya* caste to buy up their landlords' confiscated farmland, but also encouraged them to attack their landlords. In one *Baraiya*-dominated village he was reported to have said: 'All suits are decided by me. I'll give judgement in your favour. This is a time for revenge. They've suppressed you up to this day. Beat any man who wears a white cap' (Brailsford 1943: 191–6).

In Madras, cap controversies revolved around an official prohibition on the wearing of Gandhi caps in the Guntur district and surrounding area. The rationale behind the legislation was that the Gandhi cap, as a symbol of sympathy with civil disobedience, was a potential disturbance to public tranquillity. A few days after the announcement (on 20 June 1930), the police raided a local press office in Guntur and seized all copies of pamphlets that had been printed by Congress volunteers, urging the public to wear Gandhi caps. A total of eight arrests were recorded relating to cap-wearing.

The Madras government soon received a critical note from the Home Department of the Government of India, warning them that 'the issue of orders of this nature against the use of such emblems or symbols is of doubtful wisdom, save in very exceptional circumstances. The Government of India hope therefore, that it will be found possible to avoid the issue of similar orders in the future' (*ibid.*: 144). A year after the prohibition was introduced, the cap was still a flourishing topic in Madras. At a meeting of the Madras council in July 1931, the local government was accused of introducing the prohibition as a convenient justification and useful cover for police violence which would have occurred anyway without the supposed provocation of Gandhi caps (OIOC: L/P&J/7/27).

The Gandhi cap illustrates the complexity of symbolic formation and interpretation. At a superficial level Gandhi must be regarded as the author of the symbol, since it was he who created the cap and tried to define its significance as a garment of unity for all Indians fighting the non-violent battle for *swaraj*. British suppression of it enabled him to heighten its significance as a symbol of political freedom. But neither Gandhi nor the British were entirely responsible for the symbolic developments of the cap.

For the British authorities, the cap posed continual problems precisely because its symbolism could not be controlled. They could, of course, have simply ignored the sudden appearance of thousands of *khadi*-capped heads in the Indian streets, but while this might have diminished the symbolic value of the cap, it would have done so only at the risk of allowing the number of cap-wearers to increase. An alternative policy, which was periodically favoured, was to stamp out the physical presence of the cap, but this only encouraged the symbolism of the garment which, under Gandhi's nurturing, became at times a cap of martyrdom. A third technique was to belittle the cap, like Beverly Nichols when he argued that the 'Gandhi cap is a very bad fit indeed for a man with a modern brain' (Nichols 1944: 176), or like a correspondent to the *Statesman* arguing that the cap was really only a cross between the Brodwick cap and the cap worn by British prisoners at Dartmoor (*Statesman* 11 Aug. 1921). But in spite of providing amusement to anti-Gandhians, such statements did little to disperse either the physical presence or the symbolic value of the cap for its wearers. Since none of these actions provided a solution to the Gandhi cap problem, the British administration fumbled around with each alternative, trapped in a symbolic bind cleverly manipulated by Gandhi.

But if the British were not able to control the significance of the cap, nor was Gandhi himself. Once the cap was in widespread circulation, its meaning could no longer be centralised. By the time Gandhi's teachings had filtered down through Congress organisations, volunteers, local leaders and distant villagers, they emerged, like 'Chinese whispers', in what were sometimes almost unrecognisable forms. Throughout this process of diffusion, individuals and groups picked up Gandhian symbols and injected them with their own specific values and desired meanings. Sumit Sarkar records an incident in Bengal in 1922 when a group of Gandhi-capped Santals (a well-known tribal group in eastern India) attacked the police, demanding the release of Santal prisoners and 'shouting all the while that they were immune from bullet wounds as they were wearing Gandhi Maharaj's caps' (Sarkar 1984: 301). Three were killed in the process. To them the Gandhi cap had taken on the role of a talisman, capable of protecting its wearer. Yet Sarkar also reveals how for the industrial workers in the area the same material symbol played more the role of an emblem of unity, like a trade union mascot (*ibid.*: 312–19). Similarly for Hindus and Muslims fighting the Khilifat[6] cause in 1921, the cap had been momentarily perceived as a garment of solidarity that cut across religious boundaries. In the Bombay riots *khadi*-capped men of both religions had attacked and been attacked by those in foreign headwear and fifty-three had died in the process. But by the

6 Khilifat was the movement to support the rights of the Muslim *khalifah*, the religious leader of Turkey who had been defeated by the British in the war. From 1919 onwards Gandhi tried to persuade all Indians, whatever their religion, to join the movement, which could be part of the more general struggle to oust the British from India.

mid-1920s, after the Khilifat issue had subsided, hardly a Muslim could be found wearing the cap, which had regained its reputation as essentially a Hindu cap in a Hindu fight for a Hindu India. Increasing numbers of patriotic Muslims began to wear caps modelled on the Turkish fez, sometimes emblazoning them with the crescent moon.

The above episodes of capping and de-capping the opposition reveal that the battle of head-dress in the 1920s and '30s extended beyond the question of British-Indian relations. Gandhi cap-wearers were not only victims of oppression but also active aggressors and participants in many of the on going disputes. An incident in Lahore in August 1947 reveals cap-wearers forcing Gandhi caps not only on fellow-Indians but also on a British official. Fred Burrows (then Governor of Bengal) was seated in an office in Government House when a large crowd of *khadi*-capped men stampeded the building and, holding their victim in his seat, forced on to his head a succession of Gandhi caps and into his hand a Congress flag (Swayne-Thomas 1981: 92).

The Gandhi cap controversy, like Gandhi's loincloth, reveals how a political symbol can be accepted by many without their necessarily sharing an idea of its meaning. In fact it has been argued that a political symbol is powerful precisely because of its ambiguity, which allows a number of different people to respond to a single unified form without necessarily sharing a single interpretation of it (cf. Elder and Cobb 1983). But while Gandhi cap episodes reveal how people projected different meanings into a single material form, *khadi* episodes reveal how people projected difference through the material artefact itself: that is, they diversified the material symbol and not merely the interpretation thereof. An examination of various sartorial disputes concerning *khadi* shows how this cloth, which Gandhi hoped would unite all Indians, in fact became a medium through which social, religious and political differences in Indian society could be subtly expressed.

KHADI: FABRIC OF UNITY OR FABRIC OF DIFFERENCE?

United in khadi

Historians have emphasised the fact that *khadi* acted as a fabric of unity, visually uniting Indian politicians and wealthy peasants with the rural poor (Kishwar 1985: 1695, Hardiman 1981: 126). This was certainly Gandhi's intention, and at some levels he was successful. Photographs of Congress meetings and political activities during the non-cooperation movement reveal that the dark European and semi-European suits worn by politicians in the past had been entirely replaced by loose white cotton garments such as *dhotis*, *kurtas* and *pyjamas*, together with turbans and Gandhi caps.

To this extent Gandhi's plan for re-Indianisation was visibly successful. Vijayalakshmi Pandit[7] claimed that she could no longer detect the social class of visitors to her home since *khadi* made all Congressmen look the same (cited in Bean 1989: 373).

This apparent visual uniformity and the choice of a traditional Indian idiom through which to express it were undoubtedly unnerving for the British, especially since the Congress Party contained some of the most educated and respected men of India who had previously enjoyed the 'privileges' of both Western education and Western dress. That anyone could reject the latter in favour of a cotton *dhoti* was both disturbing and farcical for many Britons. A journalist on the *Times of India*, horrified at the image of the eminent Motilal Nehru dressed in homespun and hawking *khadi* through the streets of Allahabad, concluded that 'even in India it must be recognised that Pandit Nehru is making an ass of himself'. He continued:

> If the British public had learnt that Lord Birkenhead, wearing a Union Jack waistcoat, had been selling true blue Tory rosettes beneath the lions in Trafalgar Square, that Mr Baldwin had been promoting empire industries by hawking trays of British toys in Piccadilly, that Ramsay MacDonald, attired in corduroys and a muffler, had been disposing of red flags among the workers in Limehouse, or that the Clydeside Bolshevists had set up a stall in Clydeside for the sale of miniature sickles and hammers, the unanimous conclusion of all classes would be that their leaders had gone mad (CWMG vol. 30: 288).

Before his sudden shift in 1920 to Congress politics and *khadi*, Motilal Nehru had been considered almost a parody of the English gentleman. Although he had always continued to wear Indian styles of dress inside his own home, the public knew him as the extravagant man of European fashion and in the early twentieth century he was frequently accused by the Indian press of 'being a foreigner' (SWMN vol. 1: 120). In 1911 he had been invited to the King's Darbar in Delhi, for which he ordered a series of outfits including full court dress (fig. 4.2), a number of lounge suits and even a *sola topi* which he requested his son Jawaharlal to post from England (*ibid.*: 164). There were few men in India with a greater reputation for a love of foreign clothes, and

7 Daughter of Motilal Nehru and sister of Jawaharlal.

Fig. 4.2 Motilal Nehru's changes of dress. *Top left*: In top hat and tails (London 1899). *Top right*: In Darbar dress (1911). *Bottom left*: In Gandhi cap, *kurta* and *dhoti* after his shift to Gandhian politics. *Bottom right*: Reading, with fine *khadi dhoti*, *kurta* and *chadar*. Courtesy of NMML.

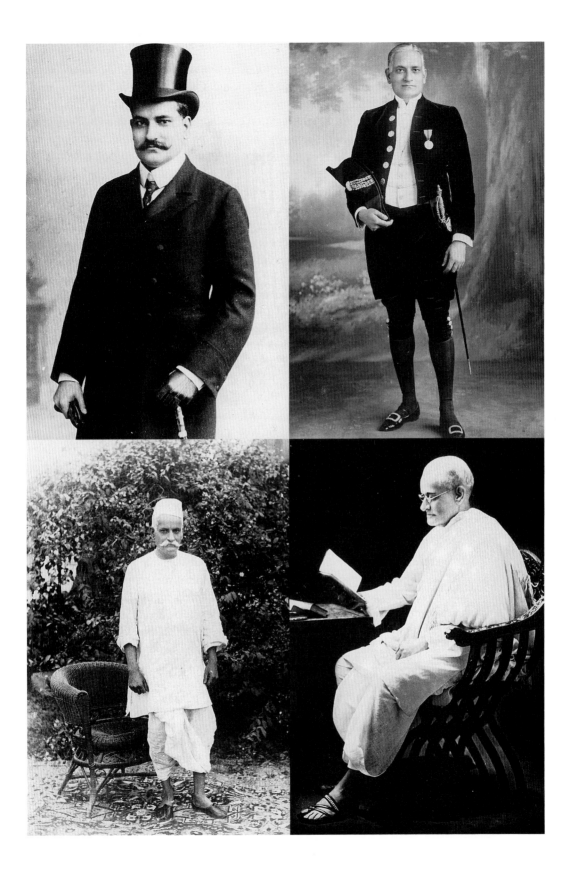

Motilal's sudden conversion to *khadi* was undoubtedly a shock to many.

From 1920–1 all members of National Congress appear to have made a similar shift, usually setting fire to their machine-spun apparel and replacing it with white *khadi* (fig. 4.3). As with the Gandhi cap, the beginning of *khadi*'s popularity was also the beginning of its oppression by the government, which tried to prohibit its use by government servants and at times forcibly removed it from certain sectors of the *khadi*-wearing population (CWMG vol. 21: 204, 240). For the British authorities, then, the sudden conversion of Indians to *khadi* did indeed provide a cohesive and threatening image. But the question is, did it provide the intended link between the many entrenched divisions of religion, wealth and caste in Indian society? Was *khadi* really capable of covering difference at an internal level?

For some men and women of the élite classes, the adoption of *khadi* clearly did bring about new feelings of solidarity with the masses. One such man was Abbas Tyabji who, inspired by the spirit of non-cooperation, flung aside his previously tailored garments along with his job and became involved in village welfare. Writing to Gandhi from a village in 1920, he exclaimed: 'God! What an experience! I have so much love and affection for the common folk to whom it is now an honour to belong. It is the fakir's dress that has broken down all the barriers' (Nanda 1989: 126). Similarly, Sarladevi Chaudhurani, whose clothing dilemma introduced this chapter, found that her final choice of a coarse white *khadi* sari was a great success among the Punjabi women whom she addressed at political meetings. It seems, however, from Gandhi's report of the events that her *khadi* dress singled her out rather than enabling her to blend with her Punjabi sisters, because the latter were not wearing *khadi*. Gandhi recalls:

> Sarladevi herself writes to say that her khaddar sari impressed her audiences more than her speeches. . . . The good ladies of Lahore flocked around her and felt her coarse but beautifully white sari and admired it. Some took pity on her that she, who only the other day was dressed in costly thin silk saris, now decked herself in hand-woven swadeshi khaddar. Sarladevi wanted no pity and retorted that their thin scarves lay heavy on their shoulders with the weight of their helpless dependence on foreign manufacture whereas her coarse khaddar lay light as a feather on her body with the joy of the knowledge that she was free because she wore garments in the manufacture of which her sisters and brothers had laboured (CWMG vol. 18: 20).

Tyabji and Chaudhurani were two members of the Indian élite who tried through their dress to identify with the masses. While Tyabji's white

Is *Khadi* the Solution?

khadi broke down social barriers, Chaudhurani's simplicity of dress made her conspicuous. One problem with the idea that simple *khadi* could bind the élite to the rural masses was that the villagers themselves, particularly the women, were by no means all dressed in plain *khadi*. But there were other problems with the idea that *khadi* covered social differences. Close inspection of the voluminous literature on the subject reveals that, despite an ideology of egalitarianism, many of the people who adopted *khadi* found, both intentionally and unintentionally, subtle means of expressing their social or religious identity. This apparent desire for differentiation was expressed in the fineness of the *khadi*, the types of fibres used, the colour, the decoration and of course the style in which the *khadi* was worn. These transformations of simple *khadi*, along with the numerous social, religious and political squabbles they engendered, reveal that through the fibres of this simple fabric of unity ran most of the major divisions of Indian society.

Divided in khadi

At a meeting in Devakkottah in 1927, Gandhi was presented with a piece of exceptionally fine *khadi* woven by a local weaver from very fine hand-spun yarn. Appreciative though he was, Gandhi found himself unable to accept the gift: 'This khadi I cannot wear for the simple reason that it would be against my profession and that I want to have no more than any of the starving millions' (CWMG vol. 35: 28). His objection was that the *khadi*, being so fine, was a luxury item such as the poor could not afford, and therefore since his duty was to represent the poor, he had no business to wear it. He hoped, however, that some wealthy and patriotic man from Devakkottah would be able to adorn his body in this delicate piece of *khadi* by buying it for the extravagant sum of 1,001 rupees. The following day he found his buyer.

The incident highlights the fact that *khadi*, intended to eliminate the distinctions between rich and poor, had become diversified according to the fineness of its weave. Those poor villagers (mainly men) who wore white *khadi* tended to wear the thick, coarsely woven variety, since it was cheaper and more durable. When wealthy townsmen adopted *khadi*, they may have appeared to be choosing the clothes of the masses but very often they found a means of stressing their own superior refinement by sporting expensive fine *khadi* which was as costly and prestigious as the famous muslins of Dacca; as we have seen, fineness of cloth denoted not only wealth but also social and ritual superiority. It was worn almost exclusively by those of high social status who could support themselves in prestigious occupations and did not need the hard-wearing clothes necessary for manual labour.

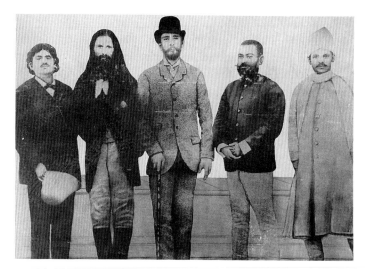

Fig. 4.3 Transformations of Political dress. (a) *Left*: Allahabad Congress, 1888, with only Madan Mohan Malaviya in Indian dress. (b) *Below*: Motley-clad delegates to the National Congress in Amritsar in 1919. Swami Shraddhanand is conspicuous in his *sanyasi's* garb, seated between Motilal Nehru and Annie Besant.

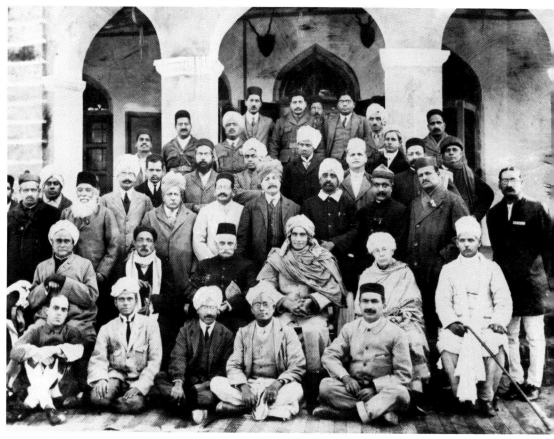

Is *Khadi* the Solution?

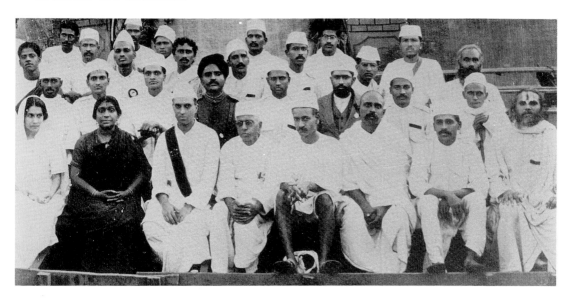

(c) *Above*: Congress workers in South India after the Congress Party had agreed to adopt *khadi* (date unknown). Saurojini Naidu, the politician and poet renowned for her rich silk saris, wears conspicuously dark colours. (d) *Below*: Members of the Interim Government in 1946, wearing mainly *khadi* in a number of different styles. Courtesy of: Anand Bhawan (a) and (c); Press and Information Bureau, Government of India (b) and (d).

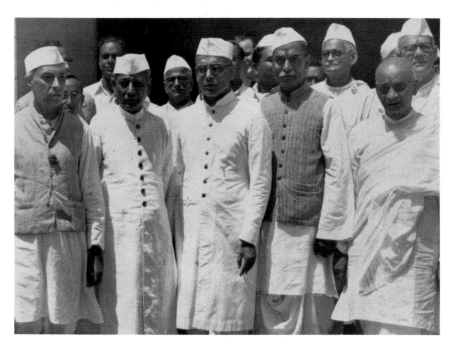

It therefore carried the secondary associations of education as well as general refinement. Some high-caste educated people even claimed that their bodies were too sensitive and delicate to support the terrible weight of thick *khadi* cloth.[8]

It is worth now taking a closer look at the *dhotis*, *kurtas* and *pyjamas* of the Nehru family (figs 4.2 and 4.4). Even in photographs, it is clear that their clothing lacks the crudity of texture characteristic of peasant *khadi*. Evidence of this may be found in the letters between father and son concerning dress. Writing from jail in 1922, Jawaharlal complained of the quality of his clothing and requested three new *dhotis* and *kurtas* of a superior variety (SWJN vol. 1: 328–31). The concerned and loving Motilal responded by sending his son a large stock of high-quality garments, for which Jawaharlal was grateful:

> Thank you for the clothes you sent me. I have an abundance of them now. I was at first inclined to return the Andhra dhotis you sent me as they were too fine. On second thoughts, I kept them. They are not as fine as some Andhra stuff. Kripalani used to wear a much finer dhoti. The dhotis you have sent are just right as regards weight. The length too suits me ... (*ibid.*: 335).

Clearly Jawarhalal was aware that the fineness of these *dhotis* consorted uneasily with the ideology of *khadi*, but even in jail it seems that he was unable to resist the luxury of well-made and finely woven garments which clearly set him aside from the average peasant. Later he further distinguished his own identity by adopting the short tailored *khadi* waistcoat, now known as the 'Nehru jacket'.

Social and economic distinctions manifested themselves not only in the texture of the weave but also in the nature of the fibres employed. Unlike Sarladevi Chaudhurani, many people were reluctant to take the full plunge into cotton *khadi*, and chose instead *swadeshi* silk. This, otherwise known as *khadi* silk, was silk which had been hand-woven and hand-spun in India, using indigenous yarn. Since silk manufacture was restricted to only a few parts of India, and silk thread was finer than cotton yarn, requiring more time for weaving, *swadeshi* silk was naturally a luxury product, restricted

---

8   This attitude was particularly prevalent among educated Bengalis, who, coming from a rich intellectual tradition, were often reluctant to identify themselves with the poor farm labourer. In letters from Bengalis to the *Statesman* we read: 'Bengalees have not got the strength to carry the weight of coarse cloth, so they will never use it' (30 July 1921), and 'Many will sympathise with Mr. Gandhi in his grief but at the same time the cultured Bengalee race should be proud of the fact that the Mahatma's teachings have not been able to take Bengalees back to prehistoric uncivilised days ... to the period of Barbarism' (9 Sept. 1921).

Is *Khadi* the Solution?

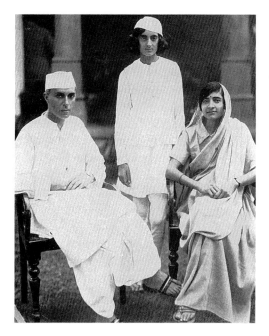

Fig. 4.4 The Nehru family in 1929. Kamala Nehru wears a plain sari (not white) while her daughter Indira is dressed like Jawaharlal in a *kurta* and Gandhi cap. He wears a *dhoti* and she wears *pyjamas*. It was very unusual for a woman to wear such clothes. Courtesy of NMML.

to élite buyers. This disturbed Shrikrishnadas Jaju, secretary of the All India Spinners Association, who wondered whether it was advisable for *khadi* organisations to sell *swadeshi* silk at all in view of the fact that it competed with cotton *khadi*, and encouraged a luxury-loving attitude in the wearer (CWMG vol. 75: 167). The question of the morality of *khadi* silk was a dominant factor in this debate. At their most lenient, khaddarites felt that the diversity of choice that *swadeshi* silk provided should be encouraged since it was all part of the *khadi* cause. At their most puritan, however, people objected not only to the unnecessary luxury of silk, but also to the process by which it was made, which, because it involved the destruction of silk worms, could be defined as a violent act (CWMG vol. 23: 462–3). This finally lead to a new division of types, even within the comparatively small category of *khadi* silk. A moral distinction was made between 'violent swadeshi silk' and 'nonviolent swadeshi silk', defined according to the degrees of violence involved in the production process (CWMG vol. 75: 166–7).[9]

These fine varieties of *khadi* cotton and silk were never in widespread use, partly because of their cost and partly also because they often did not reach the open market: it seems that Congressmen and other important

---

9 Gandhi felt that 'service to the millions is possible only through cotton *khadi*' but that nonviolent *swadeshi* silk was preferable to foreign cloth (CWMG vol. 75: 166–7).

notables often found means of reserving such pieces for their own use by making special arrangements with people who worked in the *khadi* shops.[10] Despite the apparent humility of Congress uniform, the sartorial link between politicians and the Indian poor seems to have been less close than it appeared to be on the surface.

There were other problems with *khadi* besides its coarseness – in particular, the question of its plainness. Male clothing in India had often bordered on the simple in colour and motif, but most women were accustomed to wearing more elaborate materials, decorated with printing, embroidery, dyeing and woven patterns. Gandhi, who sometimes referred to bright colours as 'ugly spots' (CWMG vol. 20: 451), was opposed to excessive decoration and accused women of being slaves both to their own whims and fancies and to their husbands. He told them: 'If you want to play your part in the world's affairs, you must refuse to deck yourselves for pleasing men' (Gandhi 1946: 195–6). White *khadi*, he thought, was a suitable means of enabling women to enter the public political sphere without appearing sexually provocative or immodest. But for most women the *khadi*-clad image had little appeal. Even Gandhi's wife Kasturba was at first so reluctant to wear the cloth that she helped other women protest to Gandhi about the unreasonableness of his expectations (cf. Kalarthi 1962: 62–3).

Women's objections related not only to the weight of *khadi* but also to the threat it posed both to their aesthetic senses and indeed to their sense of identity as women. Aesthetically, some feared that it would stamp out many of the decorative arts which women enjoyed. Certain types of embroidery, for example, required the use of Chinese silk, which was clearly contradictory to Gandhi's philosophy (CWMG vol. 31: 321). More generally, women feared the dull uniformity and sombre unattractive image that *khadi* represented. Kamala Das has recorded her childhood memories of seeing her *khadi*-clad family. 'I thought Gandhiji a brigand', she recalls, 'I thought it his diabolic aim to strip ladies of their finery so that they became plain and dull' (K. Das 1976: 12). Nehru's sister, Vijayalakshmi, also bemoaned the drabness of *khadi* and felt deprived when the men of the family persuaded her to wear it for her wedding (Bean 1989: 372). One woman even expressed the fear that by wearing *khadi* she might be guilty of leading her husband to 'lose his character' since he might be attracted to other more glamorous women wearing foreign or mill-cloth (CWMG vol. 26: 185). Yet perhaps more poignant than any of these aesthetic considerations were

---

10   The association of extra-fine *khadi* with politicians is recognised today in government stores where fine cloth is often sold under the name of 'politician's *khadi*'.

Is *Khadi* the Solution?

the negative associations that plain white *khadi* evoked. For white was essentially a colour worn by men and, worse still, by widows. Since widowhood was the most feared and least respected state a woman could attain, most young women seem to have been reluctant to embrace so grim an image however much they sympathised with Gandhian sentiments. As a result, few but the most devout ashram dwellers and some old women adopted plain white *khadi* saris in their simplest form. Even the most politically motivated women like Kamala Nehru[11] (Jawaharlal's wife) and Sarojini Naidu[12] retained at least some form of decoration in their saris.

There soon grew up a wide variety of coloured, printed and decorated *khadi* saris, sometimes embroidered, sometimes bordered with silk, which saved *khadi* from monotony but which simultaneously increased the possibilities of betraying social and economic differences. The National Council of Women, founded in Bombay in 1921, began making embroidered ready-made garments and items of household use which they hawked from house to house and displayed in *khadi* exhibitions (Kalhan 1973: 58–9). These of course sold for considerably higher prices than plain undecorated *khadi*, which was already expensive compared to mill-cloth. Rural women, like urban women, were reluctant to adopt white *khadi* and generally could not afford the elaborate decorated *khadi* worn by a small urban élite.

Although Gandhi wanted to build *swaraj* on a 'white background' (CWMG vol. 20: 451), dyeing *khadi* became a common means of differentiating not only individuals but also various groups within the freedom movement. A special female volunteer corps adopted black saris with orange, green and red borders. These were later replaced by plain orange[13] ones at the instigation of Kamaladevi Chattopadhyaya, who found the previous colour combination distasteful (Brijbhushan 1976: 29). These women became known as the 'Orange Brigade'. Meanwhile the male Congress volunteers in some cities

---

11 Kamala Nehru usually wore a simple *khadi* sari with a decorative border. Even so, she was severely rebuked by her mother-in-law for her simplicity of dress and lack of jewellery, which was inappropriate to a married woman (Kalhan 1973: 89). Kamala, an unusually independent woman, sometimes even dressed herself and her daughter in the men's outfit of *kurta pyjama* and Gandhi cap (see fig. 4.4 for Indira Nehru – later Indira Gandhi – in men's dress).

12 Sarojini Naidu, despite playing a major role in the nationalist movement, refused to sacrifice her feminine dress for plain coarse *khadi* (fig. 4.3c). She wore rich Indian silks 'except at times of grave political crises' and even during such critical times she beautified her *khadi* by dyeing it (Sengupta 1966: 259). When she accompanied Gandhi to Buckingham Palace in 1931, she wore heavily embroidered white silk, rather than plain cotton. She believed in the economic benefits of *khadi* but not in its aesthetic merits – nor in the benefits of austerity.

13 Orange is the colour normally worn by Hindu ascetics. It is possible that it was chosen as an attempt to retain the theme of renunciation without the horrors of whiteness (associated with widows). But orange probably alienated Muslim women.

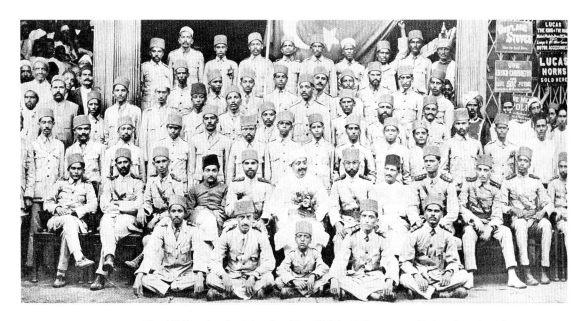

Fig. 4.5 Dressing for Diversity. *Top*: Khilifat Volunteers in khaki-coloured uniforms (courtesy of NMML). *Bottom*: Members of the Congress Party at the inauguration of a hospital in Allahabad, wearing a motley array of different colours and styles (courtesy of Anand Bhawan). *Opposite top*: Shaukat and Mohamed Ali, after their conversion to long green *khadi* robes with woollen fezes, one with the Islamic crescent moon symbol (courtesy of NMML). *Opposite bottom*: The so called 'Orange Brigade': women protesters wearing orange *khadi* saris in Bombay, 1937 (courtesy of Pierre Dupuy).

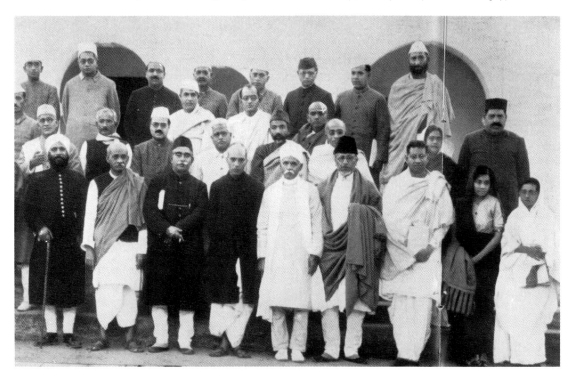

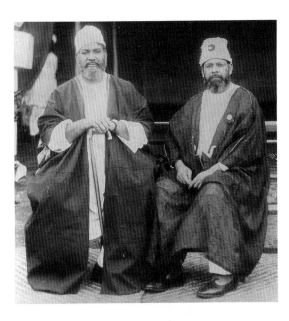

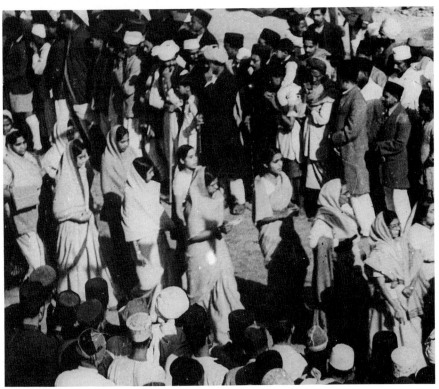

distinguished themselves by wearing khaki-coloured *khadi* uniforms. A volunteer corps of Muslims who joined non-cooperation sported either khaki uniforms with the Turkish fez and crescent armbands or else the long green[14] Arab-style robes popularised by the Ali brothers (Minault 1982: 119–20). The Muslim Pathans, on the other hand, wore a distinctive red uniform, and were even named 'Red Shirts' after their dress.[15]

Even when people adopted plain white *khadi*, they were still able to differentiate themselves if they wished through the style in which they made up their garments. Gandhi hoped that *khadi* would help to unite 'Hindu-Muslim-Sikh-Parsi-Christian-Jew' (CWMG vol. 23: 59), but he did not insist that everyone adopt the same style of dress. As long as it was a simple Indian style, he was content. Yet the acceptance of different styles allowed the expression of different interests. Some felt that this prevented *khadi* from being a symbol of national unity:

> The Musalman by putting on khaddar in Muslim fashion may feel that he is injuring British interests but he will never feel that he has become one with the Hindu. That is, he begins to feel politically but not a bit nationally. Pictures of political leaders bunched together appear in newspapers. They are so dressed that the Muslim eye selects the Muslim leader, the Sikh the Sikh. Under these circumstances it is impossible to educate the mass mind nationally (Kumria 1941: 19–20).

On the whole, Hindus who adopted *khadi* wore *dhotis*, *kurtas* and Gandhi caps; Muslims wore *kurta pyjamas* with a cap or fez, and Sikhs retained their distinctive turbans. Some Hindus, far from uniting with Muslims in

14 Green was the favourite colour of the Prophet and is worn by those who mourn his death.
15 The adoption of red shirts by volunteers in the North-West Provinces provides an interesting example of how an accidental phenomenon attains symbolic importance. The volunteers, led by Abdul Ghaffar Khan, were originally dressed in white clothes until one day a man, wishing to cover the dirt on them, threw his white turban, trousers and shirt in a vat of pine bark solution at a local tannery. Others liked the colour and followed suit. When they moved on to other villages, they found that crowds came out to see them, attracted by the strange red colour of their clothes. It became a useful instrument for attracting attention, so the red colour became institutionalised (Zutshi 1970: 51–2) and the volunteers themselves became known as 'Red Shirts'. When the British tried to stamp out the movement in 1930 the red colour became a potent sign of patriotism (cf. Khan 1969). In one town British soldiers arrested all those wearing red shirts; when they demanded if there were any left, a local resident wearing white dress rushed into his house, threw his clothes in a dye vat and, dripping with wet red dye, cried 'Here are the Red Shirts.' Tendulkar writes: 'His chivalrous act infused such spirit in the people that no amount of repression could banish the red uniform' (Tendulkar 1967: 71). The British frequently mistook this accidental redness as a sign that Pathans were Russian-style communists (Bernays 1931: 326). The 'Red Shirts' movement was founded in Peshawar in 1929 by Khan, and by 1931 was an integral part of the Congress struggle. Khan became known as the Frontier Gandhi and he encouraged his followers to ensure that their red shirts were made from *khadi*.

Is *Khadi* the Solution?

khadi, actually refused to wear the cloth because the *khadi* available in their region was made by Muslim weavers (CWMG vol. 24: 426). Parsis and Christians, on the other hand, rarely adopted *khadi* because they found it primitive and preferred to stick to Western styles. This led one Parsi man to suggest that *khadi* should be made up into European as well as Indian styles (CWMG vol. 35: 263). Even as early as 1921, when *khadi* was still a comparatively new cause, there were reports of people making it up into Western-style suits, shirts and trousers, and even dyeing it black to make it visually indistinguishable from European dress (*Statesman* 18 Aug. 1921).

Where *khadi* threatened to cover difference, there were often traditionalists ready to object. An interesting example of this was the dilemma of a Maharashtran woman who wrote to Gandhi in 1928, explaining her difficulty in adopting *khadi*:

> A year ago I heard you speaking on the extreme necessity of everyone of us wearing khadi and thereupon decided to adopt it. But we are poor people. My husband says that khadi is costly. Belonging as I do to Maharashtra, I wear a sari of nine yards long. Now if I reduced the length of my sari to six yards, there would be a great saving, but the elders will not hear of such a reduction. I reason with them that wearing khadi is the more important thing and that the style and length of the sari is absolutely immaterial, but in vain (CWMG vol. 35: 504).

In this case the objection to *khadi* was that it threatened regional rather than religious identity. The desire of the Maharashtran elders to preserve local traditions stood directly in the way of national unity. When Gandhi harped back to India's mythical past when all had worn *khadi*, he failed to consider the extraordinarily diverse clothing traditions that had always coexisted among different social, religious and ethnic groups in India. For *khadi* was in danger of blanking out local Indian traditions just as much as it sought to stamp out British influences. Gandhi's response to the woman's dilemma was that she should sacrifice her provincialism for the wider benefit of nationalism (CWMG vol. 35: 504–5).

The above examples reveal that despite the notions of voluntary poverty, equality and national unity which Gandhi attributed to *khadi*, there was a tendency among many *khadi*-wearers to retain visible signs of their social, economic, regional and religious identity. This is not altogether surprising since many of the people who adopted it did not actually agree with much of what Gandhi attributed to it. Some, for example, believed only in its political value and its ability to hasten *swaraj*, while others emphasised its power as the counterpart to the boycott on foreign cloth, and yet others believed chiefly in its ability to stimulate cottage industry or to promote a more humane economy. Furthermore, mingled with these various personal beliefs and motivations was the feeling of an *obligation* to wear it, which loomed large on the political horizon for believers and non-believers alike; as the examples at the beginning of this chapter show, the pressures to adopt *khadi* were enormous, ranging from subtle encouragements, blatant propaganda, regulations and family pressures to threats of physical violence. But perhaps the greatest pressure of all lay in the explicitly moral association that Gandhi himself attributed to it: his countless speeches on its virtues and the sinfulness of foreign cloth made many people embarrassed to be seen in anything other than *khadi*.

This pressure led to a bizarre sartorial paradox: the greater the stress on the idea that clothing was an expression of integrity and moral worth, the greater the increase in the use of clothing as a form of disguise or as a mask for a person's actual beliefs. For there were those who found that the combination of moral pressure to wear *khadi* and moral condemnation if they did not was more powerful as an inducement to *khadi*-wearing than their actual beliefs in the cloth itself. Furthermore, there were not merely the negative consequences of being seen in foreign cloth to consider, but also the positive benefits of wearing khadi. For as the Rev. C. F. Andrews pointed out to Gandhi, *khadi* was 'a cheap method of gaining popularity' (CWMG vol. 25: 235). That the mere act of wearing *khadi* could earn a person a reputation for honesty, self-sacrifice and integrity undoubtedly made it a tempting clothing option for those with little belief in its ideology.

It was the combination of Gandhi's moral emphasis and the apparent hypocrisy it engendered in others that caused men like C. F. Andrews and Motilal Nehru to contemplate giving up the wearing of *khadi*. In 1924, Motilal even accused Gandhi of being 'systematically duped by unscrupulous liars who have ingratiated themselves into your favour by the simple device of pretending an abiding faith in khaddar to the exclusion of all else' (SWMN vol. 4: 72). An equally disillusioned *khadi*-supporter wrote from Purulia informing Gandhi of the shallowness of people's *khadi* faith:

> As you are expected to come to Purulia, all the people are buying khadi just to wear it during your stay. Your visit has reminded some of these men of their promise to use khaddar, and some are buying it just to escape public criticism. Now, if a man uses foreign cloth as a rule, but only wears khaddar on certain occasions, he is a hypocrite. And if your visit increases the number of hypocrites, what is its use? (CWMG vol. 28: 143).

Is *Khadi* the Solution?

Even Gandhi was forced to acknowledge that 'many self-seeking "workers" have exploited khadi dress. Wearing khadi and having made people believe that they were men of self sacrifice, such workers deceive society and refuse to make any amends. Such khadi wearers disgrace khadi' (CWMG vol. 31: 57).

In particular, it was Congressmen who came under frequent criticism for their 'insincere' use of *khadi*. But if there were wolves in sheep's clothing in the Congress Party, there were also sheep in wolves' clothing in the Indian Civil Service, for the same fear of recrimination that persuaded Congressmen to wear *khadi* in public also persuaded some *khadi*-lovers to hide their *khadi* beneath a public façade of foreign cloth. Indeed most of the sartorial antics popular in the nineteenth century resurfaced in the Gandhian era with a somewhat changed emphasis and an explicit moral overtone. No longer were people preoccupied with the problem of how much foreignness to allow into their clothes. Rather, it was a question of how much *swadeshi* they ought to integrate into their clothing and lifestyles. Like westernisation, *swadeshi* was usually a matter of degrees rather absolutes (fig. 4.6).

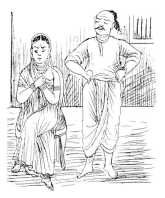

THE NON-CO-OPERATIONISTS
AT THE PHOTOGRAPHER'S.

(During the Divali holidays.)

Alo, a non-co-operationist and a Swadeshi to the core, boycotting his cycle cap, russian leather boots and German broad-cloth coat, stands in his native garments by the side of his Ali, dressed in a Sholapori saree, ready to be taken. And a good photo it is. Genuine Swadeshi! Taken by a Swadeshi, non-co-operationist photographer too. But the camera, the materials, the chemicals &c. &c. ? ? ? ? ? ?

Fig. 4.6 Reproduced from *Hindi Punch*, 1920. Courtesy of OIOC.

Khadi transformations of the problem of what to wear

In the pre-Gandhian era many men and women found a relatively uncontroversial solution to the problem of what to wear by wearing foreign cloth in Indian styles. But with the new Gandhian emphasis on *khadi*, this solution was now considered unpatriotic and immoral. Whereas in the past the style of a garment had been the most important criterion for judging patriotism, this was now the cloth itself, its production and origin. The result was that some Congressmen, being officially obliged to wear *khadi*, concealed their lack of *khadi*-faith by wearing mill-made imitations that were mass-produced in both India and Japan. By choosing simple white cloth they could continue to enjoy the comforts of the cheaper softer mill-cloth, while simultaneously reaping the benefits of a sanctimonious *khadi*-clad image. Some such imitations were pure fake while others were what Gandhi called 'half khadi', i.e. fabrics that were hand-woven but with machine-spun yarn (CWMG vol. 28: 144). In Simla Congressmen not only bought and wore *khadi* imitations, but actually sold them in so-called *khadi* shops (*Harijan* 19 Nov. 1938). The All India Spinners Association tried to control these developments by introducing its own stamp consisting of a spinning-wheel motif, which guaranteed that their *khadi* was 'certified'. But 'uncertified' *khadi* remained a constant problem and there were even reports of dealers sending specimens of 'certified' *khadi* to Manchester with the intent of obtaining cheap *khadi* imitations on which they could print the image of the *Mahatma*'s head to attract custom (*Statesman* 30 July 1921). The inevitable consequence of these developments was that some people who actually intended to wear *khadi* were clothed in fake *khadi* without even knowing it.

Another sartorial option, popular in the nineteenth century, was to wear a combination of Indian and European garments. Photographs of crowds in the 1920s and '30s reveal that this remained a common choice. Gandhi was irritated by the sight of foreign jackets worn over *khadi* outfits by children in National Schools. 'They should be saved from this miserable condition', he argued (CWMG vol. 26: 551).

Just as in the nineteenth century Indian headwear was often worn with European dress, so the Gandhi cap was often adopted without the wearer Indianising the rest of his clothes. The cap was cheap and easily obtainable and, as we have seen, people were often coerced into wearing it. But a mere *khadi* cap was not enough to satisfy either Gandhi or his Muslim co-worker Mohammad Ali. Confronted by a crowd of white caps and assorted clothes at a meeting in Sholapur, the latter proclaimed: 'Personally I don't find anybody clad in khadi. . . . You must, you have to, bear the burden that full khadi dress entails' (M. Desai 1968: 291).

For many who were not prepared to bear this 'burden' but who none the less wished to appear patriotic, the solution was to maintain two alternative sartorial images through changing their clothes to suit the situation. Always a popular solution, this enabled people to distinguish their public from their private selves. Gandhi's intention, as we have seen, was to abolish the public/private dichotomy altogether by suggesting a permanent sartorial solution corresponding to a person's inner self. In theory this should have ended the necessity of changing clothes, since *khadi* was the Indian expression of a constant unchanging truth. But far from discouraging constant changes of dress, Gandhi's preaching had the effect of reinforcing the necessity of changing clothes. For with the new Gandhian emphasis on the morality of dress, public appearances were interpreted as realities. This meant that the clothes of the public self were under more rigorous scrutiny than ever before. Whereas in the past people judged one another's loyalties ultimately by the clothes of the private self, they were now encouraged to interpret the dress of the public self as an explicit expression of belief, national allegiance and moral worth. This inevitably tempted people to present acceptable external images regardless of whether or not they corresponded to their personal beliefs.

The threshold of the house remained an important border for conversion. Those who did not fully believe in *khadi*, and who retained the idea that

Is *Khadi* the Solution?

European dress was more civilised, cast off their *khadi* on entering the house and replaced it with mill-cloth or European dress (cf. fig. 4.7). Many, like Sarojini Naidu, wore *khadi* only in periods of intense non-cooperation or when attending political meetings. In particular, Congress politicians developed a reputation for wearing *khadi* only for ceremonial purposes in public events. According to Gandhi, such men had 'become the laughing stock of all', creating an 'atmosphere of cant hypocrisy and humbug' (CWMG vol. 32: 523). Some Congressmen restricted their *khadi*-wearing exclusively to the election period, buying *khadi* clothes at the last minute to bolster their political image. But worse still were those politicians who refused to invest their money in *khadi*, yet who, wanting the political benefits, borrowed clothes from the All India Spinners Association solely for election purposes and returned them once the elections were over, at which point they reverted to foreign cloth (*Harijan* 16 July 1938).

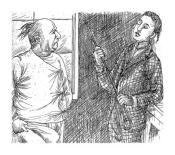

IRATE FATHER—You num-skull ! What do you mean by going in this European dress in these Divali days ? Be a pucca Swadeshi like me and wear khadi—

FASHIONALLE SON—That I do, pa, when I've to attend n. c. o. meetings But my fiancee does not like to see me in the dress of a Parsi corpse-bearer ! She considers it so ill-omened !

Fig. 4.7 Reproduced from *Hindi Punch*, Bombay, Oct. 1921. Courtesy of OIOC.

To Gandhi it was vital for *khadi* to remain at the centre of all political activity. Advising someone on how to select a candidate for the Legislative Council, he wrote:

> I shall tell you what I should do. I will first of all scan the candidates from top to bottom and if I find that among all the candidates there is not one man who is dressed from top to bottom in khaddar, I will retain my vote in my pocket absolutely sealed. And if I am satisfied there is at least one man who is dressed from top to toe in khaddar, I will go to him in all humility and ask him if he is dressed in this style for the occasion or if he habitually at home and out of home wears hand-spun and hand-woven khaddar. If he returns an answer in the negative, I should again retain my vote in my pocket. If positive, I would ask, 'It is extremely good that you always wear khaddar, but do you also spin for the sake of the masses at least for half an hour [per day]?' (CWMG vol. 26: 375).

Yet even with such elaborate screening, it was not impossible for some stealthy politicians to satisfy their love of foreign cloth. Locating the boundary between inner and outer selves somewhere between their inner and outer clothing, these men retained the comfort of their silky-textured mill-made underwear, safely submerged beneath a coarse external layer of *khadi*. Reversing the formula, there were other men working in the British administration who put on, beneath their smooth-textured Western suits, coarse *khadi* underclothes which remained close to their hearts and their inner beliefs both at home and in the workplace.

The only time when Gandhi considered it admissible for someone to change his sartorial image was when that person was going abroad; then it was acceptable for a patriotic Indian to wear European styles as long as they were made from *khadi*. Advising Dr Gurudas Roy about what to wear on his trip to England, Gandhi wrote:

> I am perfectly confident you can do without any European clothing in England and Scotland provided that you take a sufficient stock of hand-spun woollen clothing. . . . You may not know that Pandit Motilalji when he was preparing to go to England as a member of the Skeen Committee had an entirely hand-spun outfit including his cardigan jackets. . . . I suggest your consulting Satis Babu of Khadi Pratishthan, and if he cannot furnish you with an outfit, I know that the Khadi Bhandar of Bombay can, because that Bhandar has provided many England-going Indians with proper outfits. . . . All your underclothings may well be cotton *khadi* (CWMG vol. 34: 273–4).

Making *khadi* up into European styles was one of the most innovative methods of remaining patriotic and loyal to the ideology of *khadi* without sacrificing one's personal liking for European dress. But although such a solution was more acceptable to Gandhi than the reverse solution of making foreign cloth into Indian styles, it was not accepted by the Indian public, who retained the old idea that the style of dress was the most important criterion of patriotism. If clothes looked European they were likely to be criticised more than Indian-looking garments, even if the former were made from *khadi* and the latter were not. For once all the Indian features of *khadi* had been masked through cutting, tailoring and dyeing, there seemed little point in wearing *khadi* at all. Those men who wore black *khadi* suits of the European cut were suspected of British bias as they appeared embarrassed by their indigenous clothing traditions. This suggested that for at least some members of the Indian public a person's physical appearance was actually more important than his or her belief in *khadi* as an economic and moral solution to India's poverty.

A final example concerning the ever-controversial question of headwear reveals this distinction between Gandhi's emphasis on the morality of the cloth and the public's emphasis on the morality of the clothing style. In 1929 a lawyer wrote to Gandhi concerning the criticism he had received for wearing a *sola topi* which had been specially made out of certified *khadi* cloth:

> I was a practising lawyer but non-co-operated in 1921. Circumstances have driven me back to law but I am a strict khaddarite. I have given up the use of trousers and ties and attend the court and local legislature in dhoti. As Chairman of my District Council I am running Famine

Is *Khadi* the Solution?

Road Works, which require my being out in the sun. Recently I got a touch of the sun and went in for a hat, which has been specially made of pure khaddar. This has started a controversy. Will you take part in it? (CWMG vol. 41: 25).

Gandhi replied in *Young India*:

This is an old controversy. My narrow nationalism rebels against the hat, my secret internationalism regards the sola topi as one of the few boons from Europe. But for the tremendous national prejudice against the hat, I would undertake to become president of a league for popularising sola hats.... But I know that national likes and dislikes are not governed by reason.... I do not expect Indians to take kindly to the sola hat. Nevertheless workers like Pandit Durgashankar need not be ruffled by criticism and may certainly wear khadi imitations of the sola hat. It is in reality an easily portable umbrella that covers the head without the necessity of one hand being occupied by carrying it (*ibid.*: 25).

Gandhi's liking for the *sola topi*, which the Indian public rejected with such vigour, reveals the distinctiveness of his personal belief in the meaning of national dress. To him a moral and patriotic outfit consisted of simple, practical clothes made from *khadi*, preferably though not exclusively in Indian styles. But for the Indian public, style remained a central criterion of Indianness. To many the *sola topi* was as much a symbol of Britishness as their own Gandhi cap was a symbol of Indianness. The British themselves were well aware of the symbolism of their *topis*. Not long after poor Fred Burrows was forcibly *khadi*-capped by zealous Gandhians, the British voluntarily removed their own hats. The ritual was described by Rupert Mayne, who was sailing with the last British regiment to leave the newly-created Pakistan: 'As we left Port Said and sailed into the open waters, everyone was paraded with their topees on deck and at the given signal we all flung our topees into the sea and that was the last of India' (cited in Allen 1985: 229). What better final victory for the Gandhi cap?

Post-independence political sartorial inheritance

Needless to say, the problem of what to wear did not end with the dawning of Indian independence. And no one suffered more from this problem than Indian politicians. The intensification of nationalist feeling and moral righteousness that became attached to *khadi* could not easily be shaken off. As Bayly has pointed out, Jawaharlal Nehru never shared Gandhi's vision of a non-industrial village-based society, yet during his years as

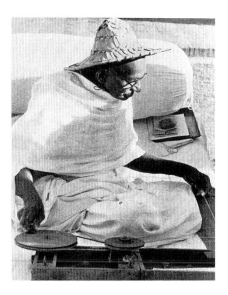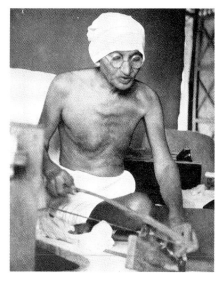

Fig. 4.8 Gandhi, unable to wear the *sola topi* which he considered 'one of the few boons from Europe', resorted to a number of alternative methods of warding off the heat. *Top left*: Wearing a Noakhali straw hat in Delhi (1947). *Top right*: Cooling his head by wrapping a damp cloth around it (Sevagram 1940). *Bottom left*: With a mud pack on his head (Sevagram 1940). *Bottom right*: With a piece of white *khadi* to keep off the sun (1930). Courtesy of NGM.

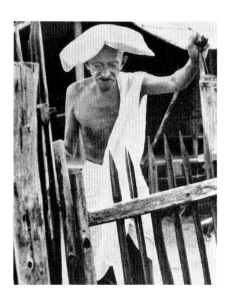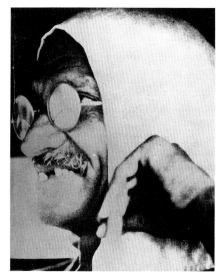

Is *Khadi* the Solution?

India's first prime minister he continued to support *khadi* production while simultaneously promoting industrial progress. Successive governments have all followed this line regardless of whether the *khadi* and craft emporiums ran at a profit or a loss (Bayly 1986: 314–15). As with government policy, so with clothes.

After fighting for freedom under a banner of *khadi*, politicians could not just turn about and forget it once the British had left India, even though the majority of the populace (excluding perhaps artists and intellectuals) did exactly that. Furthermore the moral stigma which Gandhi had so cleverly woven into imported fabrics could not be unravelled any more than the moral integrity which he had so neatly woven into *khadi*.

Nehru's solution was to carve himself a highly tailored but noticeably non-Western image, while retaining *khadi* as the fabric of his dress. He therefore opted for the stitched tight *pyjama* which he wore with either the long *sherwani* or the short, now famous 'Nehru jacket'. It was more or less a return to the pre-Gandhian version of respectable dress,[16] with the difference that Nehru's version was made from *khadi*. He sometimes wore foreign dress on foreign visits but in India his clothes remained essentially Indian.

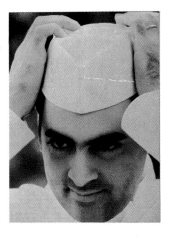

Fig. 4.9 Rajiv Gandhi, photographed by Raghu Rai. Reproduced from India Today June 1991. Courtesy of Raghu Rai.

Concerned by the post-independence sartorial confusion around him, Nehru wrote an official note on dress, advising those in high grades of government office to steer clear of European clothes 'which marked them out as a privileged, denationalised, and out-of-date class, and to adopt such clothes as would take them closer to the people' (cited in Chaudhuri 1976: 131–2). He passed on his own chic notion of *swadeshi* to his daughter Indira Gandhi, who usually dressed in handloom cotton saris, at least when she was in India. Similarly, her son Rajiv Gandhi threw aside his European dress and aviator's uniform in favour of *khadi* when he entered political office in 1984 (see fig. 4.9), and his wife Soniya is still seen in public in handloom saris. In the run-up to the 1991 elections, most political candidates were wearing white *khadi*, and one New Delhi candidate was even dressed as Mahatma Gandhi himself. But despite the efforts made to keep politicians in touch with the humble masses, the modern-day politician remains a remote and conspicuous figure for most villagers. Fig. 4.10, published in the run-up to the 1989 elections, shows the distance between the *khadi*-clad politician and the rural masses who wear a motley array of European clothes. The irony is heightened by his words: 'Tighten your belts ... roll up your sleeves ... pull up your socks....' A sockless,

---

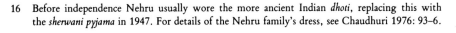

16 Before independence Nehru usually wore the more ancient Indian *dhoti*, replacing this with the *sherwani pyjama* in 1947. For details of the Nehru family's dress, see Chaudhuri 1976: 93–6.

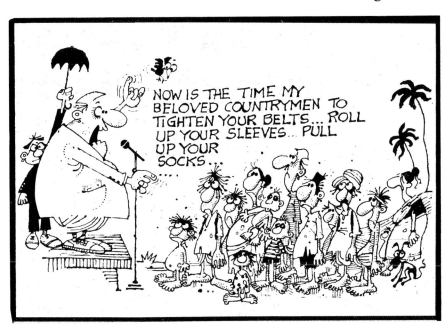

Fig. 4.10 Cartoon by Mario Miranda for the *Illustrated Weekly*, Nov. 1989. Courtesy of Mario Miranda and Penguin Books India.

beltless, partly-sleeved village population stares incredulously at this strange, prosperous orator who proclaims his message from beneath the comfort of a black umbrella, held by an assistant in a European suit and shoes. For many politicians *swadeshi* remained, as always and perhaps more than ever, a matter of degrees (fig. 4.11) and a useful election stunt.

It is the long-term association with morality and patriotism that has enabled and indeed forced plain white *khadi* to remain in politics. No longer everyday dress, it is an obligatory appendage whenever the public political self is most on show. Modern-day sceptics tend to view this phenomenon as a sign of degeneration, of the shallow integrity of contemporary leaders who lack the sincerity of their freedom-fighting ancestors. But, as we have seen, strategic *khadi*-dressing was born in the Gandhian era itself, even at a time when Gandhi was preaching a virtual religion of *khadi*. It merely intensified after independence when the moral pressure to believe in *khadi* dissipated, leaving only the fabric itself to stand as an anachronistic but emotive symbol of the humble, caring politician. Most people know that the *khadi*-clad politician is no more humble than the rest of them, but then, as fig. 4.12 reveals, it is sometimes difficult to do things without *khadi*!

Is *Khadi* the Solution?

Post-independence political heads

A discussion of post-independence political dress would not be complete without reference to the age-old saga of headwear. Jawaharlal Nehru, India's first prime minister, often wore a Gandhi cap, a relic of the freedom struggle, and the same cap continues to sprout on Indian heads today, primarily at times of political intensity or at nationally important funerals. But Nehru had always disliked Gandhi's peculiar way of over-simplifying things, sartorial or otherwise. While Gandhi tried to condense all Indian diversity into a single item of headwear, Nehru instead put into practice his favourite maxim 'unity in diversity', and wore a variety of different things on his head. In the desire to communicate with other nations and ethnic groups, he developed a habit of dressing up in other people's clothes when on political tours; this was 'dressing up' because it was an attempt not so much to adopt the identity of the other as to greet others on their own terms and thus accept their otherness. To this end he generally retained his *sherwani pyjama*, adding some foreign appendage to his dress, and it was often the headwear of the other that he chose to wear on his visits (see fig. 4.13). It was a means of expressing acceptance of ethnic diversity, even when the ethnic group he was visiting did not look so ethnically diverse (fig. 4.14)! Nehru initiated his daughter Indira Gandhi in the same sartorial practice, and through her it passed to her son Rajiv (see fig. 4.15). Indeed accepting the headwear of the people has now become a common feature

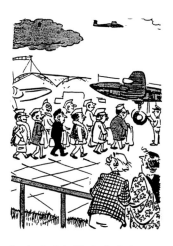

Now, that chap in the dark suit—how has he managed to go abroad with all these restrictions on travel!

Fig. 4.12 Cartoon by R. K. Laxman. Courtesy of R. K. Laxman in the *Times of India*.

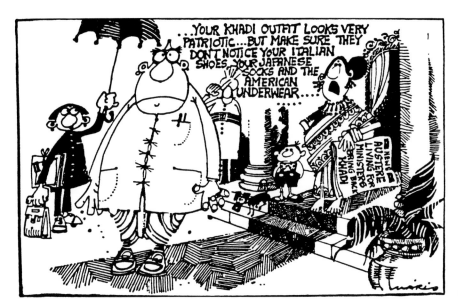

Fig. 4.11 Cartoon by Mario/Sapre (1988). Courtesy of Mario/Sapre and Penguin Books India.

125

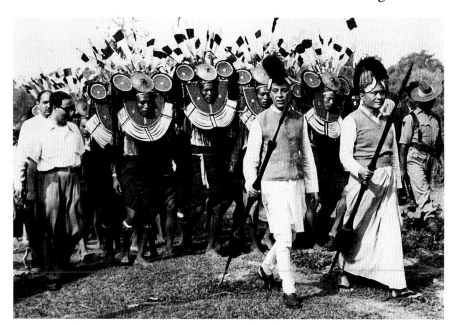

Fig. 4.13 Jawaharlal Nehru greeting others on their own terms, pictured here wearing Naga head-dress and accompanying the Prime Minister of Burma in Singkaling. Courtesy of the Press and Information Bureau, Government of India.

of Indian ministerial tours, thereby reversing the traditional practice whereby the ruler bestowed authority on his subordinates through the distribution of headwear. The reversal of the gesture serves as symbolic acknowledgement of the fact that in democratic India it is the people who have the ultimate power to legitimise the authority of their elected leaders.

Despite their practice of using different forms of headwear, the Nehru men did not abandon the Gandhi cap, which they continued to wear for certain official occasions. And the cap has remained an important feature of election campaigning although its popularity has waned somewhat in recent years. It is also worn by some Indian men at funerals or for important religious rituals when many who normally go bare-headed cover their heads. As we have seen, the Gandhi cap was never quite the symbol of national unity that Gandhi hoped. This is reflected today in the wearing of different coloured caps to represent different interests: some Hindu fundamentalists have taken to wearing orange Gandhi caps, and certain sections of the protesting peasantry green ones. Meanwhile the old-style Gandhian with his white *khadi* cap has become an increasingly rare sight.

Some reflections on khadi's limitations
Having considered the strengths and limitations of *khadi*'s appeal primarily in relation to educated urbanites, it is interesting to reflect on how villagers

Is *Khadi* the Solution?

might have confronted the problem of what to wear in the 1920s and '30s. Unfortunately there is not the same level of documentation here. Only the educated could pour out their sartorial anxieties in diaries and letters to Gandhi, and thus it is their dilemmas that are on record. Yet even if one takes Gandhi's speeches as a means of judging the popularity of *khadi* in rural areas, it becomes clear that villagers were not as responsive as Gandhi expected. Of course there were pockets of supporters in rural India, such as the Kaira peasantry and the Santals of Bengal, who felt that *khadi* represented their interests. But the rural response seems to have been muted. Gandhi acknowledged this when he wrote in *Young India*: 'So much is town life now dominating the villages that, unless towns set the fashion in *khadi*, it becomes most difficult to persuade the villagers to spin even in their own interests and just enough for their own use' (Gandhi 1959: 234). And if the urban-influenced villagers were difficult to convince, how much more must this have been true of conservative villagers, tenacious of their local clothing traditions?

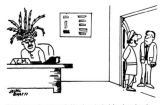

'He has started wearing tribal headgear in the hope that when the Prime Minister visits his State he might be able to meet him!'

Fig. 4.14 Cartoon by Jaspal Bhatti. Reproduced courtesy of Jaspal Bhatti and Penguin Books India.

Clearly the rural response to *khadi* must have varied from region to region, influenced perhaps by the extent to which it blended with existing traditions. But Gandhi, as we have seen, had little patience with the problem of region diversity, and even less with the social and aesthetic aspects of local traditions. This must have made his *khadi* policy particularly unpalatable to those rural women used to wearing elaborate clothes, the style and colour of which expressed not only their regional identity but also their social position and marital status. In such areas *khadi* threatened literally to blank out the fabric of social life.

There is not, as far as we can ascertain, any record of how the inhabitants of a single village responded to Gandhi's clothing policy earlier in the century. But even an analysis of contemporary clothing issues in an Indian village can provide a context for understanding the basis of rural resistance in some areas. In the following chapters, we take the problem of what to wear to a village in Gandhi's native Saurashtra (in Gujarat), where it is clear that even today questions of local hierarchy and identity rest uneasily with the notion of sartorial uniformity. This conservative nature of the Saurashtran people clearly irritated Gandhi, who criticised many of the local customs to which he had been subjected as a child. Later, when he returned to Saurashtra for political meetings, he was disappointed by the absence of *khadi* in the area (CWMG vol. 26: 174) and complained that the spinning-wheel was still a 'stranger at the door' in the Kathiawar states (CWMG vol. 26: 254). At other times he was critical of local women's jewellery, referring to their glimmering foot ornaments as '*unbearable* heavy ankle hoops' (CWMG vol. 28: 328). But while Gandhi was irritated by the Kathiawadis' powers of sartorial resistance, it was of course this same conservatism that had prevented many local women from adopting foreign cloth. By advocating the shedding of jewellery and the wearing of *khadi*, Gandhi was trying to save such women not so much from the bonds of colonialism as from the bonds of local tradition. While he was critical of traditions which advocated elaborate adornment, others praised the women of Saurashtra for continuing to wear their colourful hand-embroidered clothes at a time when other Indian women had converted to mill-cloth (cf. Billington 1973 [1895]: 186).

The image of the 'traditional' Saurashtran woman, glowing with embroidery and jewellery, with her husband dressed in a white cotton smock and colourful turban, is today a favourite in both tourist brochures and books about Indian craft where conservatism is often promoted as authenticity. But descriptions, like photographs, are selective. The image is today outliving the reality. The people of Saurashtra, like people all over the globe, are developing new tastes and habits. For young men this means wearing trousers, shirts and plastic sandals, a transition already well advanced. For young women it means rejecting previous regional styles in favour of the comparatively uniform machine-made sari. But the change in women's dress has been gradual and the transition often painful, as the following chapters show.

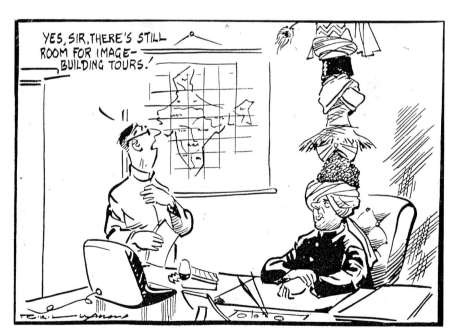

Fig. 4.15 Cartoon of Rajiv Gandhi by R. K. Laxman. Reproduced courtesy of R. K. Laxman in the *Times of India*.

5   Questions of Dress in a Gujarati Village

Prologue: an anthropologist's clothing dilemma

I first visited Jalia[1] village in April 1988, accompanied by a Gujarati professor and an English woman who was interested in textiles. The professor, a man in his late fifties, was greeted with all the respect and reverence that surrounds the educated city man, and we were greeted by all the staring, pointing and laughing that foreigners inevitably attract when they first appear in unexpected parts of rural India.[2] Being so conspicuous, we were immediately surrounded by a crowd of women and girls who seemed to alternate between staring in wide-eyed bemusement and giggling coyly into their veils. We were both wearing loose cotton dresses that fell well below the knee, but took care none the less to pull these down over our ankles while sitting in people's courtyards. For my part, I felt somewhat uncomfortable among these women who were covered from head to toe, and many of whom swiftly disappeared behind their veils whenever the professor looked in their direction. Some went into total silence behind their colourful mobile screens. Others spoke when addressed from beneath their veils with a shy giggle. Their shyness and sense of modesty did not make me feel immodest so much as over-exposed and, above all, inappropriately dressed.

The members of one family were particularly friendly since it was through their youngest son who studied in the city that we had made our initial contact. When the professor had to leave after only an hour, this family invited the two white strangers to stay in their house for the night. We soon found ourselves alone in the kitchen with the women of the household – in this case, a mother and a daughter – who bombarded us with questions: 'Why are you wearing such funny clothes? Why this rough cotton cloth? Why aren't you wearing bangles? Why no nose-rings? You

---

1   In response to requests, I have changed the name of the village and given all villagers fictional names. There are in fact a number of villages in Gujarat with the name Jalia, but the Jalia of this book is not any of them.

2   There is nothing new about Gujarati women laughing at peculiar-looking foreigners. Marianne Postans records women's reactions when she visited the Roa's palace in Kutch in the early 1830s: 'I was greeted by whisperings, gigglings, and other demonstrations of amusement, at what they thought remarkable in my dress and manner' (Postans 1838: 51).

don't even have holes in your noses? No anklets? No earrings? Nothing. Nothing at all? Are you married? Not married? Is that why you are not wearing bangles? So, what kind are you? What is your caste?' I heard mother explain to daughter: 'You see. They will put on nose-rings and bangles after marriage. Then they will wear nose-rings, bangles, earrings, anklets, sari, everything.' I tried to explain with my then extremely limited knowledge of Hindi and Gujarati that we would not wear all of these things, not even after marriage, and that in our country women generally did not oil their hair or wear nose-rings; it was not the custom. The only aspects of our appearance that were approved of were the whiteness of our skin and my cheap plastic watch, which was immediately identified as good once it was known to be foreign.

The next morning Ramanbhai,[3] the youngest son, handed us towels and saris and ordered us to wash ourselves. The women wanted our clothes for cleaning. Since they were filthy from long bus journeys, we could not refuse. I returned from my wash somewhat embarrassed, with a sari swathed precariously about me. I thought it strange that they had not even given me a petticoat or blouse to put on underneath. But it soon became apparent that this was only temporary apparel, for mother, daughter and son were in the throes of discussing what clothes they should give their new guests. It was apparently not a simple matter. The problem revolved around the fact that as 'unmarried girls' we should not really be wearing saris, but on the other hand we were much too old and too big to be 'unmarried girls', which seemed to suggest that saris were most suitable. The other possibility was a *shalwar kamiz* (trouser and knee-length tunic), the dress worn by the daughter of the house when she went to school in the city. A fitted pale blue polyester version of this outfit was given to my companion while I was dressed in a long petticoat and tight synthetic *kamiz* (tunic), also belonging to their nineteen-year-old daughter. We found the clothes uncomfortable and physically restrictive but were willing and even amused to wear them for the day. But it was soon clear that our hosts were taking the ritual of dressing us up more seriously than we thought. They began to get out their bangles and tried to force them on to our over-large wrists. They oiled our hair, screwing it back into tight

---

3   In Gujarati, the names of adults are rarely spoken without a kinship term being added as a suffix. Here, the term *bhai* (brother) has been added to the name Raman as a gesture of respect. Suffixes such as *bhai*, *ben* (sister), *dada* (grandfather) and *kaka* (uncle) are frequently attached to names, and although they are kinship terms they can be used to refer to both kin and non-kin. A respected old man is therefore likely to have *dada* attached to his name whether or not he is the grandfather of the person addressing him.

Questions of Dress in a Gujarati Village

smooth buns. They stuck red *bindis* (spangles) on our foreheads. And finally the mother looked pleased, announcing in triumph: 'Now you are *real* Gujaratis. Now you are *our* people. You are my very own daughters. Now I have three daughters, no longer one, but three!' The reality of being '*real* Gujaratis' and '*our*' people' became apparent when Ramanbhai began to introduce us to people in the village not only as *Brahman* girls, but actually as his mother's aunt's daughters who lived in 'Foren'.[4] This explanation seemed to satisfy the general curiosity. Somehow, through our clothing, we had been transformed, at least temporarily, into people comprehensible in local terms. The whiteness of our skin, the peculiarity of our speech, our very origins were submerged by a heavy layer of cultural dressing. Brief though the victory was, it was the triumph of dress over descent; of culture over the body; of the collectivity of caste over our peculiarly Western sense of individuality.

Looking back on the incident, I realise that I was by no means fully aware of its significance at the time. Yet I was strangely relieved to get back into my own apparel at the end of the day, even though I knew it to be inappropriate; this was not simply because it was more comfortable, but also because their clothes gave me a sense of restriction as though I was somehow expected to move and act differently. Dressed in their long and cumbersome garments, not only did I no longer look my normal self but I did not feel it either.[5]

When I returned to the village after some months, I was alone and equipped with a better knowledge of Gujarati and what I considered 'appropriate clothing'. This consisted of a *shalwar kamiz*, the dress worn not only by Indian Muslims but also by college girls in the nearby city and by a few educated village girls. The *Brahman* family were pleased that I was wearing Indian dress and approved of my choice of style, which they said was suitable for an educated unmarried girl. But they were angry that I had purchased my own cloth and disappointed in my choice of fabric which,

---

4 'Foren' was the general term used for the place where foreigners live. It had wide and varied application according to where the flexible boundary was drawn between the indigenous (*deshi*) and the foreign (*videshi*). Where the boundary was narrowly drawn, any place outside the immediate neighbourhood could be labelled 'Foren'. Where the boundary was drawn more widely, the term could be used, as here, to refer to places outside India. Ramanbhai's mother's maternal aunt had in fact emigrated to Kenya and later settled in Leicester, which Ramanbhai's family assumed to be in London.

5 In a brief but pertinent article entitled 'Lumbar Thought', Umberto Eco has explored this idea that clothes impose demeanours. Reflecting on the effects of his tight denim jeans, he concluded that they reduced his sense of interiority by forcing him to 'live towards the exterior world' (Eco 1986: 191–5).

being cotton, was much too coarse and plain for their taste. They told me they would have provided clothing for me, and would have chosen much more suitable synthetic, shiny cloth and a better-fitting style. They felt I should not have purchased anything myself, and they were annoyed too that I had arrived with a few vessels of my own. They wanted me to eat their food, wear their clothes, in short to 'be' one of them. I for my part was anxious to maintain some degree of independence for I realised that 'being one of them' was going to place insurmountable restrictions on my movements. I had already seen that unmarried *Brahman* daughters scarcely stirred outside the house.

The problem of how I should be dressed was, of course, linked to the much more fundamental problem of my identity at large. It was a cause of great concern that an 'unmarried girl' could stray so far afield without her parents, and it also seemed inconceivable that any university could allow such irresponsible behaviour. Ideally, a respectable girl of marriageable age (though at twenty-five I was pushing the limit) should stay inside the house as much as possible, and if my studies took me outside I should at least be accompanied by a male family member. For I must surely feel both scared and shy to venture out alone; I needed male protection. My situation was made all the more miserable in their eyes because my 'sister' had gone back to 'Foren' and found 'service' (a job) while I was left in India on my own.

The immediate, and indeed considerate, response of this *Brahman* family was to put right my shameful and apparently lonely position by incorporating me into their own family structure, and providing me with clothes was a natural familial duty. It was, after all, the obligation of the head of the house to provide both clothes and food for his wife and daughters. What would neighbours say if I seemed deprived of my due? And just as this responsible father sought to provide for me, so he sought to 'protect' me from the prying eyes of the outside world of the village; it was his paternal duty. For the first few days of my stay, I could not stir outside the house without the protective companionship of my 'Gujarati brother' who tried to control both whom I spoke to and what we spoke about. He too was fulfilling his 'duty'. His presence made conversation difficult, for the farming women and girls with whom I was talking were not accustomed to visits from a twenty-year-old *Brahman* boy, and seemed to find his serious and masculine presence even more disturbing than my own. This was not aided by the air of distinct superiority he had adopted towards these, his social inferiors. He was standing guard. When after a week his father ordered him to buy new cloth for me from the town and get it stitched at the tailor's, I quickly refused the offer and assured them that I had

Questions of Dress in a Gujarati Village

enough clothes of my own. I was never to accept clothes from them again except as a parting gift on leaving the village, for wearing their clothes seemed tantamount to accepting the identity they wished to confer on me, with all its attendant benefits and constraints.[6]

This refusal was part of a more general attempt to shed my new Gujarati identity and preserve my own. I soon informed the family that I did not wish to be presented either as their relative or as a *Brahman*. Finally we settled on a compromise identity. I was to be introduced as the friend and neighbour of their relative who lived in 'Foren', thus providing a good explanation for why I had chosen their particular village and family with whom to stay. This would satisfy the curiosity of other villagers who might be jealous or suspicious of my presence. For my part, it freed me to some extent of the obligation to act like a *Brahman*, although the role of daughter remained with me throughout my stay.

This initial experience gave me a taste of the problem of what to wear: the feeling of exclusion and peculiarity engendered by being inappropriately dressed, and the feeling of group inclusion with all the apparent limitations and restrictions that being appropriately dressed seemed to embody. Finally, I had searched for a garment sufficiently neutral to allow me to circulate among the maximum number of people, decent without being confining, female without being too 'feminine', and Indian without being associated with any particular caste.[7] It had the added benefit of being reasonably comfortable for a Westerner, accustomed to wearing trousers. I chose cotton because it seemed the coolest material and I restricted myself to comparatively simple designs.

Often women would remark on my lack of jewellery and suggest that without it I looked like a man. But this ambiguity of gender was something that worked in my favour. For the shapeless *shalwar kamiz* which

6 Cohn has demonstrated how sets of clothes (*khilats*) were given by Moghul rulers to their inferiors as a gesture of authority. Receiving a set of clothes implied a person's inferiority and subordination as well as his/her entitlement to protection. In their attempts to escape being placed in this position, the British tried to avoid receiving such 'gifts' (Cohn 1989: 316–18). The idea that receiving clothes implies a relationship of dependence and indebtedness is a recurrent theme of Indian culture. Saurashtran rulers, for example, used to give turbans to leading peasants in order to guarantee commitment and ratify agreements which, if broken, incurred a fine (cf. Spodek 1976: 28).

7 The *shalwar kamiz*, though introduced to India by Muslims, has been worn for centuries by both Hindus and Muslims in parts of northern India (see chapter 2). It has recently become the acceptable garb of female college students of all religions throughout the subcontinent. However, once married, Hindu women often revert to saris unless they either live in the far northern states or belong to a cosmopolitan urban élite. In most rural areas, the *shalwar kamiz* has retained its Islamic associations more strongly than in cities and is worn only by the educated few.

de-emphasised the female form, combined with the lack of jewellery, seemed to enable me to circulate in the village with the mobility more commonly experienced by men. This did not mean that I mixed equally with men and women, for my contact with the former was always secondary to my contact with the latter. But the fact that my dress distinguished me from identification with any particular social group enabled me to talk with a variety of people from all different castes, to visit other villages and to ride a bicycle without being too much restricted by the normal constraints on female behaviour. It was both desexualising and freeing.[8] Interestingly, villagers were not unaware of this. Sometimes old women informed me that I was wise not to wear jewellery since it meant I had nothing to fear and was free to move around; their young women, by contrast, were afraid to go out alone for fear that thieves might snatch their large gold earrings. More often men would acknowledge my 'freedom' and preach to their wives: 'You see. She does not bother with all these things [jewellery]. She can progress.' As the providers of ornaments they saw in me the idea of escape from this financial burden. But, in reality, men dared not skimp on gifts of jewellery, for they feared the censure of other villagers and the crushing accusation of being miserly.

My search for appropriate clothing was, of course, very different from village women's clothing dilemmas. I could select my own option, a compromise between how other people wanted me to dress and how I wished to dress myself. Furthermore, I was able to refuse their offer of clothes and in doing so could to some extent avoid the role being ascribed to me with those clothes.[9] But the experience of being temporarily dressed and

8   Young educated women in cities often cite this as the reason for the increasing popularity of the *shalwar kamiz*. A dress designer in Ahmedabad told me: 'It has offered a new ease of movement to women and a sense of liberty. Its popularity is part of the changing role of the upper middle class woman today.'

9   Ann Grodzins Gold's account of her reception in a Rajasthani village illustrates how another anthropologist has dealt with this issue. Her position differed from mine in that she was considerably older and married. She had chosen to wear a *shalwar kamiz* but since this was worn only by local Muslims and college girls in towns, it was considered inappropriate by all but the Muslim villagers. She therefore bought some material which was sewn up into ruffled skirts by her Rajput landlady's daughter. She wore these with a loose blouse and veil. She writes: 'When I donned these clothes, it turned out that I looked like a Rajput, for the daughter had sewn them in her caste's distinctive style.' The *Brahman* women thought she looked ridiculous and told her to wear a sari. Muslim women said she was better off in a *shalwar kamiz* which afforded her good protection from men, and peasant women teased her by suggesting she adopt their briefer style of skirt and blouse. In defiance, she appeared one day in jeans which, being 'men's dress', met with unanimous disapproval. Finally, after struggling with the discomfort of a veil for a while, she decided to keep her head uncovered and to settle for a long skirt and cotton blouse which did not directly identify her with any particular

Questions of Dress in a Gujarati Village

presented as a *Brahman* relative gave me some insight into what it is both to wear and to receive apparel which simultaneously defines identity and places expectations on behaviour. Village women never had my kind of choice, nor did they contemplate it, but neither did they blindly accept the expectations of caste and family tradition. My attempt as an outsider to avoid being drawn into the minutiae of their traditions could perhaps be seen as the reverse of their attempts as insiders to reach out from those traditions to a changing environment and to incorporate aspects of modernity into their clothing and behaviour. This chapter explores the relationship between clothing and identity in the village.

Historical background of the village

Jalia is in Saurashtra, the peninsula that juts out from western India into the Arabian Sea. It is a region with a long and chequered history of invasions, wars and territorial disputes, making it for centuries one of the most politically fragmented regions of India. Centralised authority was to some extent imposed by the Moghuls in the late sixteenth century, but even then the land of the peninsula was principally in the possession of rival Rajput, *Kathi* and *Koli* chiefs who established their claims to territory largely by force. As the Moghul empire declined, the situation of extreme instability increased and was compounded by regular tribute-raising expeditions by the Maratha forces. The latter encountered such opposition from *Kathi* chiefs in the area that they named the peninsula 'Kathiawad' (land of the *Kathis*), a name which many Saurashtrans continue to use today.

It was in trying to settle tribute relations between the Gaekwar (Maratha ruler of Baroda in Gujarat) and the Kathiawad chiefs that the British became involved in the peninsula. In 1807, Major Alexander Walker drew up a settlement which not only defined revenue payments but also crystallised the territorial rights of the Kathiawad chiefs. By the 1820s, the British had expanded their role in the area to that of administrators and were ruling over a motley political patchwork consisting of more than 200[10] separate

---

community. She avoided the heavy silver anklets worn by villagers but agreed to don the bangles appropriate to a married woman, without which she was considered inauspicious (Gold 1988: 13–14). Like me, she had found a neutral compromise somewhere between personal discomfort and social expectation. Some ethnographers have opted for a fuller identification with the women with whom they work. Sarah Hobson (1978) and Doreen Jacobson (1970), for example, both wore saris for their fieldwork in Indian villages.

10   The precise number was in constant dispute. Walker initially identified 153 states when he visited the peninsula in 1807. By 1860 eighty of these had disappeared and 300 new ones had sprung into being (Copland 1982: 99), demonstrating the general confusion in the area.

princely states. These varied from a few large and well-organised states which, by the late nineteenth century, had full powers of self-jurisdiction, to numerous petty feudal states which were non-jurisdictional and might cover little more than a few square miles of land each. All states, great and small, were merged after independence; the ancient name of Saurashtra was then restored to the peninsula, which later became incorporated into the modern state of Gujarat.

Although Saurashtra has been part of Gujarat since 1956, it has maintained a distinctive sense of regional identity. Rural Saurashtrans still tend to refer to themselves and their language as Kathiawadi rather than Gujarati. Their cultural distinctiveness is clearly manifest in their dialect, food and dress, all of which combine to encourage mainland Gujaratis to view the peninsula as a somewhat 'traditional', if not 'folkloric' place.

Jalia is in one of the more progressive districts of Saurashtra, which for the purpose of this book is called Larabad.[11] It is a large village with over 8,000 inhabitants. It is just off a concrete highway and a now disused railway line, and thus within easy access of the district capital – it is not in any way remote. As the largest village in the immediate neighbourhood, it attracts people from smaller surrounding villages, who come to make purchases or catch a bus or truck to the city. With a bank, a post office, a selection of temples, three medical dispensaries and a primary and secondary school, Jalia has many of the facilities of a small town. Its main street is lined with shops selling foodstuffs and a variety of household items ranging from steel utensils to soap, cloth, jewellery and school notebooks. Interspersed with these are goldsmiths' workshops, tailoring units and stalls selling *pan* (betel nut), *bidi* (local cigarettes), tea and the ubiquitous cold drinks. Spare parts for farming equipment and kerosene are also available, though in limited quantity and supply. For major purchases of clothes and other large items, most villagers prefer to make the one-hour bus trip to Larabad city where produce is cheaper and the choice more varied.

Jalia is linked to other villages and towns, not only through its strategic position on the roadside but also through extensive kinship ties. The practices of village exogamy and virilocal residence ensure that women from other towns and villages marry into it, and Jalia women marry into other towns and villages, thereby providing networks of familial links throughout the area. The practice of exchange marriage is common among many of the poorer castes, in which case women literally exchange villages and homes when they marry.

11 Because of the personal nature of some incidents in the following chapters, the names of the district and its capital have been altered and their exact whereabouts left vague.

Questions of Dress in a Gujarati Village

Despite its size and proximity to a large and prosperous city, Jalia remains a village by official definition.[12] Surrounded by fields and hills, it continues to be dominated by an agricultural and pastoral economy. A high proportion of the working population engages in farming activities for all or part of the year, the main crops being groundnuts, onions, millet, barley, wheat, sesame and lemons. Many landowning farmers also own at least a pair of bullocks and a buffalo or cow, from which they obtain sufficient milk to fulfil their own needs.

More important than the official definition of Jalia as a 'village' is the local perception of it as such. The explanations 'But this is only a village' or 'In the village only the village way goes' were frequently invoked by both men and women to describe patterns of expected behaviour. Women, in particular, were conscious of the need to act in accordance with 'village custom' (*gamno rivaj*). As in many parts of North and Central India, most married women were expected to veil their faces when stepping outside their homes into the public space of their marital villages. The ability to remain out of view and within one's own home was considered the privilege of the wealthy few. Once outside, a woman was generally conscious of what 'people of the village' would see or say. And although the village was large, heterogeneous and in the process of expansion and change, people often invoked its name as if it had some sort of fixed autonomy and moral code. Stepping into 'the village' was like mounting a stage where an audience (real or imagined) was ready to assess your performance.[13]

The people of Jalia
The people of Jalia are predominantly Hindu and belong to various *jatis* (caste groups).[14] Table 5.1 lists the main social divisions of the village,

12 To qualify officially as a town, at least 75 per cent of its male working population would have needed to be engaged in non-agricultural activities.

13 There are many parallels here with Ursula Sharma's discussion of Harbassi village in the Punjab. With a population of 6,000, Harbassi was neither so small that it had no public space nor so large that public space predominated. Inhabitants described it as 'our own place' (*apni jegeh*), as opposed to the city where there was a certain anonymity and reputations did not need to be so closely guarded. Sharma notes that married women were more restricted in their movements in the large village of Harbassi than in either smaller villages (with little public space) or cities (with predominantly public space) (Sharma 1980: 230–9). This observation accords with my own observations in the district of Larabad.

14 There is not space here to enter into the growing debates about the inadequacy of the term 'caste' as applied to the Indian context. The term is used here to refer to those groups whose members are willing to intermarry, accept cooked food from one another and identify with a shared caste name. It should, however, be recognised that social identity is not a rigid phenomenon and that, as has often been pointed out, there is a certain blurring and fluidity at the boundaries of caste (cf. Cohn 1955, Pocock 1972). Furthermore, discrepancies in wealth

classified according to traditional occupational type. These correspond somewhat to local perceptions of hierarchy, although the criteria by which status is judged vary considerably according to whether wealth, land-ownership, ritual purity or a mixture of these and other factors is emphasised. In many ways it is social differentiation rather than hierarchy as such that is stressed. The *Bharwads* (shepherds), for example, are best seen as 'different from' artisan and service castes rather than 'above' them, particularly since the status of the latter varies considerably according to the actual professions in which they are engaged.[15] Similarly traders, priests and ex-ruling aristocrats, whose value systems are to some extent at variance, should be seen more as representing different facets of the village élite rather than as heading any single hierarchical order.[16]

SOCIAL COMPOSITION OF JALIA

TRADERS, PRIESTS AND FORMER RULING ELITE
Vaniya (traders), *Brahman* (priests), *Darbar*[17] (land-owners of the previously ruling local *Rajput* clan)

MAIN FARMING GROUPS
Kanbi and *Kharak* (cultivators and cattle-owners), *Koli*[18] (usually farm labourers)

PASTORALISTS
Bharwad (shepherds, keeping mainly goats and sheep)

ARTISAN AND SERVICE GROUPS
Soni (goldsmiths), *Sutar* (carpenters), *Darji* (tailors), *Luhar* (blacksmiths — Hindu and Muslim), *Teliwala* (Muslim oil pressers), *Kumvar* (potters), *Dhobi* (washermen), *Vanand* (barbers), *Mochi* (cobblers)

LOW-RANKING GROUPS
Vaghri (sellers of sticks for cleaning the teeth and players of the *saranai*, a wooden wind instrument), *Jogi* (mendicants), *Harijan* (previously divided into *Dhed/Vankar*, weavers, and *Bhungi*, sweepers)

---

between different members of the same caste ensure that shared caste identity does not necessarily guarantee shared social and economic standing locally.

15 As an extreme example, the wealthy goldsmith who works with prestigious metals has little in common with the cobbler who works with polluting substances like leather.

16 Tambs-Lyche's doctoral dissertation (1992) discusses this issue extensively and is recommended to those interested in the social, cultural and religious composition of Saurashtra.

17 The term *Darbar* is used in Saurashtra to refer to the ruling, land-owning élite, who in Jalia were *Rajputs* rather than *Kathis*.

18 The *Kolis* are often considered to have been the ancient rulers of Saurashtra, although evidence of their hegemony has long vanished (cf. Copland 1982: 4). In Jalia many *Kolis* used to be servants to the *Darbar* élite. Today they are poor and work mainly as agricultural labourers.

Questions of Dress in a Gujarati Village

A high degree of occupational specialisation persists in the village today, with many older and some young men continuing to pursue their caste professions. Of the crafts cited above, only weaving is entirely extinct, although pottery is unlikely to endure into the next century. But the existence of artisans continuing to ply their 'traditional crafts' cannot mask the fact that rural Saurashtra has undergone major economic and political changes since independence, and that these changes have greatly altered the lived experience of individuals and groups in the village and region.

While the abolition of princely rule formally dissolved the political authority of the ruling *Darbar* princes and their families, it was post-independence land reforms which most radically altered the economic power-structure of the peninsula. In particular, the transference of full ownership rights from the previous owner to the tiller of the soil in the early 1950s resulted in the emergence and expansion of a new class of land-owning peasants, many of whom had previously been tenants at will in what was essentially a feudal régime.[19] These peasant castes benefited not only from their new ownership rights, but also from government schemes for irrigation and for the availability of credit facilities, improved seeds and fertilisers. Such measures, combined with the substantial lowering of rural taxes, opened up new opportunities for the small-scale cultivator throughout the peninsula.

In Jalia, the main groups to benefit from these changes were the *Kanbis* and the *Kharaks*. Both of these castes were numerically strong in the village and had long farmed much of the surrounding land. Today most *Kanbi* and *Kharak* households own at least a small landholding and some have fairly substantial farms. But whereas the *Kharaks* have adhered almost unanimously to their role as agriculturalists and milk-producers, the *Kanbis* have diversified their interests and re-invested much of their new wealth in the prosperous industry of diamond-cutting. This industry was developing and expanding in Surat and Bombay in the 1950s and '60s. At that time, many *Kanbi* families of Jalia, utilizing their extensive kinship networks, would send their sons to stay with relatives in Surat and to take up apprenticeships in the craft. Soon the trade was established in Larabad itself, and by the mid-1980s *Kanbi* entrepreneurs were setting up diamond-cutting units in rural areas. Cutting and polishing diamonds was not only better paid than

---

19 In much of the peninsula tenants were entirely at the mercy of their landlords, losing a high proportion of their crops in taxes which were paid in kind. However, Larabad state was unusually progressive in introducing the cash payment of taxes in the late nineteenth century. These taxes were assessed by officials of the state and were therefore more regulated than in many other parts of Kathiawad.

agricultural labour but also provided an alternative resource in times of scarcity. Indeed it was during the drought of 1985–8 that eleven such diamond-cutting workshops were established in Jalia. Of these, ten were owned by *Kanbis*, who mainly employed their own caste members.[20] So today most *Kanbi* households in the village have one or two sons employed in diamond-cutting while the rest of the family works in the fields, thereby providing a dual source of income.

Like the *Kanbis* of central Gujarat, described by Pocock (1972), the *Kanbis* of Saurashtra have accompanied their economic upliftment with efforts to upgrade their social standing.[21] In Jalia, new wealth has been invested in prestigious concrete houses, built in an area known as 'the plot'. Previously outside the village boundaries, the plot now contains some of the most modern and luxurious housing of the village and is reserved almost exclusively for *Kanbis*. Members of the caste have also begun to adopt high status values in food, dress and other social customs. In so doing they distance themselves increasingly from other farming communities with whom they used to share common traits. Changes in dress have been important in this differentiation process and are discussed in a later chapter.

Other groups which have experienced radical changes since independence are those who were previously engaged by the *Darbars* as servants (mainly classified as *Harijans*). The term *Harijan* (people of God) was popularised by Gandhi to refer to those groups whom other castes considered highly polluting. In Jalia, the term applies technically to both sweepers

20 This is true even in Surat where, according to a survey carried out in 1987, 59 per cent of diamond factories are managed by *Kanbi Patels* who also make up 70 per cent of the labour force. The report also stresses that 80 per cent of the workforce claim to have found employment through 'personal ties'. The rapid expansion of the industry in Surat, which grew from employing 500 people in 1962 to an estimated 40,000 in 1987, is attributed partly to the fact that India imports low-quality rough diamonds that European countries reject; its cheap but highly skilled labour force then cuts and polishes them to 'export-quality' standards. Expansion is also aided by the rising demand for diamonds in Belgium, Japan, the United States, Hong Kong and the Middle East (cf. Kashyap and Tiwari 1987).

21 Pocock's famous work *Kanbi and Patidar* (1972) shows how certain sections of the *Leva Kanbi* caste in central Gujarat rose to positions of importance through their role as tax officials under the British and Baroda authorities. Such '*Patidar*' families accompanied this improved economic position with an upgrading of their social customs to such an extent that, in certain contexts, *Patidars* now consider themselves a separate caste in their own right. But, as Pocock shows, the difference between *Kanbis* and *Patidars* is one of degree as more and more of the former try to define themselves as the latter (cf. Pocock 1972). The prestigious name of *Patidar* was never used by the *Leva Kanbis* of Jalia, who regarded the *Patidars* of central Gujarat as 'higher' than themselves in status. None the less, the *Kanbis* of Jalia, and indeed of Saurashtra more generally, were clearly an upwardly mobile group, as was evident from their successful attempts to improve their economic and social position.

('*Bhungis*') and ex-weavers (*Vankars*). But in practice only the latter have been accepted under the new name. Despite the official abolition of untouchability in 1955, fear of being polluted by the touch of a '*Bhungi*' persists in the village even today. Ex-weavers, on the other hand, occupy a more ambiguous position. While they are still considered ritually impure, some have made good use of government support both in education and employment and now hold relatively prestigious white-collar jobs which are reserved for *Harijans* in the city of Larabad. But if these jobs, combined with the money they have generated, have made these *Harijans* slightly more respected in the village, they have also made them more resented. Leaving aside the prejudice of other groups, they have considerably improved their standard of living and have a fairly comfortable life-style compared to the few sweeper families, whom they shun as ritually impure.[22]

In general, there is a discrepancy between the educational standards and occupations of different generations within the same caste. Among wealthy families education for boys is usually admired, and the younger generations are more literate than their parents. Female education remains poor and is rarely pursued beyond the level of minimal literacy except by a few high-caste families (usually *Vaniyas* or *Brahmans*). Some castes, like the *Bharwads* and *Kharaks*, have shown almost no interest in educating their girls and very little in educating their boys. Education and wealth are two important factors that combine with ideas of ritual purity to effect notions of hierarchy in the village.

Clothing and identity

This outline of the social structure of the village provides a background for understanding the relationship between clothing and identity at a local level. There can be no doubt that clothing has been important in establishing, maintaining and altering the image of different social groups in the area. Indeed it is often said that in the past each caste had its own distinctive form of dress that was easily recognisable by others. Clearly throughout Gujarat and neighbouring Rajasthan there was more social differentiation in dress than in many other parts of India.[23] Yet rather than assume that there was once an age when time stood still and the ethnographer could sketch out clear-cut definitions of who was who, it is also worth recognising that there has always been some flexibility in the system. Even the

---

22 For an account of attitudes to untouchability in rural Gujarat, see I. Desai 1976.
23 E.g., in Madya Pradesh particular patterns and styles of dress were more often related to region than to caste (cf. Chishti and Sanyal 1989, 20).

notion of regional styles cannot be taken as a watertight category since there were always factors to challenge the boundary between the clothing of one region and another. First, most villages were never self-sufficient, and relied on trading contacts with other villages or towns in order to fulfil basic needs like clothing. In particular, the houses and dowry chests of Saurashtran village élites were often stocked with luxury items from far afield, such as Chinese silks and Venetian beads. Secondly, even where villagers produced most of their own clothes, this did not prevent an influx of new designs entering the village through the trousseaux of new wives, who by definition came from outside their husbands' villages. This must have led to networks of designs and ideas being exchanged between villages and regions even in the relatively peaceful period after Walker's settlement of boundary rights in the nineteenth century. It is likely that in earlier times, when the peoples of Saurashtra were frequently in battle and retreat, demographic mobility and, with it, the circulation and possible interaction of local styles must have been important features of everyday life.

While there was little to prevent the horizontal spread of designs from one village and one region to another, there was also little to prevent the vertical spread of designs between different castes within a single village. Unless wealthy élites imposed sartorial restrictions[24] on those socially beneath them, they could not prevent the latter from adopting imitations of élite forms of dress. So although the notion of caste-specific dress remains important in Jalia today, it is questionable whether clothing ever formed the clear-cut system of identification that people often imply. Those women who embroidered their own clothes, for example, tended to share the same design sources and often ended up wearing the same motifs and colours as members of other castes. In Jalia this was clear in the *Kanbi* and *Kharak* case where the women of both castes embroidered identical motifs, colours and stitches on to their skirts. These designs were also shared by those poor women who could afford the time and money to embroider. Where the embroidery was successfully executed, a low-caste woman could end up looking very similar to a wealthy peasant. This could be permanent if the women concerned had the time and money to maintain such standards, or temporary, as with *Vaghri* women who are said to have adopted elaborate disguises that enabled them to mingle with the wealthy on festive occasions and so pocket their

---

24   There are cases recorded of high-caste men actively preventing low-caste people from wearing certain types of clothes (cf. Hutton 1946: 74–5), but I did not hear of any such instances in contemporary Jalia.

jewellery.[25] In short, although dress is one of the means by which a caste defines itself, it is not necessarily a straightforward 'indicator' of caste. And while dress does to some extent 'indicate' regional identity, there is and always has been a certain blurring of local styles.[26]

Yet clothing has undoubtedly been important in defining different sectors of the rural population, often revealing both the wealth and occupation if not the actual caste of the wearer. For example, it can be asserted that in the early twentieth century probably all Hindu women in Jalia were wearing the regional style of Kathiawad.[27] This consisted of some form of skirt (stitched or wrapped) with a backless bodice (embroidered or plain) and half-sari. But while small details of decoration and jewellery may have revealed the finer distinctions of social status, broader differences were more clearly expressed through a hierarchy of fabric types (cf. Bayly 1986). The most prestigious and expensive materials worn by village women were silk and gold and silver brocades. Silk was not only considered a luxury material, but it was also the least permeable to pollution, giving it high ritual value (ibid.).[28] Wealthy, high-caste women wore long gathered silk skirts (chaniyos), often embroidered or with a decorative brocade border. These skirts were sometimes made from enormous quantities of cloth, depending partly on the financial circumstances of the families concerned.[29] With her

---

25 Recorded by the Deputy Inspector General of Police in his catalogue of 'Criminal Classes', this description of *Vaghri* behaviour may be somewhat biased, although the full account is sufficiently detailed to be convincing (cf. Kennedy 1908: 160–5). Furthermore, there are numerous other accounts of people dressing up in other people's clothes, including tales of *Dhobis* (washermen) hiring out those of their wealthy clients, without the knowledge of the latter (cf. Russell 1916).

26 Shelagh Weir, when collecting material for a museum exhibition and book entitled *Palestinian Costume* (1989), found that she had to reject her initial hypothesis about well-defined regional styles in favour of a more dynamic approach which corresponded to the constantly changing reality of Palestinian dress. She defined her change of emphasis as a shift away from the 'museum anthropologists' approach (Weir 1989: 17–20).

27 This has much in common with the styles worn in Rajasthan and mainland Gujarat and can therefore be defined more broadly as the regional style of western India.

28 The ritual value and the social value of silk were of course complementary. The fabric was available to those who could afford it, who were generally the wealthier members of a caste. Johnson records how in the 1860s, the *Vaniya* women who lived east of the Sabarmati river in Ahmedabad wore silk, whereas those west of it wore cotton and were looked down on by the others (Johnson 1863, vol. 1: 43). This is another example of how members of the same social group sometimes dressed differently.

29 Crooke describes a skirt made from 75 feet of cloth, worn by women in Kutch (Crooke 1906: 159). In general it was chiefly the women and men of ruling *Rajput* clans who expressed their status through the quantity of cloth used in their skirts and turbans. A turban worn by one of the Roa of Kutch's ministers apparently weighed 15 lb. (Postans 1838: 35).

Fig. 5.1 A Kathiawadi princess (c. 1912). She wears a hand-embroidered bodice (*kapdu*) and a full silk or satin skirt (*chaniyo*) with an embroidered border. Her half-sari (*sadlo*) is worn in the Gujarati style with the end of the cloth drawn over her head from behind and falling forwards over her right shoulder and the front of her body. It is made from fine material. This is the type of dress worn by women of the local élite in the early 20th century. Private collection.

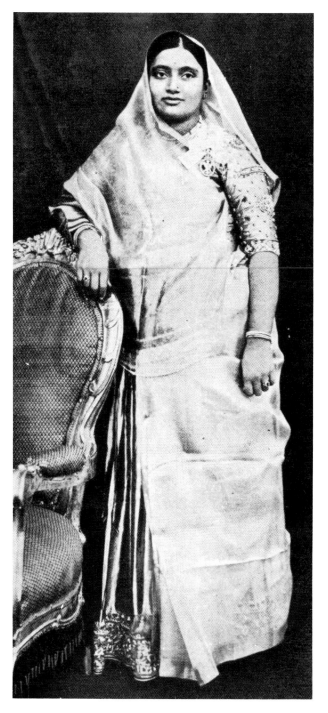

skirt, a woman would wear a backless silk and brocade bodice (*kapdu*), embroidered by herself or a professional, and a long half-sari (*sadlo*) of fine textured cloth. Today, village women rarely wear silk, but high-caste women have maintained their preference for fine textures and now wear full-length synthetic saris in a variety of thin materials with blouses (*cholis*) and petticoats (*ghaghris*) underneath. They have entirely rejected their old bodices, which they now regard as embarrassing and immodest owing to the complete exposure of the back. A few unmarried educated girls in this group now wear the *shalwar kamiz*.

Next in the hierarchy of fabric types was the embroidered cotton worn chiefly by the farming communities. This consisted of a brightly coloured and heavily embroidered *khadi* skirt (*ghaghro*), worn with an embroidered bodice (*kapdu*) and a dyed or printed cotton half-sari (*sadlo*). This embroidery was done by village women themselves, using silk threads and mirror inserts which made thick rough red *khadi* look luxuriant and glowing.[30] Even so, high-caste women were often disparaging about the clothes of the cultivators, which they thought thick and heavy, thereby indicating the coarseness and crudeness of their wearers (cf. Parmar 1969: 44). Even today, they often refer to those who wear embroidered *khadi* as 'the thick-wearing castes' (*jada lok varan*). *Jada* (thickness) was a metaphor for lack of refinement. Even the bread eaten by farmers was criticised for being *jada jada* (extremely thick). But the peasants themselves (*Kanbis* and *Kharaks*) were, till recently, proud of their skirts partly *because* of their *jada* quality. The denser and heavier the embroidery, the more they valued the cloth. Some old women in Jalia still extol the strength of thick embroidered *khadi*, which can be worn for farmwork and does not disintegrate quickly or look faded and old like poor women's cloth. Still today, if embroidery is carelessly executed or sparse, it invites comparison to 'lower' castes. Hence a *Kharak* woman rebukes her daughter: 'Why is your embroidery so patchy and bare? Are you a *Vaghri* girl?' And another tells her child she will look like a *Koli* if she does not embroider neatly and closely. Thus, good embroidery was a means by which the wealthy cultivators differentiated their appearance from that of poorer castes. As Schneider has suggested in the Greek context, embroidery can be an efficient means of building up the layers which separate the wealthy peasantry from the proletariat (Schneider

---

30 It has been suggested that mirror-work embroidery developed as an attempt to imitate the precious jewels and metallic threads used by the ruling élite in past centuries (Gross and Fontana 1981: 1). Writing of the Middle Eastern context, Wace also suggests that peasant embroidery developed as a substitute for luxurious and precious silks (in Schneider 1980).

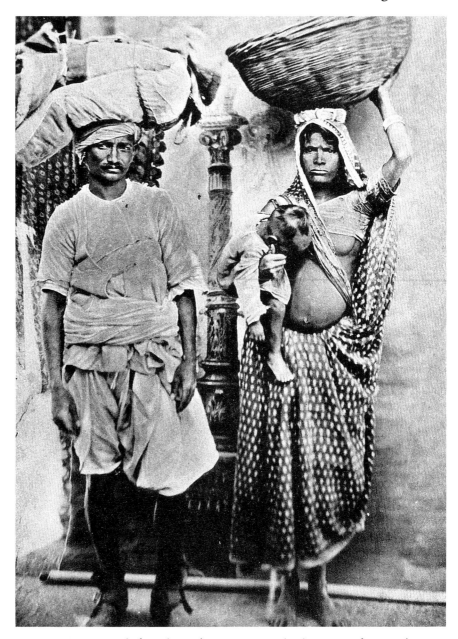

Fig. 5.2 A Gujarati couple from the *Vaghri* caste (1920). Like the princess (fig. 5.1), the *Vaghri* woman also wears a bodice, skirt and half-sari, but her clothes are not silken and are considerably more skimpy, revealing large portions of flesh. The man is wearing a short *angarkha* and *dhoti* with a cummerbund and small turban. Reproduced from Enthoven's *The Tribes and Castes of Bombay*, vol. 3. Courtesy of SOAS.

1980: 100). Today most *Kharak* women in Jalia continue to wear embroidery while *Kanbi* women have converted to synthetic saris as part of their quest for upward mobility.

Most artisans and labourers were never able to compete with the embroidery of the cultivators owing to lack of both time to embroider and money for silk threads. None the less it seems that many, like the *Kolis*, wore more sparsely embroidered skirts and bodices while others made do with plainer cotton clothes for daily wear. Today the young women from these castes have mostly converted to mill-made saris or half-saris which they wear with blouses and petticoats. These are not only cheap and easy to maintain, but also allow a woman to wear bright and decorative cloth without having to spend time embroidering. Cheap cotton or synthetic saris provide such women with a means of looking both colourful and modern, something which was probably a struggle for many in the past.

The *Bharwads* (shepherds), who are divided into the two divisions of *Motabhai* (big brother) and *Nanabhai* (little brother),[31] are generally considered the most *deshi* (local, and by implication here, backward) people in the village. Early in the twentieth century their dress seems to have consisted mainly of coarse woollen garments, woven by local *Harijans*. These consisted of a long unstitched black or red woollen waist-cloth (*jimi*) with a tie-dyed black woollen veil (*dhablo*).[32] Like the women of other castes, they embroidered their own bodices. Today *Bharwad* women no longer wear predominantly woollen clothes, but they have retained the distinctive colours and styles of their caste. Specialist shops in Larabad city stock machine-made polyester and cotton versions of shepherd dress designed especially for the *Bharwads* and *Rabaris* (another local pastoralist group). Even the embroidered bodice is now available in polyester, embroidered by machine using synthetic gold threads and brocades. The *Bharwads* are the only caste in the village where young women continue to wear open-backed bodices without embarrassment. Their style of dress is highly

---

31 Members of *Motabhai* and *Nanabhai* divisions describe their relationship by the phrase, 'bread we can exchange, but daughters we cannot'. They also refer to themselves as 'thick cloth' (*jada pachedi*) and 'thin cloth' (*nana pachedi*). Some attribute these phrases to the fact that *Motabhai* women used to wear thicker woollen wraps than *Nanabhai* women. The most popular tale of the origin of the two divisions runs as follows: Lord Krishna told two shepherd brothers to take their flocks in different directions. The elder went one way and married a *Bharwad* while the younger went the other way and married a *Koli*. This was polluting, so from that day the descendants of the elder brother (literally *mota bhai*) were ritually higher than the descendants of the younger (*nana bhai*).

32 *Motabhai* women wore veils with yellow dots, whereas *Nanabhai* women wore veils with red dots.

Fig. 5.3 The Prince of Panna, wearing a long *angarkha* with tight *pyjamas*, an outfit worn by some élite village men at the beginning of the 20th century. Private collection.

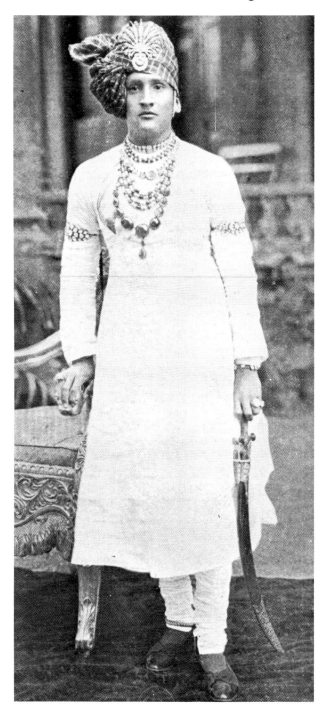

distinctive in the village, though very similar to the dress of other shepherd groups in the district.

Finally, poor and previously outcaste communities seem to have made do with whatever combinations of clothes they could get. If they performed tasks or acted as servants for wealthy families in the village, they were sometimes given clothes by the latter and therefore wore a variety of styles. One old *Bhungi* (sweeper) woman, whose task was to prepare the bodies of the dead for the funeral pyre, told me that she used sometimes to wear the clothes of the deceased, which other people considered highly polluting. The *Vankars* (weavers), on the other hand, would sometimes receive an item of clothing as payment for weaving cloth for other castes. Enthoven was surprised to find that 'a well-to-do *Dhed*[33] woman wears a bodice equalling in the fineness and price of those worn by high caste Hindus', although the bulk of the caste were 'ill-clad' (Enthoven 1920, vol. 1: 323). Similar observations on the diversity of a poor person's clothes have also been made by the Saurashtran folklorist, Khodidasbhai Parmar. He remembers seeing in his childhood an extravagant wedding procession where a richly-clad *Darbar* man flung his clothes at a *Bhungi* drummer at the end of the celebration. The poor sweeper went about dressed like a wealthy *Darbar* until the clothes fell apart. Such incidents suggest that the relationship between clothing and caste was never straightforward, although in most cases there was a clear correlation between the fineness of the fabric and the status of the wearer.

Women's dress was not only a matter of expressing wealth and social status, but also a means of beautification. The conjunction of these three aspects of adornment was most clearly expressed in a woman's jewellery, which was as lavish as her family could afford or would allow. The principal items worn by a married woman were ivory bangles, gold or silver necklaces, a gold nose-ring, a variety of gold or silver earrings, heavy silver anklets and silver toe-rings. These have changed considerably in recent years and are becoming lighter and finer. According to Parmar, caste identity used to be expressed more clearly in jewellery than in dress (Parmar 1969: 47). Nowadays differences in jewellery are related more to differences in wealth than to caste status, but jewellery remains a vital aspect both of a woman's attire and of her property.

Men's dress was and continues to be much less varied than that of women. By the early twentieth century *Vaniya*, *Brahman* and some *Soni* men were wearing long or short coats or waistcoats with shirts and finely

---

33 The *Vankars* are members of the *Dhed* who have changed their name.

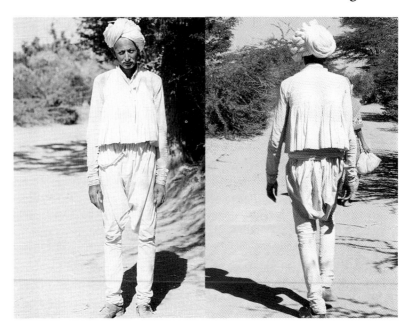

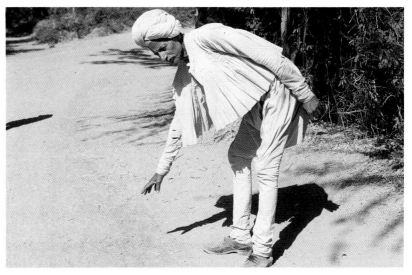

Fig. 5.4 A farmer of the *Koli* caste (1989), wearing the white smock (*kediyun*), pantaloon (*chorni*) and turban combination, worn by most Kathiawadi men earlier this century. It is noticible that Gandhi's so called 'Kathiawadi peasant dress' bore more resemblance to the long *angarkha* worn principally by the élite than to the short *kediyun* worn by many Kathiawadi peasants.

textured *dhotis*, a style which associated them more with urban than rural fashion. Many had replaced their turbans with simple black caps and some wore Gandhi caps during the 1920s and '30s. Temple portraits of important men reveal an intermingling of individualist and caste styles as new types of tailored jacket combine with more distinctive forms of local dress. However, most village men from peasant and artisan groups wore the distinctive regional style of *chorni* (pantaloons tight from the knee down) and *kediyun* (smock top with multiple gathers) (see fig. 5.4) with a turban, waist-cloth, silver bangles, gold earrings and heavy farmer's shoes. Writing of Gujarati men's dress in 1884, the author of the *Gazetteer of the Bombay Presidency* argued: 'Higher in the scale coarse hand made cloth changes to calico ... and the turban and waist-sash become more voluminous and of better material and richer colour' (vol. 8: 171).

Today the *kediyun*, *chorni* and turban combination is still seen as typical Kathiawadi dress although many Kathiawadi men no longer wear it. Some argue that the cut of the garments used to reveal a man's caste, but the evidence is unclear since the older-generation tailors in the village were unable to come up with more than a few variations and could not entirely agree on which cut was worn by which caste. Furthermore, men used different quantities of cloth according to what they could afford and to whether the clothes were to be worn every day or at festivals. One distinctive feature of *Darbar* dress seems to have been the length and width of the sleeves of the upper garment which, when not the *kediyun*, was a long coat or shirt. Since those in service often adopted features of their masters' dress, there were apparently some barbers and tailors who dressed similarly.

At the turn of the century, the *Bharwads* were probably the only village men who worked out of doors but who did not necessarily wear the *kediyun* and *chorni*. Like their women, *Bharwad* men seem to have worn three woollen blankets, one wound around the waist, another round the head and a third round the shoulders (Enthoven 1920: 119, J. Jain 1980: 67).[34] Today many *Bharwad* men wear the cotton *kediyun* with a *chorni* or *dhoti*, and they continue to wear jewellery. Most young men of all other castes have abandoned their jewellery and now wear European-style trousers with fitted shirts and shoes, sandals or flipflops. A few high-caste men change into more Indian styles on entering the house, but this is no longer considered obligatory. With the exception of the *Bharwads* (shepherds), all communities in the village have accepted the wearing of European dress by young men and no longer see it as controversial. The only feature which

---

34   According to Khodidasbhai Parmar, this was the dress mainly of *Motabhai Bharwads*.

continues to distinguish members of high castes today is the sacred thread, a sign of initiation into Vedic education; it is worn under a man's upper garments but is usually partly visible beneath his shirt.

It was a man's headwear which in the past was the most distinctive feature of his caste, region and rank. *Darbar* men wore a highly distinctive style of turban, built high and often concealing a protective brass head-plate. Most young farming men seem to have tied coloured turbans or head-wraps,[35] which in old age they replaced with white ones. But today it is impossible to establish a catalogue of earlier turban types, since many men have abandoned the turban altogether. Even as early as 1909 the author of the *Imperial Gazetteer* was forced to admit that it had not been possible to determine a person's identity from his 'costume' for fifty years and that 'even types of *pugris* [turbans]' were 'losing their significance' (1909: 49). Whether it was ever possible, or whether turban differences were as ambiguous as other clothing differences, remains unclear. But it is important to remember that clothes were only one aspect of a man's appearance, which included different styles of facial hair, jewellery, objects carried[36] and general deportment, all of which no doubt combined more or less to establish a man's identity in the eyes of a local onlooker.

A brief examination of clothing change in Jalia reveals that the jewellery and dress of both men and women have undergone considerable changes since the beginning of the century. Some men attribute this to the political and economic changes that have been disrupting the old caste-dominated hierarchy since independence. Caste differences, they argue, were previously more apparent, whereas 'nowadays anything goes'. But although this helps to explain the apparent breakdown of the social differentiation of clothing traditions, it does not explain the diverse directions that developments in men's and women's clothes have taken. For whereas most Jalia men, except for the *Bharwads* and the older generation of cultivators, have changed from local Indian styles to European styles, all Jalia women have either retained local styles or adopted alternative Indian styles. Not a single girl past the age of puberty wears European dress.

These differences cannot be attributed either to economic factors or to the differential availability of European styles for men and women, for in the nearby city of Larabad both dresses and skirts are sold at a variety of prices, from the cheap to the expensive. Jalia women buy these for their

---

35 Some farming children, both male and female, used to wear embroidered headscarves and caps, a custom which has long died out in Jalia.
36 Shepherds, for example, are rarely seen without their staffs and *Darbars* often used to walk about with their weapons over their shoulders.

children, but never for themselves. Since all Jalia families prefer to make major purchases of clothing in the city rather than the village, where prices are higher and the selection more limited, it cannot be argued that women do not have access to European styles. And if there are more shopkeepers stocking European men's styles than women's, that is because there is much more demand for the former than the latter. Despite the easy availability of new alternatives, women have been relatively slow to change their dress. This is true not only for Jalia but for most of India, where it is still extremely rare to see married women in European dress except among a fragment of the educated urban élite. The question of why Indian women in general have retained such a powerful allegiance to Indian styles is too vast an issue to tackle here. Rather, what follows is an exploration of how women's sartorial conversatism is lived out at a local level and how certain factors have served to constrain the clothing choices of Jalia women without affecting their men's choices in the equivalent way.

Clothing and the female life-cycle
Like most Indian women in rural areas, Jalia women are expected to abide by certain sartorial expectations which accord with their position in the life-cycle and which help to define not only their role within the family, but also their sense of gender awareness. While women of different caste backgrounds do not, as we have seen, share identical clothing, they none the less share certain ideas about how a woman should look in childhood, adolescence, married life, widowhood and old age. As Fruzzetti has shown in the Bengali context, a woman's entry into different states is marked by a change of clothing and adornment (cf. Fruzzetti 1982). The idea that a woman's position in the family should be clearly delineated through her dress remains important in Jalia today.

Early childhood. Childhood is the time when gender roles are least clearly delineated – also, interestingly, the only time when girls wear ready-made European-style clothes. In early childhood clothing is often minimal and not necessarily gender-specific; young girls are found wearing anything from skirts and dresses to shorts and vests like their brothers. Girls and boys play freely together and there is little to distinguish between them except for the ring in the girl's left nostril.[37] Noses and ears are pierced

---

37 The importance of the nose-ring (*nath*) was brought home to me by my being sometimes mistaken for a man without it, despite having long hair and women's clothes. More than once I was asked: 'How can people tell if you are a man or a woman if you do not wear a *nath*?' That the nose-ring should have become a repository of female identity is surprising considering that it does not

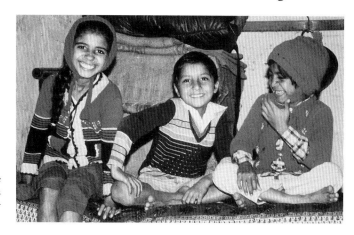

Fig. 5.5 Children playing in the author's room (1989). At this age both boys and girls wear European styles of dress.

by itinerant *Vaghris* who perform this task on children as young as one or two years old. Earlier in the twentieth century young boys also had their ears pierced and some wore bangles, but these customs have ceased among most castes. Today it is mainly girls who wear jewellery.

Tattooing is also performed by *Vaghris* and till recently most girls had a small round tattoo mark on their chin, known as *ladva* (sweet), and a cross on their left cheek, known as *makhi* (fly). Rows of tattoos were added later in childhood all the way up the lower arms, legs and neck, although these are increasingly rare for children nowadays since most groups now see them as a sign of backwardness.

Late childhood and adolescence. The comparatively asexual clothing of childhood is usually replaced by more specifically feminine clothing around the age of ten or eleven. This involves increased covering of the body. It is the time when girls are taught strict body awareness and responsibility in preparation for the more elaborate sense of covering which they must develop after marriage. Usually clothing consists of a light full-length skirt (*ghaghri*)[38] and a blouse. Those who work outside in the fields usually adopt a half-sari (*sadlo*) at this time and learn to keep their heads covered with the cloth. Everyday clothes are supposed to be plain and should not

---

appear to be an ancient Hindu ornament and features neither in Sanskrit literature nor in ancient sculpture (Altekar 1962). Altekar thinks that Hindus adopted the ornament from Muslims, while Crooke describes it as a high-caste Hindu ornament (Crooke 1906). These may both be correct, since it was mainly high-caste Hindus who adopted features of 'Muslim' dress.

38 The term *ghaghri* is used to refer to a skirt of thin cloth, and *ghaghro* to one of thick cloth.

attract unnecessary attention since this is thought dangerous and threatening to an unmarried girl. Girls of this age are expected to withdraw from the public eye as much as possible and to stick largely to female company. Covering the head signifies the beginning of awareness of the more general need to keep out of sight and out of sound. It affects not only the appearance of girls, but also their behaviour and deportment. Young girls new to the veil find it difficult to keep on their heads and have to learn to manipulate it; it becomes like an extension of their bodies and they have to restrain their movements to accommodate its requirements. Suddenly they find it difficult to run about the village and play, and this is thought inappropriate for anyone wearing a veil. Girls from wealthy families who do not work outside the home are encouraged to stay inside as much as possible. For them, the *sadlo* is not thought necessary before marriage, and such girls usually wear a long 'maxi' (like a nightdress) at home during the day.[39]

Plastic bangles, cheap earrings, anklets and nose-rings are worn before the engagement and wedding ceremonies, when more valuable jewellery is presented to the bride by both her parents and her in-laws. The marriage age for girls varies from six in some *Bharwad* families to the early twenties in high-caste groups. Most girls marry after puberty and do not live with their husbands before their middle to late teens.

Wife and mother. The movement of a young woman from her parental home to her conjugal home after marriage is accompanied by the greatest of the changes in her lifestyle and clothes. For the first time she becomes the owner of a large selection of clothing and valuable jewellery. Before this, few girls have more than three or four outfits, whereas they may own as many as twenty-five or even thirty-five when they move into their conjugal homes. This event is marked by a sending away ceremony (*anu*) when clothes and other trousseau items, given to the bride by her parents, are displayed in the courtyard of the house and viewed by friends and neighbours – an occasion on which the new wife herself remains inside the house and is dressed in green clothes by her brother's wife,[40] green being

39   Where girls are educated, they usually adopt the school uniform, which is loosely defined as a white blouse and green skirt. Many families are reluctant to educate their daughters beyond primary school, not only because they think further education unnecessary but also because they fear the public attention their daughters might attract wearing such skimpy clothes.

40   The version of the ceremony described here is practised only when there is a gap between a girl's marriage and when she begins conjugal life. This was common in the past when the age of marriage was much younger, but today most high-caste families do not marry their daughters until they have reached their late teens, in which case a woman usually joins her husband's family immediately after the marriage ceremony.

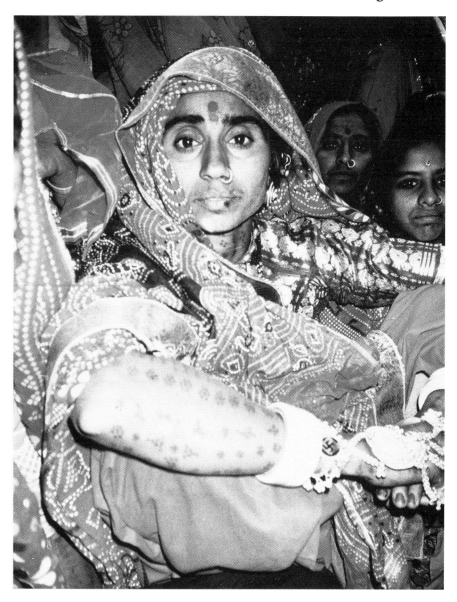

Fig. 5.6 A *Bharvad* woman in festive dress (1989). She wears the symbols of *saubhagya*, including the ivory bangles (*boloya*) and lower and upper earrings (*porkhani* and *vedla*) which most farming women used to wear. A black beaded *mangalsutra* is just visible. The studded gold collar (*daniyu*) above is today a distinctive *Bharvad* ornament. The hand and foot ornaments are worn only for special occasions. As a young married woman she wears a red waist-cloth (*jimi*) and bright red and green veil with a gold border as opposed to the black clothes worn by older women of the caste.

associated with fertility in ritual contexts and a favourite colour with young girls. Her hair is parted and vermilion is smeared in the parting; vermilion is considered the most important symbol of *saubhagya* (the auspicious state of having a living husband) and the girl will regularly apply it to her own parting in her new home. The young wife also wears whatever jewellery her in-laws offer her at this time, usually consisting of ivory bangles, a necklace, toe-rings and new ear ornaments. After tearful farewells with the women of her family, the young wife's *sadlo* is pulled well over her face and upper body and she is led, fully veiled, out of the house and taken to her conjugal village by a party of in-laws.

When a girl remains at her parental home in the time between marriage and joining her husband, she rarely wears the symbols of married life except perhaps for festive occasions. Once in her conjugal home, however, she is expected to demonstrate her married status through her jewellery and clothes. She is meant to wear bright colours[41] to differentiate her from the other women in the house and she will put on the ivory bangles, silver toe-rings, *mangulsutra* (black and gold necklace)[42] and vermilion in the parting that are only worn by women whose husbands are alive.[43] These visual marks of marital status are associated with beauty, joy, prosperity and the approbation of society. Becoming a wife, therefore, entitles a woman to be richly and beautifully adorned, but it is an entitlement dependent on her husband's existence. All the symbols of *saubhagya* are detachable, and in the event of her husband's death a woman loses her entitlement to wear them. The widow's bangles are smashed and she is expected to abandon her jewellery.

Although young married life is the time when a woman wears her brightest and most elaborate clothes, it is also when she must be most heavily concealed beneath her veil. The custom of veiling and the ideology

41 Luschinsky describes a custom in Senapur in Uttar Pradesh where young wives dip their new saris in washable dye before wearing them for the first time: the colour runs out with a few washes, after which their saris look like those worn by other women in the village (Luschinsky 1962: 348). Fruzzetti, on the other hand, describes how all married women wear saris with red borders as opposed to the plain saris of widowhood (Fruzzetti 1982: 104). Clearly the distinct form which the new wife's clothes take is open to considerable variation according to region and wealth, but the idea that the new married woman should be distinctive and wear colourful clothes seems common throughout much of India.

42 This particular style of necklace used to be worn only by high-caste women but is now popular among the women of many different castes.

43 The forehead spangle (*bindi*) was also a symbol of *saubhagya* but today it is worn throughout India by girls of any age and from any religious group.

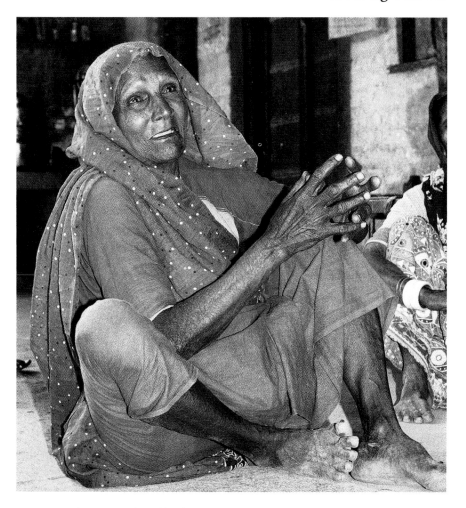

Fig. 5.7 An old woman of the *kharak*, caste, 1989. Being old, she no longer wears embroidery, and as a widow has abandoned her jewellery. To the right of the photograph it is possible to see the edge of an embroidered *ghaghro* and ivory bangle belonging to a married *kharak* woman.

of femininity associated with it have had a profound influence on the development of women's dress and is discussed below.

Old age. There is no category equivalent to the Western idea of middle age. Jalia women call themselves old as soon as their first *vau* (daughter-in-law) comes to live in their house. There are no fixed rules about how the *sasu* (mother-in-law) should dress, but it is thought no longer appropriate for her to dress up in bright and alluring clothing, which is the privilege of her new *vau*. Most women therefore tone down their colours at this stage and some reduce their number of earrings, either handing them on to their daughters or the new *vau*, or selling them for family funds. If they reach extreme maturity, as for example when a grandson's wife arrives in the house, they will usually wear entirely plain clothes without any pattern. It is only widows who are actually prohibited from wearing their ivory bangles, although some old women cease to wear them anyway.

How a woman dresses in relation to her position in the life-cycle is closely linked not so much to her biological development as to her social role, especially in relation to men. Men's dress, on the other hand, is not dependent on their relationship with women.[44] In the days when all farming men covered their heads, they usually replaced the coloured turbans they wore when young with white ones in old age. But this sartorial change was related to ideas of seniority and was entirely independent of marital status. Usually a man adopted a white turban when most of his hair had turned white. Thus while changes in female apparel are linked to gender relations, those in male apparel are independent of them.

The differential importance of clothes in the life-cycle of men and women reflects the different cultural constructions of male and female identity. Whereas a man's identity is established through birth into his father's lineage and remains consistent throughout his life, a woman's is established first at birth and then a second time at marriage when she becomes a member of her husband's lineage and moves to his village. She therefore has a dual identity as daughter of her father's lineage and wife of her husband's (cf. Fruzzetti 1982). Thus while for men the transition from son to husband is comparatively gentle, for women that from daughter to wife is drastic. Furthermore women can never play the two roles simultaneously. They are *either* daughters in their natal village *or* wives and later mothers in their marital village. This dual aspect of female identity is marked by veiling restrictions which apply to women whenever they are in their conjugal village but not in their natal village.

---

44 In her analysis of clothing prescriptions in Sanskrit texts, J. Leslie has argued that both male and female clothing prescriptions had a religious basis. Whereas a man's dress and facial marks indicated his class and sectarian allegiance, a woman's clothes and make-up indicated the living presence of her husband whom she worshipped as her personal god (Leslie 1993: 210). It is interesting that many of the ancient clothing prescriptions that Leslie cites still hold true for women in Jalia, but, with the exception of the sacred thread, they do not hold true for men, except perhaps on certain ceremonial occasions.

Veiling (ghunghut)

A married girl still living in her natal village may, as we have seen, cover her head with her *sadlo* but only in her conjugal village will she learn to pull the cloth forward, thereby obscuring her entire face. This custom, known as *ghunghut*, is a form of deference and respect performed by women largely to men.

The *ghunghut* system in Gujarat is similar to that described by Jacobson (1970) and C. Thompson (1981) in Madhya Pradesh. A woman is expected to cover her face, if not her entire upper body, in front of all men senior to her husband in her conjugal village. The obligation to veil is most rigorously felt in the presence of her father-in-law or her husband's elder brothers. It is extended to other senior males in the village through the belief that all men of the village are relatives (cf. Sharma 1978b).

A number of anthropologists have put forward explanations of the custom of veiling. Jacobson, following Murphey, interprets it as a distancing mechanism through which tensions in the joint family are reduced (cf. Jacobson 1970). Sharma extends this argument to show how veiling structures relations within the entire village, preventing married women from gaining access to all those with power. She points out that the veil does not make a woman unrecognisable so much as 'socially invisible', the point being that once veiled a woman is unable to participate in public debate (cf. Sharma 1978b). These observations have provided valuable insights into the functions of veiling in relation to the social structure of Indian society. The aim here, however, is to examine how the veil is used in Jalia in order to discuss the degree to which it discourages change in women's dress.

There is no simple dichotomy between being veiled and unveiled in Jalia. The cloth is in almost constant motion, being drawn, adjusted, withdrawn and redrawn in such a variety of ways that it seems almost like a part of the female body. And so long as a woman is in her marital village, she must move her veil with the same self-consciousness that she moves her body. It becomes in short an extension of the female space and a portable means of maintaining the possibility of shifting from the public to the private sphere at any moment. In Jalia only wealthy high-caste married women are actually secluded within their homes. Most women work out of doors where, as Sharma points out, the veil provides a means of limiting their social effectiveness without at the same time limiting their economic productivity (Sharma 1978b: 229).

In Jalia women refer to veiling as *laj kadvu* or *laj karvu* (lit. 'doing shame'). There are a number of different degrees to which *laj* can be per-

Questions of Dress in a Gujarati Village

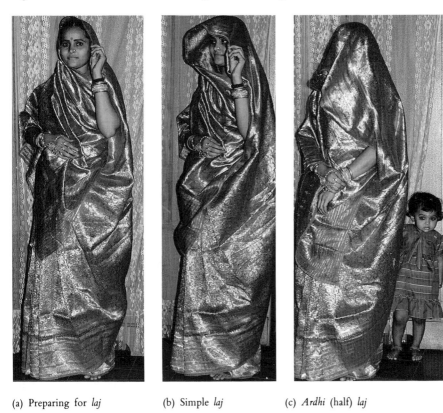

(a) Preparing for *laj*   (b) Simple *laj*   (c) *Ardhi* (half) *laj*

Fig. 5.8 A high-caste woman demonstrates different veiling (*laj*) positions, 1988.

formed. Simple *laj* consists of taking the veil by the hand and pulling it rapidly sideways across the face; this is the type of *laj* typically performed when women are out of doors in an apparently secluded spot, and a man unexpectedly walks past. It sometimes acts as an intermediary stage before going into a more complete form of *laj* if the person approaching is someone who must be avoided. In situations where women have to walk through the village or fetch water from the village well, they generally leave their veils hanging forward, covering only their face and neck so that they can see where they are walking. If carrying heavy loads, they sometimes keep one hand on the veil so that they can lift it slightly without allowing people to see in.

The term *ardhi laj* (lit. 'half shame') refers to the custom of drawing the veil over the face down to waist level, which is often performed in the presence of a senior relative within the home. Most refined women will never speak when they do this type of *laj*. Ideally they are expected to absent themselves completely if a senior man is about to enter the room;[45] they are usually given warning signals both by the man, who will make some deliberate noise, and by other women who will comment on his imminent approach. Once warned, a woman pulls her veil into the 'half shame' position and either turns her back on the approaching man or leaves the room, taking care not to face him even when veiled. Ideally he should never see her or hear her voice. In practice, however, there are often occasions when she cannot leave the room or courtyard because she is performing some task, and in this case she simply turns her back and quietly continues with it. In those families where women maintain partial seclusion, they also maintain strict rules of silence beneath their veils. Those *Darbar* women who can afford it keep the most rigorous form of *ghunghut* in the village. A *Darbar* woman, making tea for her husband and his friends, will leave it just outside the male quarters of the house where it will be collected and served by her husband. She avoids being seen, even though totally veiled. In the past such tasks would have been performed by servants, but the *Darbars*' declining wealth, combined with the unavailability of cheap labour, has forced *Darbar* women to have more contact with their men than in the past. In families and castes where women work outside the home, they are less strict about rules of silence and deference. Wives who have lived in their conjugal village for some time will often speak from beneath their veils, though taking care not to address the men they are meant to avoid.

The strictest form of *laj* observed in Jalia is referred to as *akhi laj* ('complete shame'). It involves pulling the veil forward at an angle so that it obscures even the arms, and its aim is to leave no part of the woman's body visible. Many informed me that all brides of the village used to maintain *akhi laj* throughout the marriage ceremony, although this custom is declining and is regarded as a sign of backwardness by some educated families who feel that the bride's face should be seen. After the marriage and the *anu* ceremony, most women do not often have to perform *akhi laj*. But those young women who live in seclusion are expected to be fully veiled on the rare occasions when they enter the public space of the village. At the Diwali festival, for example, young *Brahman* wives could be seen being led by other family members to visit their relations. They were totally veiled and resembled large bundles of expensive cloth, with only their toes and the tips of their fingers visible from beneath their saris.

---

45 *Vaniya* women are exceptional in being relatively unrestrained by veiling customs (cf. Tambs-Lyche 1992: 160).

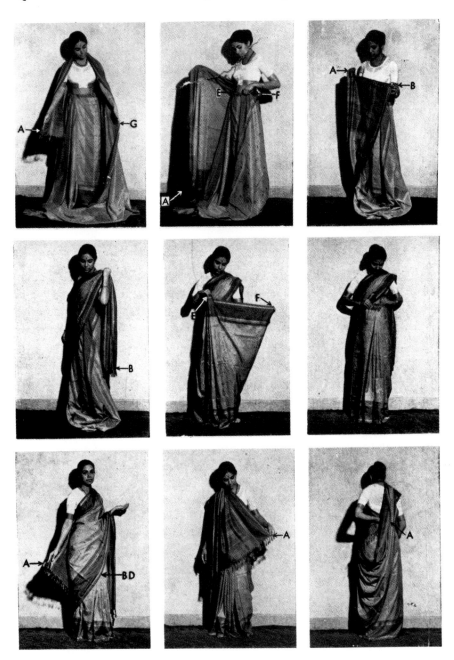

Fig. 5.9 Diagram illustrating different ways of tying the sari. Nos 1–7 demonstrate what Jalia women call the 'Bengali style' but which Dongerkery calls the 'Nivi' or 'National' style. Nos 8–9 demonstrate the Gujarati style where, instead of throwing the end of the cloth (*pallaw*) back over her left shoulder, the woman throws it forward over her right shoulder. Reproduced from Dongerkery's *The Indian Sari* 1960. Courtesy of the Ministry of Textiles, Government of India.

The degree to which different individuals and groups of women practise *laj* varies greatly, but few can afford to ignore the custom. Furthermore, women often blame the veil for their inability to wear other forms of dress. This first became apparent at Diwali time when I agreed to wear a sari for the day. Some *Brahman* women seemed in agreement that I should tie it in the so-called 'Bengali style', with the sari end thrown back over the shoulder, rather than forwards in the Gujarati style. This was not because they wished to mark me out as a foreigner but rather because they considered the Bengali style more fashionable and sophisticated. Some told me that they too wore the Bengali sari if they had to attend a wedding in some far-off place or if they ever went to Ahmedabad. But when asked why they never wore it in the village, they replied: 'How can we change our dress when we have to do *laj*?' and 'This is a village so *laj* is necessary'. The fact that the Bengali sari was thrown back rather than forward made it more difficult, they argued, to perform the type of *laj* expected of them in the village. The same explanation was given for why it was impossible for a woman to wear a *shalwar kamiz* after marriage, even if she had worn one before. Without a veil that could be pulled well over the face and body, the married woman appeared to be deprived of sartorial choice. The veil, then, seemed to provide the outer limit within which change in a married woman's dress could take place.

However, it is not enough to argue that the veil prevents change in women's dress in some deterministic way. Rather it is necessary to examine some of the reasons why women veil and why they do not seriously contemplate relinquishing the custom. This involves not only the behavioural aspect of the veil, but also the feelings and emotions associated with it. That veiling is associated with a sense of shame and modesty is evident from the fact that women use the word *laj* (shame) to refer to it. The latter is appropriate because the act of veiling is merely an expression of the female feeling of shame or embarrassment; more general feelings of shyness, modesty and shame are referred to as *sharum*. *Sharum* differs from *laj* in that it refers to the emotions themselves rather than the behavioural response to them, and therefore has a wider application and is used in all sorts of situations where people feel shy or embarrassed. A woman is expected to show more *sharum* than a man and failure to do so risks damaging the honour of herself, her family and her caste (cf. C. Thompson 1981).

It is tempting to argue that the difference between *laj* and *sharum* is expressed in the linguistic structure of the phrases associated with the terms. *Laj* is something that women 'do'; they are therefore considered the responsible agents of their own actions and if they fail to 'do' *laj*, then they are blamed for disobedience. *Sharum*, on the other hand, is never 'done', but is a feeling that comes to you or overcomes you. This is expressed in the phrase so frequently reiterated by women, *sharum lage che* (shame manifests itself). Being overcome by *sharum* is something that is supposed to occur to women in a variety of situations (cf. C. Thompson 1981). While response to it is learned, there is the idea that the feeling itself should be natural and intrinsic to all women – although some, it is recognised, have a more refined sense of it than others. While failure to perform *laj* is considered a disgrace, failure to feel *sharum* is actually thought unnatural or inhuman in the same way that failure to feel hunger or thirst is thought abnormal. In situations where I had visited another village alone or spoken to men in the village, I was frequently asked by women: 'Does not shame come to you, sister?', and 'Does not fear come?' The fact that I lacked both *sharum* and fear was treated more as a thing of surprise and bewilderment than of disgrace.

Although *sharum* overcomes women and is meant to be natural to them, this does not entirely exempt them from taking responsibility for their personal displays of it. If a young married woman had been seen taking the bus alone as I was, then this would indeed have been a matter of disgrace. Like other emotions, *sharum* was at once spontaneous and learnt. It might be compared to the emotions of love and sorrow expressed at an *anu* ceremony I attended among the *Kharaks*. Here all women related to the girl who was about to leave the village for her in-laws' house were expected to cry violently for a short space of about thirty seconds each. When I failed to burst into tears, I was met with the response: 'Don't you have any feelings in your country? Just look how much we cry. Look how much we love our sister.' A group of women then explained that crying was an expression of love; thus it was important that they should all cry well, for if they failed to do so people would accuse them of not loving their sister. Their crying, which began and ended with what was to me disconcerting abruptness, was clearly quite natural to them but at the same time it was a definite social obligation.

The fact that *sharum* is thought natural and obligatory for women is important since it makes the practice of veiling, which is but one expression of *sharum*, seem natural also. This prevents women from questioning the custom and encourages them to uphold it. Furthermore *sharum*, with its associated behaviour, is one of the feminine qualities most venerated and admired, particularly in young women. For a new wife, who has just arrived at her conjugal home, not only is her veil a useful refuge from the prying eyes of strangers (Jacobson 1970: 485), but it is also a means of gaining approval from her new in-laws. It is on the basis of her *sharum*, obedience and hard work that her character will be assessed. For women there are therefore certain positive benefits associated with the veil.

Finally there is another aspect to veiling which makes women in Jalia reluctant to drop the custom, even if it means that they must remain in Gujarati saris when they would rather be wearing 'Bengali' ones. Veiling not only structures relations between men and women, but also acts as a means of expressing different levels of social refinement (cf. Jacobson 1970). Just as the fineness of a woman's fabric indicated her high social, ritual and economic status in the past, so her ability to be as invisible as possible also indicated her family's position. When a caste or family upgrades itself, withdrawing its women from the fields and/or introducing stricter veiling practices are among the means by which it proves itself worthy of its new position (cf. Srinivas 1976, Cohn 1955, Pocock 1972). Veiling, then, is a means of both maintaining and creating the reputation of a woman, her family and her caste and this encourages women to uphold the custom.

A brief survey of the various ways in which clothes define and differentiate people within the village of Jalia reveals that the relationship between clothing and identity is highly complex, involving a number of factors. First, there is the question of regional style: the clothes that people define as *deshi* or intrinsically Kathiawadi. For women this was the three-part combination of skirt, bodice and veil. For men it was the pantaloon, smock, waist-cloth and turban. Within these regional styles, however, differences of material further differentiated groups within the village and the area. A hierarchy of fabric types corresponded broadly to a hierarchy of social groups, with fine ones suggesting social refinement and coarse ones suggesting crudity. Finally, smaller differences in the cut of the clothes, the quantity of embroidery, the way of tying the turban and the styles of jewellery suggested a person's particular caste identity, although, as we have seen, these differences were sometimes ambiguous.

While men's dress, with the exception of the *Bharwads*, has become fairly standardised, women's dress remains important in the differentiation process. It is suggested that village women are conservative because for them clothes are also important in defining their position in the life-cycle and differentiating the roles of daughter, wife and widow. Furthermore the custom of veiling is so interlinked with the cultural construction of modesty, which is seen as *natural* to women, that it acts as a sartorial constraint, preventing change beyond a certain level. When Gandhi tried to convince all Indians to wear plain white *khadi*, he threatened not only regional identity and caste hierarchy but also the separation of the roles of daughter, wife and widow which are central to perceptions of female identity.

The following chapters focus on how members of different caste groups tackle the problem of what to wear and analyse the extent to which their clothing dilemmas are characteristic of the particular social groups to which they belong. My choice of caste communities with which to work was influenced by sometimes random factors which need to be explained. First, living in a *Brahman* family automatically brought me into its social world and gave me immediate links with other *Brahmans* in the village. Their clothing disputes form the basis of the next chapter. Secondly, following my original intention to study embroidery, I worked closely with *Kanbi* and *Kharak* families who were the main embroidery producers of the village (their clothing dilemmas feature in chapter 7). The *Bharwads*, on the other hand, proved interesting as the only group which seemed entirely reluctant to follow mainstream fashion, and where even young men continued to wear local styles. Finally, I worked with *Harijans* so that my discussion would span the major social divisions of the village. *Bharwad* and *Harijan* clothing dilemmas feature in chapter 8. Prejudice against *Harijans* from some groups in the village forced me to work with them at the very end of my stay when my own reputation was no longer of great concern. Each chapter begins with a specific clothing dilemma and then proceeds to a discussion of its ramifications in relation to wider issues.

6 Some *Brahman* Dilemmas

The problem of Hansaben's cardigan

It was midwinter, January 1989, and cold. Those who could afford it draped themselves in shawls and provided cardigans, jumpers and woolly hats for their children. The whole of Jalia took on a wrapped and huddled appearance. Hansaben, the only daughter-in-law in the house of a *Brahman* schoolteacher, opened her cupboard of trousseau gifts, took out a thick warm cardigan given her by her mother, and put it on over her sari, continuing her kitchen chores. Her mother-in-law sat close by, huddled in a sari and a woollen shawl and drinking tea from a china saucer. Leriben, daughter of the house, helped Hansaben with the cooking.

At mid-day there was a customary creaking sound from below and a loud and elongated cry of 'Ram' projected up the stairway, reaching the women in the kitchen above. Leriben warned Hansaben in urgent haste that HE was coming and Hansaben swiftly turned her back, sweeping her sari over her head as she swivelled, and pulling it down till it hung well over her face and neck in *ardhi laj*. Crouched in the corner of the kitchen, her back turned, her face covered and head tilted downwards, she continued to roll out *roti* (bread) as before.

Sureshkaka, her father-in-law, entered the room and sat cross-legged on the floor while his daughter supplied him with water followed by a large selection of food. A constant supply of hot *rotis* was drafted from Hansa's hot plate to Sureshkaka's *thali* (steel plate) by the intermediary and attentive daughter and wife. But Sureshkaka soon noticed the figure of his veiled daughter-in-law stooping over the fire, dressed in an unfamiliar garment. He demanded with annoyance just what she was wearing and where it had come from. Hansa herself remained mute beneath her veil, but her mother-in-law explained that it was cold and Hansa was wearing a cardigan ('jeket') that she had brought in her trousseau. Sureshkaka, unimpressed, pointed out that the folds of Hansa's sari were interrupted by this unnecessary addition and that it looked untidy and improper. 'No village girl would think it proper to wear such a thing,' he remonstrated. 'Has she no respect for our traditions? How can she do real *laj* when she looks such a sight with her sari half hidden under her "jeket" like that?' He instructed his wife to order Hansaben to get changed. She must put the cardigan underneath her blouse. He did not want to see such a disgraceful sight again. With that he stomped out of the room and went for his rest. His wife and daughter immediately set about telling Hansaben to change her clothes. Hansaben defended herself by saying that her blouse was too tight and the cardigan was too bulky — how could she wear it under her blouse? It was not possible. She could not even fit it beneath her sari, never mind the blouse. Her two advisers reminded her that her father-in-law had ordered it and this alone should make her obey. Hansa stubbornly refused and went on with her tasks.

The next day Hansa continued to wear the offending cardigan as before and her father-in-law lost his temper. He delivered an angry tirade about disobedient daughters-in-law and their lack of respect for their elders. His anger scared all members of the household who knew his short temper, and his wife and daughter scolded Hansaben for her stupid disobedience and for deliberately causing trouble to everyone in the house. Intimidated by the situation, Hansaben removed her cardigan, still maintaining to the other women that she could not fit it beneath her sari or her blouse and that she would just have to suffer the cold instead. She would freeze. For the next few days she went about the house shivering and refusing to speak or eat. She did her tasks silently and obediently with the air of a much-abused martyr.

Hansaben was three months pregnant at the time and still breastfeeding her first child, a girl of one and a half years. The family was anxious that she should eat well lest the new baby's health should be affected. When Sureshkaka heard that she was eating virtually nothing, he lost his temper yet again, this time with all the women, leaving the three of them disputing among themselves in the kitchen late at night. Hansaben was crying out in her own defence, saying that her mother had given her the cardigan and that she should be allowed to wear it since it was her own trousseau gift from her parents. Sureshkaka heard this from the next room and flew into the kitchen in an uncontrollable rage. Never before, he claimed, had he heard his daughter-in-law speak. How dare she raise her voice? Had she no *sharum* at all? This was it. He ordered her to leave the house there and then. She caused only trouble to his family. He never wanted to see her again. She should go back to the city if she wanted to behave with so little respect for their revered customs. In Larabad, at her parents' house, she could no doubt wear such a fancy 'jeket', but not in Jalia.

By now the whole family was involved in trying to placate Sureshkaka's rage. Hansaben's husband (Sureshkaka's eldest son) tried to calm him but to no avail; he was joined by Ramanbhai (the youngest son) who was a little more successful. He pointed out that Hansaben, who spent her days secluded in the house, could not be expected to leave the village alone at midnight. Sureshkaka must rest and think with a cool head in the morning.

Hansaben spent the night in tears, refusing to speak to anyone, including her husband. The next day she continued her tasks of cleaning, washing and cooking in total silence with downcast, tearful eyes, and shivering without her cardigan. When no one was looking she slipped across the courtyard and told the neighbour that if it were not for her child, she would kill herself. There was kerosene in the kitchen. How quick and easy it would be to set herself alight. She had thought of it many times.

The neighbour, who was sure to gossip, quickly reported this back to Sureshkaka's wife and soon the whole family was anxious about the threat of a suicide in the household. Everyone knew that Sureshkaka had gone too far this time. Even Sureshkaka himself seemed to realise that. He agreed to send a message to Hansaben's family in Larabad, saying that Hansa was unhappy just now and needed encouragement to eat. The next day her brother arrived from the city and she was able to confide her problems and explain how her father-in-law had ordered her out of the house in the middle of the night just because she had worn her cardigan when she was cold. Her brother left after a polite and strained saucer of tea with his in-laws, but the next day a short note was delivered to the house by a stranger who used the local bus. It was from Hansaben's father, saying that he was currently ill and required his daughter to look after him for one month. His son would arrive to fetch her from the village the following morning and escort her back to her parental home in Larabad.

There was no protest. Hansaben packed three saris and her controversial cardigan and left the house with her young daughter in her arms and her brother by her side. The female in-laws and her husband waved her good-bye and told her to come back soon. They hoped her father was not too ill.

The incidents described here were spread over a period of seven days. But it was eight months before Hansaben was to return to the village, much to the consternation of her in-laws. During these months another minor dispute arose, this time concerning Hansaben's saris.

Hansaben's saris

Hansaben had been gone three months, already far longer than the initial request in her father's note, and long enough to set other villagers gossiping and speculating about this errant daughter-in-law, when a letter appeared written by Hansaben herself and addressed to her husband. In it she greeted

Some *Brahman* Dilemmas

other members of the family politely and gave news of her daughter's well-being. But she proceeded to say that her father was still very ill and needed her assistance. She was therefore writing to request that they send her saris to Larabad as she had to attend a wedding and had nothing suitable to wear. All her best saris were in Jalia, and besides she needed her ordinary ones too since she had only taken three of them when she left the village.

This letter was met with grim resentment and much discussion among her in-laws. Three points emerged. First, Hansaben's father was not really ill, for only three days earlier the goldsmith's son had met him in the city and he seemed fine. Secondly, Hansa's request showed her intention to remain at her *pir* (natal home) for longer still, humiliating her in-laws in the process and forcing her mother-in-law to do the cooking and household chores which were Hansa's duty. It was argued that if she asked for her saris one day, then she would be demanding her jewellery the next, then her cupboard, her vessels, the ceiling fan, the bed. In short she would try to win back the whole of her trousseau. Then she would never return to the village. It was therefore decided that not one sari would be sent to her, for with her saris still in the village, she would be forced to return to Jalia soon.

The third objection was to the idea that she should be allowed to dress up and attend a wedding at all in the circumstances. This was only proof of her lack of *sharum* and her desire to wander aimlessly about, which was inappropriate to her married status. It also highlighted the irresponsibility of her parents in allowing their married daughter to go out and enjoy herself. What business did she have to go to a celebration? How could she be a good mother to her child when all she wanted was to dress up and wander about? How could she pretend that her father needed looking after when she was going off to weddings? That only showed the type of cunning and dishonest people her family were.

The Jalia family therefore decided to ignore Hansaben's request for her saris altogether and their bitterness was expressed in the fact that her mother-in-law began to wear Hansa's saris during the day. These were stored in Hansa's personal cupboard, also a trousseau gift from her parents. Her mother-in-law had ensured that Hansa handed over the key to the cupboard before leaving on the grounds that a few communal things were stored there. This gave her access to Hansa's saris, though not to her jewellery which was locked in a separate compartment from her clothes.

A second letter requesting Hansa's saris arrived a fortnight after the first, and seemed only to aggravate the mounting tensions between her and her in-laws, making reunion difficult. As the months passed the Jalia family became more and more desperate for her return, yet personal pride and cultural etiquette prevented them from lowering themselves to demand it.[1]

Family delegations: how to get Hansaben back

Late one evening in the fifth month of Hansaben's departure some surprise visitors arrived at Sureshkaka's house. They were his two elder brothers (a priest and a trader), his eldest brother's son (a doctor) and a cousin (a teacher). Although they all lived in Jalia, they rarely visited Sureshkaka's house owing to long-term family tensions. The priest's wife and Sureshkaka's wife claimed not to have spoken to each other for twenty-six years and had lived separately for more than twenty. The trading brother and Sureshkaka had remained together for longer but now blamed each other, and in particular each other's wives, for the split in the joint family some eight years before. A visit from these men could not be interpreted as a casual call, nor was it. They had come with a purpose. They wanted Hansaben back. A lengthy and heated discussion ensued between these five men (Sureshkaka, his two elder brothers, his brother's son and his cousin). Hansaben's husband was excluded from this and fell asleep outside on the verandah. However his mother, well wrapped beneath her veil, was straining to hear the discussion and posted her daughter just outside the main room to convey the gist of it.

It seemed that rumours were circulating via the goldsmith's son and his family that Hansaben would only return if she could live alone with her husband, separate from her mother-in-law, who caused her sorrow and treated her badly. The family delegation was concerned and horrified that such gossip should be conveyed by other people in the village and not even through personal relatives. Hansa, it seemed, was talking to her neighbours in Larabad, some of whom had relatives in Jalia who were talking in the village. One rumour claimed that her in-laws had threatened to burn her. The delegation was concerned about the ramifications of all this for both the family and the caste reputation. It was disgrace enough that Hansaben had left, bringing shame on them all, and now these rumours made it worse. It was time, they felt, for direct action. Hansaben must be recalled and must be well treated.

This led to a second, highly sensitive issue which was raised by Sureshkaka's eldest brother, the priest. If Sureshkaka were not so lax in maintaining old

---

1 According to beliefs widespread among high-caste Hindus in northern and western India, wife-takers are superior to wife-givers at least during the marriage ceremony, if not in everyday life (cf. Van der Veen 1972, Parry 1986, Vatuk 1975, Werbner 1990). Apologising to Hansaben's family and asking for her return would therefore have seemed like an act of humiliation that Sureshkaka's family, as superiors, were not prepared to take.

traditions, he argued, then this type of behaviour in a daughter-in-law would never have occurred. But Sureshkaka had tried to improve himself too far and by 'becoming a *Vaniya*'[2] he was losing sight of their own caste traditions. Most respected families in Jalia were content to educate their daughters up to seventh standard in the village school. This meant they could read and write, and why should they need more? But for Sureshkaka this was not enough. He sent his daughter to high school on the bus where 'anything might happen'. Then there was the question of her being dressed in a *shalwar kamiz*. It was not right for a Hindu girl to put on the trousers of a Muslim. Did he know how people talked when they saw her at the bus stop? Only the other day their cousin the *panwala* (betel-nut seller) had exclaimed at the sight: 'See, the *Vaghran*[3] is coming. Look, the prostitute!' Sureshkaka owed it to his family and his caste to keep up his standards. His daughter should cease her education right away and this would save her from the disgrace of using the bus, roaming alone in town and dressing in clothes that were unsuitable for any Hindu village girl. But most important of all, Sureshkaka must send his son to fetch Hansaben back at all costs, even if this meant a split in the household. For just now Sureshkaka's family brought disgrace on all his brothers in the village.

The meeting ended with Sureshkaka losing his temper and the delegation leaving in haste. He did not want a split in his own household, particularly since he had another son and a daughter whose marriages were yet to be arranged. These would be costly affairs for which he required the financial assistance of his eldest son (Hansaben's husband), who ran the shop. Hansaben's husband in fact hoped to escape this burden, particularly in the case of his brother's wedding. Not only did he want the financial independence of running his own house, but he also felt resentment that his younger brother was more respected by their father; for the elder brother this seemed unjust, since it was he who contributed to the family income while his younger brother merely 'played around at college', costing them money and contributing nothing.

A few weeks after the visit of the first family delegation a second family delegation was planned. This time, much to my surprise, it involved my

2   This was a reference to the fact that Sureshkaka, though a schoolteacher and part-time priest, had also entered the trading profession and owned one of the village shops which his eldest son now ran. The *Vaniyas* were not only the principal traders of the village but they were also considered the most fashionable and urban in their ways, partly owing to their extensive links with Bombay. By accusing Sureshkaka of 'becoming a *Vaniya*', his elder brother was referring both to the trade and to the reputation of the *Vaniyas* as a social group.

3   This was a reference to the *Vaghri* caste, who have a bad reputation. The term is often used in Gujarat as an insult, implying that the person so called is immoral, disreputable and ill bred.

own family. My parents had come to visit Jalia for one day and, shortly after their arrival, it became clear that they were to be sent with me and Ramanbhai to Hansaben's house in Larabad as a gesture of reconciliation. As older-generation white educated people, they were greeted with considerable respect in Jalia, and by sharing the honour of their brief visit the Jalia family were making a gesture of goodwill to Hansaben's family without having to lower themselves to actually asking for her return. My parents, who were entirely unable to communicate in linguistic terms, were essentially to act as peace envoys. They sat obediently on a bed drinking tea and smiling at appropriate moments while I was beckoned into the kitchen by Hansaben, who was keen to hear what havoc her departure might be causing to her in-laws. When I asked about her plans, it soon became clear that her problem was not so much *whether* to return as *when*. She explained her position as follows:

> 'I am married and must stay married. It is my misfortune to be married with those people, but what can I do? I know my life is there in the village and all my trousseau things are there. I asked them for my saris and they sent not one, not even one. My jewellery, my vessels, everything is there. I have nothing here in my parents' place. My life is not here. Soon things will get better in Jalia. Ramanbhai will marry and a new wife will come to the house. She will help me with the work and she will judge who is honest in the house. She will know that I am good.'

Hansaben never feared that her in-laws would not take her back for, as she explained, they needed her not just for the housework but for their reputation. Ramanbhai, their youngest son, would never be able to find a really good wife if there was already a divorce in his family. Even at this moment their reputation was being discussed because, according to Hansaben's interpretation, everyone always wanted to know who was treating their daughter-in-law so badly as to make her leave. Hansa perceived her sojourn with her parents not merely as a refuge but also as a good revenge for her in-laws' unpleasantness. She demanded to know how difficult her absence had made things in the village and expressed particular pleasure that her mother-in-law, who disliked cooking, was now doing so every day. Hansa would play hard to get. She wanted her in-laws to apologise and ask her back but her own parents would not make the approaches. They were waiting for her in-laws to call her and in the mean time she was enjoying the comfort and pleasure of being in her parental home.

When, one day, her husband finally visited her in Larabad, requesting her return, she refused to speak with him and denied him access to their daughter, but her parents told him that Hansa would return to the village for a two-week trial period. Her husband refused this humiliating offer and left. As far as he was concerned this was a sign that she was intending to return and he was not going to receive her on *their* terms. If she was coming back to Jalia, she must come and she must stay.

Hansaben's return

In the sixth month of her departure, Hansaben gave birth to their second child, another daughter. Two months later her father wrote to Sureshkaka saying that Hansaben was ready to return, having recovered from the birth. Since it is customary for women to give birth to their first child and occasionally their second at their parents' house, the birth provided a suitable time for her reappearance in the village, giving it some façade of normality. She arrived with her daughter and new baby girl and was greeted with much affection and lavish displays of love from her mother-in-law and sister-in-law. The family was back to its customary state of precarious stability and the cardigan returned to the cupboard.

At first sight it might appear that the seemingly exaggerated response of Sureshkaka to a mere cardigan tells more about the temperament of one particular man than it does about the significance of clothes. The cardigan might, for example, have been simply a random catalyst which happened to spark off flames in what was already a tense relationship. But closer investigation of the meaning and value of clothing to the people of Jalia suggests that the nature of the catalyst was by no means arbitrary. To gain some insight into the labyrinth of tensions which this clothing dispute seemed to evoke and embody, it is necessary to examine briefly certain aspects of the giving and receiving, wearing and possessing of clothes.

Giving and receiving clothing and adornment

Giving and receiving gifts forms a vital element of every major life-cycle rite in Jalia. The most important of these rites is the giving of a virgin daughter (*kanyadan*) in marriage.[4] Around this central rite a whole series of other gift-giving obligations is organised. Clothing and jewellery are, along with food, the most important components of these gift-giving rituals, accompanying marriages, pregnancies, births, deaths, arrivals and departures. Werbner has shown how Pakistani migrants from Manchester, visiting their relatives in Pakistan, often pay excess luggage charges owing to the enormous quantities of clothing they carry back and forth as gifts

---

4   For detailed accounts see Fruzzetti 1982, Parry 1986 and Van der Veen 1972.

for kinsmen and women (Werbner 1990: 270). Such gifts tie immigrants to their natal homes and objectify social relations between families (*ibid*.: 283). In Jalia, gifts of clothing hold a similar importance, binding together individuals and groups, ratifying agreements, confirming commitments, ascribing social roles and protecting future interests. As Evans-Pritchard once commented in the African context, 'material culture may be regarded as part of social relations, for material objects are the chains along which social relationships run' (Evans-Pritchard 1967: 89). In India the major links of such chains are often forged in cloth.

Although both men and women give and receive clothes, these gifts have a special and particular importance for women. Large stocks of clothing are accumulated in preparation for a daughter's wedding, and after marriage a wife usually keeps her trousseau clothes in her personal dowry chest or cupboard to which she generally keeps the key. Men never acquire the large stocks of clothing that women receive from their parents. Nor do they discuss clothes with the same enthusiasm and eye for detail. Clothing is for women a frequent topic of conversation as they compare and inspect each other's apparel and even display their entire clothing collection to visitors and friends (Gold 1988: 13–15).

For women clothing is not merely a question of adornment but also a form of property, particularly in a village context where women's rights of inheritance to other forms of property such as land are rarely recognised (Goody 1973: 17). If they get the opportunity, women hoard clothes, often in excess of their apparent requirements (Chaudhuri 1976: 42). Clothing, carefully locked away, and jewellery, worn or safely stored, are often the only parts of a new wife's trousseau over which she has primary access and control. It is not therefore surprising to find that women take more interest in accumulating and comparing clothes than men who inherit other, more permanent forms of wealth.

A brief examination of the gifts of clothing and adornment given to a woman in connection with her marriage reveals her gradual assimilation into her in-laws' home:

Betrothal (*sagai*). Following the agreement between parents that their children should marry, the father of the prospective groom offers the future bride a veil-cloth (*chundadi*), one outfit of clothes and a selection of jewellery, usually comprising a nose-ring, anklets and earrings. He paints a vermilion mark (*chandlo*) on her forehead and places the veil over her head.[5]

---

5   The precise details of the betrothal ceremony vary from caste to caste and according to whether or not a priest is involved. In all betrothal ceremonies, however, the offering of the *chundadi*

Some *Brahman* Dilemmas

There is no written contract at the time of betrothal but the offering of the veil and the painting of vermilion are seen as a concrete agreement on the part of the groom's parents to take on responsibility for the girl's future. It is a contract written, as it were, on the girl herself.

This became clear in the case of a *Brahman* girl who suffered rejection by her future husband only one week after the engagement ceremony had taken place. This caused great outrage among her relatives who had witnessed the offering of the *chundadi* and *chandlo* and who remonstrated that the groom's father had already given the veil and therefore could not 'cut it now'.[6] Broken engagements, although they sometimes occurred, were rare and considered highly inauspicious. The offering of the *chundadi* usually served as a formal acknowledgement of the intention of the groom's family to accept the gift of the bride.

Marriage (lugan). During the marriage ceremony the bride is dressed in a new set of clothes given by her parents, consisting usually of petticoat, blouse and *paneter* (special red and white tie-dyed wedding sari). As she enters the marriage booth, however, one of her in-laws (usually the mother-in-law) covers her face and head with a *gharcholu*, a special marriage veil, usually green with yellow and red tie-dyed dots. She therefore simultaneously wears the veil given by her parents and that from her in-laws, symbolising her passing from the protection of one household to another. The colours red and green are associated with fertility and auspiciousness and are worn mainly by young women, married or unmarried.

Along with the *gharcholu*, a bride also receives jewellery from her in-laws, including the *mangalsutra* and ivory bangles which she will wear throughout her married life.[7] As the ceremony begins, the bride's brother declares in Sanskrit: 'This maiden, decorated with ornaments and robed in twin apparel, I give to you.' The priest joins together the hands of the bridal pair and leads them to the central marriage square (*chori*). Here their upper garments are tied together and the couple take four turns around the sacred

---

    and the painting of the *chandlo* form the central rite. These are usually accompanied by the gift of a coconut and 1 rupee.

6   The incident was unusual since the parents of the groom had come to Jalia to ratify the betrothal without the groom's knowledge or his consent. He had in fact already stated his refusal to marry the girl after seeing her photograph. His parents had ignored his wishes and gone ahead with the engagement, which the angry son later refused to acknowledge.

7   In cases where the bride is young and will not accompany her husband at the end of the ceremony, she does not wear permanent marriage bangles at this stage. These are sent by her in-laws some years later just before she leaves her parental home to embark on married life.

fire, physically united by the knot in their clothes and a long cotton thread (*mala*) which binds them together. The knotting of garments and the tying of thread are a metaphoric enactment of physical union and it is through these actions that the permanence of the union is stated.[8]

The sending away (anu) ceremony. The customs surrounding sending away (*anu*) ceremonies vary greatly according to the community and the age of the bride at the time of marriage. If she is young and there is a gap of some years between the marriage and the main *anu* ceremony, then the groom's parents are often expected to send one outfit of clothes to the bride every year to reaffirm the wedding contract. Often they are also expected to give money to the bride's parents to cover the stitching charges incurred at the tailors during the preparation of the bride's *anu* clothes.

The number of *anu* ceremonies may vary from one to three according to the particular preferences of different individuals or castes. The main *anu*, however, takes place when the mature girl first goes to live in her husband's home, rather than simply visiting it. On this occasion she receives a large collection of clothes from her parents, consisting usually of at least twenty-one outfits and a few items of jewellery.[9] After being carefully displayed to friends and neighbours, these are placed in a cupboard or dowry chest, along with a selection of steel kitchen vessels contributed by all her near relatives, and small items of household furniture and ornaments which vary considerably according to family wealth and caste expectations.

The final *anu*, called *jianu*, occurs when a woman returns to her marital home after giving birth to her first child at her parental home. When she returns to her in-laws' house, she receives from her parents a few outfits of clothing and a number of outfits for the baby, along with a baby's cot and quilt. For the rest of her life she will usually receive a gift of clothing from her parents each time she visits her parental home. She will also be

8 In the same way that the act of knotting symbolises union, so the act of ripping symbolises the dissolution of social bonds. In some poor communities, such as the *Vaghris* and the *Bhungis*, the marriage tie itself can be broken through ripping cloth. Enthoven described a *Bhungi* divorce earlier in the twentieth century as follows: 'The husband tears a piece of cloth from his headdress and gives it to his wife and the wife takes off her glass bangles and puts them into her husband's lap. This done, the divorce is complete' (Enthoven 1920, vol. 1: 104).

9 The number of outfits naturally varies according to the wealth of the families involved but there has been a marked increase in recent years in the amount of clothes even poor parents are expected to provide for their daughters. Most families try to give at least fifteen outfits, each consisting of a petticoat, blouse and sari or half-sari. Many mothers reported having received only three outfits at the time of their own *anu* ceremonies. The wealthiest families in Jalia today usually give thirty-five outfits. Until recently outfits were always given in odd numbers, these being thought more auspicious than even numbers. Nowadays, however, even numbers of outfits are sometimes given.

expected to provide gifts for her in-laws, but these are secondary to those she receives herself.[10] Her in-laws will in turn provide her with clothes and jewellery from time to time, particularly on festive occasions; thus a woman can accumulate clothes even after marriage.

Social relations between two families are therefore expressed and reconfirmed through a series of gifts of clothing and adornment which bind the two groups together through the conversion of daughters into wives.[11] The knotting of garments acts as the central pivot around which such gift-giving takes place. In the case of Hansaben and her in-laws, the contractual aspect of these gifts was particularly apparent. They belong to a *Brahman* subgroup[12] that is numerically small, with a severe shortage of marriageable girls. When Sureshkaka first discovered Hansaben, she was only fifteen and her parents had considered her too young to marry for at least another three years. She was pretty, fair-skinned, intelligent and well-bred, which had made Sureshkaka particularly anxious to procure her for his son. One of her strongest attributes was that she came from the city of Larabad, where he himself hoped eventually to settle. This, he felt, made her refined and greatly preferable to the less educated girls found in villages. All in all, Hansa had seemed too good to lose and the Jalia family had wanted to fix the betrothal straight away. Hansa's family had been apprehensive because this meant a three-year gap between betrothal and marriage. Finally they were persuaded by Sureshkaka's offer of twenty-one saris which would be given to Hansaben at the engagement ceremony. These revealed his family's commitment to the future marriage. They also acted as a deposit which guaranteed that Hansaben would be reserved exclusively for them, even if other more appetising offers presented themselves in the three years before the marriage.

---

10   I do not propose to discuss the full complexity of gift-giving in India, a subject already covered extensively in anthropological literature (cf. Parry 1986, Van der Veen 1972, Vatuk 1975, Werbner 1990).

11   There is also a complex series of monetary payments that are an important part of the marital union but tend not to be discussed or emphasised during the actual marriage ceremony, which should ideally appear like the gift of a daughter, freely offered without expectation of reward (Parry 1986, Van der Veen 1972). In Jalia, as elewhere, poor families often paid brideprice whereas wealthy families tended to pay dowry money.

12   They are *Saracharsau Brahmans* (lit. '400' *Brahmans*) who, along with the *Agyarasau Brahmans* ('1,100' *Brahmans*), belong to the wider category of *Audichya Brahmans* who originated in Uttar Pradesh. According to caste traditions these *Brahmans* were called to Sihor in Kathiawad by Siddharaji Jaysinghji to assist in a ritual which was to rid the king of his leprosy. After the worship was completed, 1,100 *Brahmans* chose to settle in Sihor and 450 settled in Jalawad where they served as *gor* (priests) for different castes and ceased to intermarry. Members of both groups live in Jalia.

When Hansaben married three years later, she received another twenty-one saris from her own parents in her trousseau, making her the owner of forty-two saris and a fine selection of gold jewellery, mostly given by her in-laws. These were her own property and were kept separately from the other women's clothes in her new home. She had, as we have seen, her own steel cupboard which was used almost exclusively by her.

In theory, the forty-two saris belonged to Hansaben, yet during her absence they were kept by her in-laws as hostages to ensure her return. When I asked Hansaben why she had taken so few saris with her to Larabad in the first place, she replied that her mother-in-law had been watching over her while she was packing and had told her she did not need to take much. Her mother-in-law was suspicious, so Hansa had left with only three saris. In other words, if she had taken too many saris with her, she would have been seen to be breaking the contract under which those clothes had been given by expressing her intention to stay away from the marital home as long as possible. But her departure, though obviously based on just such a desire to get away, had to be made to look like a departure of necessity, an obedience to her sick father's wishes rather than her own.[13]

During Hansa's absence, the topic of the twenty-one saris given at betrothal was frequently raised by the Jalia family. Their deposit seemed to have proved worthless and they felt cheated. It was apparently in a spirit of bitterness and vindictiveness that the mother-in-law began to wear the saris herself. When I first saw her dressed in one of them, it was not entirely obvious that they were not her own since she had selected a fairly subdued colour. But she seemed self-conscious and immediately confessed, with a laugh, that she was dressed in Hansa's clothes which were really more suitable for a younger woman. Wearing Hansa's saris seemed a way of reclaiming the remnants of a broken agreement.[14]

13　One striking feature of this entire dispute was the indirectness in which it was couched. Hansa rarely expressed her opinions to her in-laws, but rather influenced events by talking to others such as her neighbour and her brother or myself. Such indirectness is common, especially among young daughters-in-law, since they are the people most constrained in their speech, visibility and mobility. But maintaining a façade of 'normal life', whatever the situation, seems an important feature of social life more generally in small Indian communities where generations of men of the same family live in close proximity and where gossip is rife. Apart from Sureshkaka, who expressed his opinions openly, other members of the family all took care to keep up appearances and restrain their opinions in public.

14　It would be interesting to know the extent to which other mothers-in-law wear their daughters-in-law's (vaus') saris. In Jalia I came across one other case of an angry woman who was wearing her vaus' saris in the latter's absence. Sharma has suggested that it is not uncommon for senior women to redistribute their daughters-in-law's saris among other family members (Sharma 1984: 65). However, this practice was not common in Jalia, where most young wives

Some *Brahman* Dilemmas

Although Hansa possessed a large collection of saris, it was clear that her rights of ownership were constrained by the context in which the clothes had been given. Owning clothes seemed to require the acceptance of certain conditions. The saris were hers so long as she was prepared to fulfil her wifely duties, but they ceased to be so the moment she appeared to step outside the role of wife, a role which, after all, justified her entitlement to the saris in the first place. It has been suggested (Jacobson 1976) that a woman's control over her own jewellery varies according to her relationship to the donor. Just as a woman's kinship bonds with her parents are strong and permanent, so her ownership over jewellery from her natal kin is absolute, but in the same way that her relationship with her in-laws is vulnerable and precarious, so too is her control over jewellery given by them. A dissatisfied in-law can reclaim jewellery in the same way that Hansa's mother-in-law reclaimed her saris. Such gifts from in-laws are conditional on the daughter-in-law's obedience and good behaviour. This raises interesting questions about what it means to own and receive clothes as a woman in Indian society.

Women as owners and recipients of clothes

Women receive and accumulate clothes more than men, and this is one of the privileges of becoming a wife. While a woman's control over the gifts from her own parents is more secure than that over gifts from her in-laws, it must be remembered that both sets of gifts are conditional on her marrying; only through making the transition from daughter to wife does a woman become entitled to a large stock of clothes at all. Girls who never marry never receive the trousseau items that their parents accumulated for them in their youth. Indeed such unmarried women, who are in themselves a rarity, do not receive more than the basic requirements of clothing from their parents. Women who are separated or widowed, on the other hand, sometimes retrieve their trousseau clothing, but this is often at the discretion of their in-laws and cannot easily be enforced. If they return to their parental home with their trousseau clothes, these are usually given in remarriage or distributed among other family members if remarriage is unacceptable. One *Brahman* woman who returned to her parents after prolonged maltreatment by her husband regained her saris yet contributed all

---

kept their clothes in their own chests or cupboards and maintained a reasonable degree of control over them. It was other trousseau items such as furniture (beds, fans, display cabinets) and vessels which were used by other members of a woman's conjugal family. But a sense of ownership was preserved by the fact that all steel vessels given to the bride were engraved with the name and village of their donors before the *anu* ceremony.

but three to her younger sister's trousseau as it was no longer thought necessary or appropriate for her to possess such clothes now that her marriage was over. She accepted this as her contribution to the parental home.

Young married life is, as we have seen, the only time when a woman is expected to adorn herself extravagantly and possess fine clothes. Great emphasis is placed on the beauty and adornment of the youthful bride and wife who symbolises prosperity and auspiciousness. The finer her clothes and the more lavish her jewellery, the greater her resemblance to Lakshmi, the goddess of wealth and prosperity. She should dress brightly, and have smooth oiled hair, lampblack round her eyes, polish on her nails, vermilion in her parting and an abundance of gold jewellery on her wrists, round her neck and in her ears. But if an unmarried girl adorns herself too beautifully, she is immediately thought disreputable, attracting unsuitable attention. Before marriage she must dress plainly except for special festivals when she can wear her finest apparel. Similarly, in old age a woman is supposed to tone down her appearance until finally, if widowed, she loses her entitlement to look beautiful altogether, casting aside the symbols of happy married life. *Brahman* widows usually wear white clothes, farming widows dull red, and shepherd widows black. Excessive adornment worn either before marriage or after a marriage has ended is associated with immorality and even prostitution.

This suggests that the adornment of women is closely related to the celebration and control of their fertility – which must not be emphasised before marriage. Nor should it be expressed in old age, even though some of the women who called themselves 'old' were only in their thirties and clearly still capable of conception. Such 'old' women risked the accusation of trying to 'be' their daughters-in-law if they dressed too lavishly. Once their daughters-in-law had come to the house, they themselves were expected to cease producing children and to begin to divest themselves of excess ornament. It is therefore only the child-producing years that entitle a woman to dress brightly, lavishly and decoratively. These are the years when her beauty can be safely expressed within the context of her relationship with her husband. Yet if a woman's freedom to dress lavishly reaches its highest expression during this period, it is also the time when her behaviour is most constrained and her physical presence most hidden. She must absent herself behind her veil, hiding her powers of allurement from other men of the household and the village, and *Brahman* wives like Hansaben usually cannot leave the house or enter the village, even when screened by their veils. The privilege of receiving clothes and displaying one's beauty is therefore closely linked with the need to conceal it. Conversely, for men the act of providing clothes for their women entitles them to expect certain displays of *sharum* and obedience from them. To husbands and fathers the obligation to give is as much a part of the masculine role as the privilege of receiving and obeying is part of the feminine wifely role.[15]

Men as givers of clothes

For parents giving clothes is an obligation, a duty and a necessity. Much time is spent on deciding precisely how much should be spent on the clothing and jewellery for a daughter's wedding. It is sometimes suggested that women control the distribution of goods while men control financial transactions (Sharma 1984: 66). This is true to some extent but the distinction is not rigid (Vatuk 1975: 191). Furthermore, while the mother of the bride does indeed play the major role in organising the trousseau and selecting appropriate items of dress, among most castes it is the father who takes the financial responsibility. And although it is women who inspect and assess a girl's trousseau display, it is the man's reputation that is at stake if her provisions are thought to be lacking. Chaudhuri sums up the situation when he writes that men give enthusiastically because their own position and prestige depend on the clothes of their women. He quotes the lines from *Manu Samhita* (ancient Brahminical legal code) which read:

'Women must be honoured and adorned by their fathers, brothers and husbands and brothers in law for their own welfare.... The houses on which female relations, not being duly honoured, pronounce a curse, perish completely as if destroyed by magic. Hence men who seek their own welfare should always honour women on holidays and festivals with ornaments, clothes and food' (Chaudhuri 1976: 42).

Often the obligation to give reaches unfortunate proportions, particularly for men with a predominance of daughters, whose marriages and trousseaux cause many families financial difficulties. But the obligation to provide, and to be seen to provide, is stronger than any purely financial consideration;

---

15 Cohn discusses Moghul rituals of cloth-giving as acts of subordination and incorporation through which something of the ruler's substance is transmitted in the act of giving clothes. These prestations were structured according to the idea that superiors give more than they receive. Receiving clothes was therefore an act which reinforced the recipients' lowliness in relation to the giver (Cohn 1989: 309). It is tempting to draw parallels between the gifts of a ruler to his subjects and the gifts of men to women. But it must be remembered that not all prestations of clothing are given by superiors to inferiors. There are, for example, occasions when a daughter-in-law may be expected to present a sari to her mother-in-law, who is clearly defined as a superior.

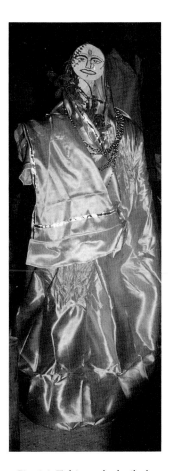

Fig. 6.1 Tulsima, the basil plant goddess, dressed in a silky sari for her marriage to Takadada (Lord Krishna). Her nose-ring (*nath*) and spangle (*bindi*) are visible but her earrings have fallen off.

it is part of the duty of fatherhood and an indicator of a man's worthiness of respect. Gifts are often given in public situations where there is a large audience of kinsmen and women to impress (Werbner 1990: 277). Displaying one's wealth and generosity, establishing and reconfirming social bonds, providing for daughters and fulfilling the duty of fatherhood are all features that are intermeshed in the giving of the trousseau.

The intensity of the obligation to clothe a daughter is expressed in the annual ritual of *Tulsi Vivah* (Basil Wedding) when Tulsima, the holy basil plant which grows in every courtyard, is formally married to Takadada (Lord Krishna) in a ceremony which marks the end of the austere monsoon season and the beginning of the more festive winter period.[16] The ceremony takes place on the eleventh day of the bright half of *Kartik* (mid-November) and only after this sacred marriage can mortals in the village celebrate their own weddings.

The marriage of Tulsima with Takadada resembles a human marriage in most ways, since it contains the essential elements of any Hindu wedding, including the setting up of a marriage booth (*mandap*), a central square (*chori*), a sacred fire (*agni*) and so on. Tulsima (the basil plant) receives all the privileges of the bride, including a full set of marriage clothing which is wrapped around her leaves. When I witnessed the ceremony, a nose-ring and earrings, provided by the substitute parents of the bride, were attached with difficulty to a paper face which had been inserted at the top of the plant (see fig. 6.1). Takadada, in the form of a small statue of Krishna, was dressed in a *dhoti* and seated beneath a canopy. The couple were linked by a cotton thread (*mala*). Responsibility for the cost and equipment necessary for the wedding is taken every year by a married couple who have no daughter. They become the parents of Tulsima for the night and give her away. It is significant that they not only provide her with bridal clothes but also with an entire trousseau of saris. The year I attended the wedding, Tulsima was promised twenty-one saris, which were to be taken by the *Brahman* priest and distributed to female ascetics.

Taking the financial responsibility for this event is considered a privilege and is meritorious to couples without daughters. It is said that a man cannot fulfil his full duty of fatherhood if he has only sons. Although sons are as a rule greatly preferred, people feel it necessary to have at least one

16 According to local tradition, the ceremony developed from the days when Krishna wished to kill the wicked demon Jalandhar. He failed to do so because the demon's wife Vrinda was so chaste and virtuous. Krishna therefore assumed the form of Jalandhar and violated his wife, after which he was able to kill the demon. She transformed herself into a tulsi plant and Krishna, now in love with her, married the plant.

Some *Brahman* Dilemmas

daughter whom they can give away in marriage. The *Kanbi* man who acted the role of father explained this as follows: 'It is only after obtaining wives for our sons and giving away our daughters with the provisions of a good trousseau that we can say we have completed our duty as fathers. Before today I had no daughter, but now I have given Tulsima, my daughter, to our god Takadada and I can become old quietly.' When I questioned him about the necessity of providing Tulsima with twenty-one saris, he looked me askance and answered: 'Who would give away a daughter without a trousseau of fine clothes? What kind of father is that?'

The nature of the relationship between the sexes is restated in the female privilege of receiving clothes and the male privilege of providing them. This is particularly true among high-caste groups. Where women are secluded, as in Sureshkaka's family, the man's obligation to provide is at its strongest but so too is his ability to control the clothing and behaviour of the women of the house. Sureshkaka's wife claimed (somewhat exaggeratedly) not to have been shopping since before her marriage some twenty-six years earlier. If she needed clothes, then she asked her husband or her son to provide them. She said she would like to shop but her husband would get angry if she left the house.[17] She only went out for funerals, weddings and special events. When Leriben, her daughter, came to marry, then she would be able to shop with her husband for Leriben's trousseau, but this would be an exceptional event for which they would make a special trip to Ahmedabad.

Leriben herself, being unmarried, was not so restricted in her movements as her mother. She was able to visit the cloth shops of Larabad with her brother and choose the material for her own clothes. It was considered acceptable for her to have clothes made by a tailor so long as he did not take her body measurements. But this 'freedom' did not exempt her from her father's criticism and overriding choice. He wanted her to look like an educated city girl, which meant wearing a *shalwar kamiz* of shiny synthetic fabric. In the sweltering heat of the summer she had tried to explain that cotton would be cooler and more comfortable, but her father had objected: 'What will people say if they see you dressed in *sada kapda* [plain

---

17 *Laj* restrictions for Sureshkaka's wife were so strict that she was prohibited from buying vegetables even though this required taking no more than two steps outside the front gate for the vegetable shop was actually located in the front of her own house. All food and clothing supplies were brought home by the men of the family and if for any reason they were delayed elsewhere, there would be a temporary panic about how to obtain chillies or aubergines for the next meal. If Leriben were absent, then a neighbour's child would have to be called, or me if I were around. Leriben was allowed to fetch milk from a neighbouring *Kharak* woman who lived nearby but was prohibited from entering the main street of the village, unless for a special purpose.

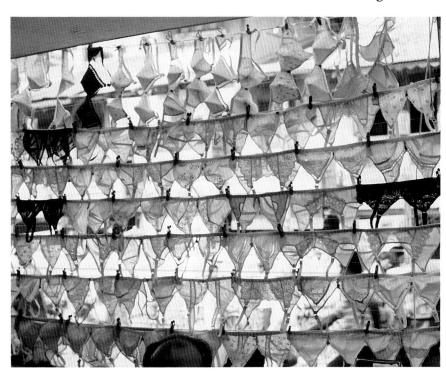

cloth]? They will say that your father is so mean and poor that he dresses his daughter like a *Vaghri*. People talk.' And people, usually relatives, did talk about Leriben's clothing. Her uncle, the priest, felt it indecent for a respectable Hindu girl to wear a *shalwar kamiz* which was suitable only for Muslims or fancy city people. His own unmarried daughter, who was more or less confined to the house, wore simple long 'maxis' and, on the rare occasions of her entering the village, a sari. The *panwala* (betel-nut seller), Sureshkaka's cousin, called Leriben insulting names as she stood at the bus stop. But Leriben waited quietly for the bus and went to college despite the objections of her extended family, some of whom thought she was dressed above her station while others thought she was dressed below it. As the heat of the summer increased, her father gave her permission to wear cotton 'maxis' inside the house and even agreed to her having a cotton *shalwar kamiz*. But these were strictly for indoor use, and she was severely chastised when an unexpected guest arrived at the house and saw her wearing cotton. Cotton was too *deshi* (local, unsophisticated); as far as Sureshkaka was concerned, it was the cloth of rough, uneducated, backward farming people.

Some *Brahman* Dilemmas

Finally, as we have seen, Hansaben had little control over her own apparel. She too relied on the choice of her husband if new clothes were required. But she resented the limitations of the village. She wanted to dress like a city woman in the 'Bengali sari' that hung down the back instead of the front. But her in-laws argued that she would not be able to perform proper *laj* dressed in that style. Why, they asked, did she feel the need to look like a *sarawala* (well-to-do person) when she was living in a village? She also wanted to wear a bra, but her mother-in-law had forbidden it on the grounds that she would not be able to feed her baby easily. Hansa resented this for there were, as she told me, front-fastening bras available in Larabad. She did not see why Leriben, who was younger and unmarried, should be allowed to wear a bra when she, who was older and married, was forbidden to do so.

The cardigan reconsidered

Examination of the importance of giving and receiving clothes helps to explain the apparently extreme reactions of Sureshkaka and Hansaben to what at first glance seems like the trivial matter of a mere cardigan. Because clothes are given in the context of specific relationships and events, they embody the relationships between individuals, families and groups (cf. Cohn 1989, Werbner 1990) with the result that each item of clothing that a person possesses has a very specific history which becomes embedded within the garment itself. Hansa's cardigan had been made by her mother and given by her parents in her trousseau and therefore evoked a whole series of associations: parents, home and Larabad, where her life had seemed happier and freer. This accounts in part for her extremely emotional attachment to the garment and her reluctance to remove it, but it cannot fully account for her persistence in wearing it even after her father-in-law's initial objection. Before addressing this particular problem, it is worth considering exactly what Sureshkaka's objections were really about. This is difficult to assess since he refused to discuss the incident in any detail, but his wife claimed that he felt the cardigan was too modern, being a city style, and one which no married woman would wear in a village. Other women, if they needed warmth, wore shawls.

The city style of Hansa's cardigan was symptomatic of Hansaben in general. She came from a well-to-do police inspector's family in Larabad city where her parents had a modern concrete house, well equipped with furniture and items of urban living. Members of Sureshkaka's family seemed at once to admire and resent this. It was in many ways what them-selves aspired to for they felt oppressed by the village and referred to 'village people' as if they were something entirely different from themselves. But Sureshkaka was unable to find work in the city and therefore remained frustrated in Jalia, hoping for a way out. That the daughter-in-law was so obviously city-bred seemed to rile the household. The women of the house would often inform me that Hansaben was a *shaher wala* (city type), used to fine things, with a high-level cooker in the kitchen, a fridge and much else besides. This would be said with an air of sarcasm and jest, and Hansa would deny it with a laugh, saying that things in Jalia were good too. In private, however, she confessed that she hated the village with all its restrictions. She wanted to be a schoolteacher, not to cook and clean all day inside the house. She had studied to tenth grade, which was four years more than her husband. When Hansa's in-laws felt that she thought herself superior and above the village, they were in a sense right. How many of these more general household tensions were evoked by the sight of that modern city-styled cardigan it is difficult to tell, but it is at least likely that they lurked in the background, adding poignancy to the event.

Thus the clothing style and what it represented were in themselves a means of provocation, which was enhanced by the fact that Hansa's sari had not hung straight on account of her cardigan. This meant that instead of being the absent, unnoticed figure draped in the corner of the room, she was noticeable and in Sureshkaka's mind unsightly. The mere fact of being so visible was, he thought, a sign of immodesty since it attracted inappropriate attention. He had immediately accused her of lack of *sharum* even though her face was properly hidden and her back well turned. In other words Hansa in her cardigan was too modern and too visible.[18]

This leads to the second question of why Hansaben persisted in wearing the cardigan even after Sureshkaka had made his objections clear. Her refusal to remove it was more than a case of personal attachment. It was, as she well knew, a denial of Sureshkaka's authority. By keeping her cardigan on, despite being fully veiled, she was showing her autonomy in a situation where she should have been meek and unnoticed. No one was more aware of this than Sureshkaka himself, who reacted with due fury, causing her finally to remove the garment and lapse into silence and resentment.

Hansa's actions are worth examining in more detail. Everything she did was indirect but highly effective, illustrating how even a daughter-in-law can carefully circumvent the apparently rigid system of senior male autho-

---

18   There has been much discussion of the importance of the veil as a means of rendering women socially invisible (cf. Sharma 1978b, R. Mehta 1976, Jacobson 1970, Papanek 1973). For a more general discussion of women as an invisible and 'muted group', see Dube *et al.* 1986 and Ardener 1975.

rity. If she had chosen a more confrontational approach, such as answering back to Sureshkaka or lifting her veil, this would have been viewed so badly that it is doubtful if she would ever have obtained her parents' sympathy or support. But in choosing the apparently innocent gesture of wearing a cardigan, she was in the advantageous position of appearing like an innocent victim, denied a basic right and forced to go cold. Her refusal either to eat or to speak played on the guilty conscience and ultimate helplessness of her in-laws, as did her threat of suicide which was delivered to the neighbour and to me, on the assumption that it would get back via one of us to the rest of the family. This it did, and she was soon able to speak to her brother and leave the house on the pretext of her father's supposed illness. Unhappy though she was with the oppressively patriarchal environment in which she lived, Hansa was by no means the helpless victim of the incident. She was carefully manipulating events in her own subtle way.

This raises interesting questions about the role of clothes in female disputes generally. Where women are confined to the house in an essentially male-dominated culture, control of their own bodies – whether through starving, becoming mute, withdrawing sexual favours or dressing in a provocative way – becomes one of the few means by which they can assert their wishes, sorrows and desires. As actors, inventive women can even find means of reworking the very institutions that stand against them. For example, their own dependence on their men for jewellery and clothes can be exploited by women who try to bribe their husbands into providing such adornment. Similarly the restrictive custom of *laj*, in which a woman is expected to withdraw herself from view, can be used at times when a woman is expected to be on display but does not wish to be seen. Although the veil conceals women, it does not deprive them of a means of expression (Sharma 1978b: 224). It can be drawn out of defiance and flirtation as much as modesty. This was beautifully illustrated by a popular song performed in a local drama in a neighbouring village. It depicted a desperate man with two wives who were denying him access to their bodies unless he gave them each the most expensive gold necklace available in the city. He was trying to approach them with offers of mere bangles and earrings, but they swivelled away from him every time, both flirting and taking refuge under their veils, swearing that they would never come out of *ghunghut* until their wish for the necklaces was fulfilled. Finally the man, exasperated by these two shrouded women, was forced to agree to the purchases.

Despite the numerous prescriptions and restrictions concerning how a woman should dress, it is clear that some women do not blindly follow the expectations of their seniors and, like Hansaben, are prepared to put up a challenge. Similarly, some women in central India siphon off money in their conjugal homes and then purchase jewellery which they later pretend has been given to them by their parents (Jacobson 1976: 165). Using such indirect methods, they can accumulate new apparel without their in-laws' approval or consent. In Hindi movies clothing often arises as a subversive issue for women, as for example when an urban girl defiantly appears in jeans instead of a sari when her undesirable prospective husband pays her a visit.[19] Just as Gandhi used clothes to shock and to challenge British authority, so Hansa from her subordinate position could assert at least a little independence by rebelling through the apparently innocent medium of dress.

Brahman considerations

To what extent are the clothing disputes of Sureshkaka's household unique unto themselves, and to what extent are they symptomatic of more general caste and village dilemmas? Certainly every household in Jalia had its own concept of acceptable and unacceptable clothing, but it seemed that in wealthy, orthodox families like Sureshkaka's men played a much greater part in deciding what their women should wear. This sartorial power was reinforced by *laj* restrictions which ensured that married women did not leave the house except for festive occasions, and which were strictest among wealthy families of the *Darbar* and *Brahman* castes.

Darbar women, if their families could afford it, were entirely secluded, living in separate quarters from their men and dressing in comparatively plain and simple clothes. As a group they were not on the whole either very fashionable or well educated. It was *Vaniya* and a few wealthy *Brahman* families who were considered the most modern and progressive people in the village. In particular, the *Vaniya* took the fashion lead. They favoured pale-coloured, flimsy textured synthetic saris, preferably from 'Foren', and the more foreign the better. In general, a Jalia-bought sari was spurned, a Larabad sari was more or less acceptable, an Ahmedabad or Bombay sari could be desirable, and one from America or Japan was highly coveted. It was usually impossible to determine the origin of a sari purely on the basis of its appearance, since patterns and prints from all over the world are successfully reproduced in India. But the point about a new sari is that people *discuss* it. They ask its price, they feel its texture, they demand to know where it was bought and where it was made, and it is usually only

19 The role of clothes in Hindi cinema is a fascinating subject that merits a study in itself. While at one time virtuous women were almost always dressed in Indian styles, the heroines of the 1980s and '90s have a chameleon-like quality and have generally worked their way through an immensely varied wardrobe by the end of the film.

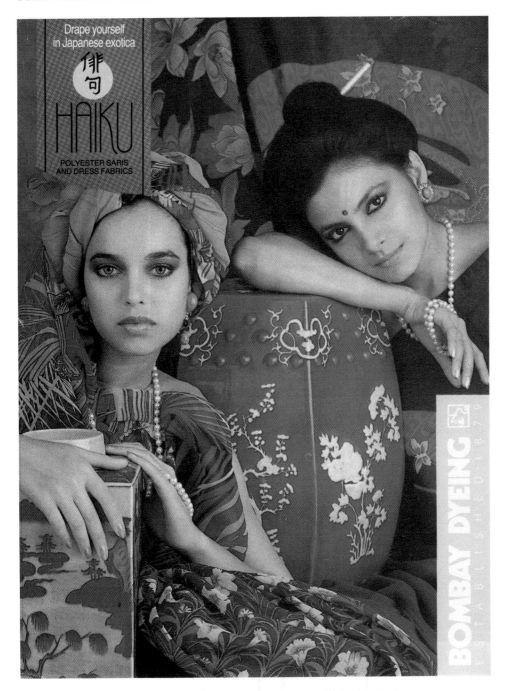

Fig. 6.3 Advertisement for 'exotic' saris from Japan, 1989. Courtesy of Bombay Dyeing.

after accumulating this knowledge that they assess its true desirability.[20] A popular fashion in 1989 was floral prints in pale greens and blues known as *angreji reng* (English colours).

For the youth of the village, *Vaniya* girls were looked on both as trendies and as trend-setters. Some went to college in Larabad and bought city fashions of shiny *shalwar kamizes* which they wore for going to town or for special events. They tended to put on make-up and nail-varnish and some even cut their hair in modern styles and spent time in Larabad beauty parlours where they learned about the latest beauty tips and had their eyebrows shaped. These were expensive, luxury pursuits with which few other people bothered. The *Panchayat* (village council) secretary's two daughters, who were *Brahman*, also followed such fashions, but they had been living in the industrial city of Rajkot until four years earlier. Rajkot was, they nostalgically explained, a 'forward-looking place'. The government doctor's daughters (also *Brahman*) wore *shalwar kamizes* for special occasions, but they too had come to Jalia only recently and had been brought up in a town. At home during the day such girls dressed simply in full-length skirts or 'maxis' which were considered more appropriate to the village.

On the whole, *Brahman* men seemed far stricter than *Vaniya* fathers about what their children should or should not wear. Comparatively few allowed their daughters to wear the *shalwar kamiz* which, as we have seen with Leriben, was considered improper by some village men. The question of whether or not a girl should be allowed to wear such a garment often boiled down to the question of how far she should be educated. At the time when Leriben had completed her seventh standard, higher education was not available in the village. Any further education meant travelling by bus to college in Larabad, and this in turn entailed a change of clothes. As Leriben explained, 'We cannot wear our maxis or skirts to the town. All the college would laugh at us and call us village people. At college almost every girl wears a *shalwar kamiz*. And those who do not wear it, dress in "midis" or frocks. If I went in a maxi, I would be the laughing-stock and people would insult my father's name.'

Sending a daughter to college entailed breaking two major village taboos, quite apart from embracing the radical assertion that female education was desirable or necessary. The first taboo was allowing a daughter to travel by bus, a risk few fathers were prepared to take for fear that it would spoil their daughter's reputation and hence that of the family. The second was

---

20 The words 'export quality' have very positive connotations in India, and are often stamped prominently on new clothing which is worn with the logo showing.

192

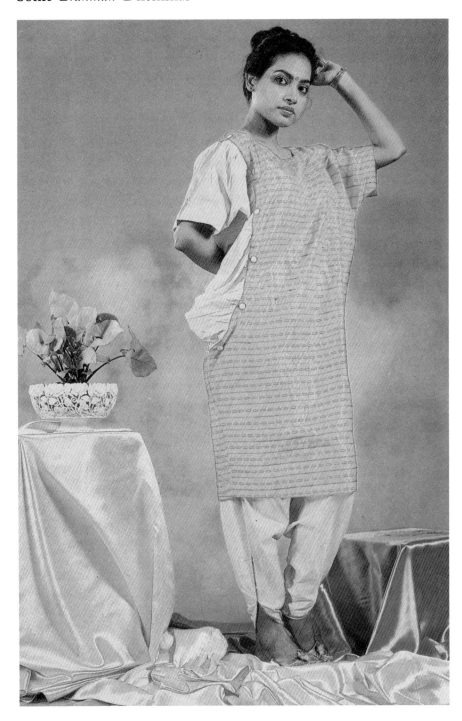

Fig. 6.4 Desirable images: shiny synthetic *shalwar kamiz* of the type worn by some *Brahman* and *Vaniya* girls, but objected to by some villagers. Courtesy of *Sweet Sixteen* fashion catalogue, 1989.

193

allowing one's daughter to wear a *shalwar kamiz*, contradicting the local assumption that only Muslims wore trousers while Hindus always dressed in skirts and bodices or saris. In theory, the breaking of these taboos should have been no more difficult for a *Brahman* family than a *Vaniya* one, but two factors combined to ensure that they were. First, the *Vaniyas*, with their long-standing trading links outside the village, were more in touch with urban attitudes and ideas. Indeed many *Vaniya* families had left the village for Bombay and other cities, leaving their Jalia homes empty for much of the year. Those who remained made frequent trips to visit relatives, and their women were expected to conform more to urban ideals in fashion and education than village ones. Secondly, the *Vaniyas* did not hold the traditional religious functions of the *Brahmans* and this gave them a greater freedom of expression. The specific dilemma of wealthy *Brahman* families like Sureshkaka's seemed to revolve around their connection to the priesthood, which still persisted at some level. And although many *Brahman* men now held professional, clerical or trading positions, there was a general feeling among ex-priestly *Brahmans* that the ritual status of the caste had to be ensured by maintaining high moral standards and adherence to a strict code of Hindu practice.[21] One means of doing this was through keeping married women in seclusion and ensuring that even unmarried girls in their teens did not venture into the streets, so tarnishing their families' reputations. Such girls should be modestly dressed and as little visible as possible. But this presented a fundamental dilemma, for such families saw themselves not merely as upholders of tradition but also as modern and forward-thinking as opposed to the more 'backward' farming and labouring castes. Being *sudharo* (progressive), however, meant educating one's women, recognising the value of literacy and rejecting certain age-old village customs such as the total covering of the bride during the wedding ceremony. Yet such enlightened attitudes entailed accepting new forms of clothing and, above all, new canons of modesty.

A fundamental problem for many villagers, but one perhaps felt most acutely by well-to-do *Brahmans*, was the clash between the conflicting values of the village and the city on the sensitive issue of female modesty in dress. This concept of modesty was in a state of flux, and those who lived in villages but harboured urban aspirations were to some extent caught between two contradictory models. In the 1930s, according to Darling, the fashionable clothes worn by élite Punjabi girls were the equivalent

21 This would not have been the case among agricultural *Brahman* groups like the *Pariwal Brahmans*, found in other parts of the district. Their women apparently dressed and behaved like farming women and were looked down upon by *Brahman* families in Jalia.

of a prostitute's garb to most other villagers (Darling 1934: 84). Similarly in Jalia the *shalwar kamiz*, which some high-caste people consider the most fashionable dress, is also considered the least reputable by other villagers' standards. For few people have adopted the criteria of modesty that the *shalwar kamiz* demands.

At the beginning of the twentieth century women in Jalia wore, as we have seen, a backless bodice (*kapdu*) which left the entire back exposed to view. This was considered desirable as it allowed air to circulate. It was only as the century progressed that high-caste women began to feel embarrassed at such exposure and took to wearing full blouses, often with long sleeves. Parsi women in Bombay were considered important trend-setters in Indian women's fashion. Billington describes them as wearing petticoats 'of white lawn or batiste, or even silk all frilled and laced, and a bodice of silk or material cut after the English or French patterns, though without the extravagances of exaggerated sleeves or high stiff collars' (Billington 1973 [1895]: 180–1). Lace and silk blouses, adopted by the Indian élite, gradually took the form of the more familiar short *choli* (blouse) which is something of a compromise between the Indian bodice and the European blouse.

The backless bodice (*kapdu*) was formerly worn by high-caste women with a long petticoat and a half-sari (*sadlo*) wrapped once around the body and over the head. Thus the modest well-bred woman had her back uncovered but her face and head concealed beneath a veil, and her legs well hidden beneath large quantities of cloth in the form of a long silk skirt (*chaniyo*). Some groups in Jalia, such as the *Bharwads* (shepherds), continue to expose their backs and cover their faces in this way, but they are considered the most *deshi* and least educated people in the village. The new model of female behaviour and appearance that is promoted among the local educated urban élite calls for precisely the opposite canons of modesty and exposure. Influenced by a Western and, more specifically, Victorian tradition, it requires that the back should be covered but the head and face exposed. It asserts that the uncovered back is naked and indecent (cf. Billington 1973 (1895): 178) but the covered face is backward and oppressive. Progressive local urban men are therefore expected to allow their women to walk in the streets bare-headed and to forswear the custom of *laj* not merely during the marriage ceremony but also in everyday life. They are also expected to condone female education and the new styles of clothes thought appropriate to the college-going girl. This, of course, includes the *shalwar kamiz* which covers the entire body and cannot therefore be considered too revealing, although, as we have seen, it can be

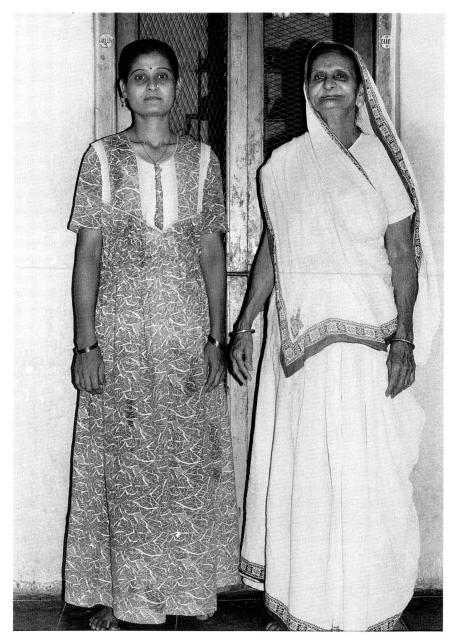

Fig. 6.5 Mother and daughter from a priestly *Brahman* family, 1989. The daughter wears a cotton maxi inside the house and a sari on the rare occasions that she leaves the house. Her father, who officiates as a priest and usually wears a fine *dhoti* and *kurta*, does not allow her to wear the *shalwar kamiz* on the grounds that it is 'Muslim dress'. The mother wears principally white saris, having taken a vow to dress plainly.

thought too masculine, too Muslim, or too much like something that the undiscriminating *Vaghris* might wear. Still more progressive local urban fathers allow their daughters to wear Western-style skirts ('midis') and dresses ('frocks') but these play more serious havoc with convention, since they expose the lower leg, which in high-caste village terms is a sign of immodesty and lack of refinement, found only among the lower castes.[22]

Sureshkaka's frustration about how the women of his household should dress arose because he sought appraisal from both the village and the city simultaneously. Yet what was socially upgrading in wider national terms was morally downgrading in local terms. This was not so great a problem for *Vaniya* families, who were more concerned with their urban reputations than with the attitidues of villagers. It was also less of a consideration with the *Darbars* or the farming castes because the identity of these women was still essentially village-based and mostly little interest was shown in their education. But well-to-do *Brahman* parents wanted their daughters to be educated and modern yet at the same time to preserve their reputations for modesty in the village. Furthermore, the more religious-minded among them regarded the *shalwar kamiz* as a minor sacrilege, not because it broke some Hindu rule about the sanctity of unstitched cloth, but for the simple reason that it was more commonly worn by Muslims.

The women of Sureshkaka's family were therefore in the difficult position of having to conform to contradictory role-models in two quite different spheres. Hansaben and Leriben occupied the opposite sides of the same dilemma. Hansaben had been reared and educated in the city and was now having to mould herself to village life whereas Leriben, brought up in the village, was expected to adapt to becoming a college girl in the city. The only solution to this problem was either to risk offending one group or another by one's choice of clothes or, like Leriben, to change one's clothes to suit the specific demands of each sphere.

Changing one's style of clothes to suit the situation was, as we have seen, an extremely popular solution for men in the late nineteenth and early twentieth centuries. This is not to say that women at that time were *entirely* unfamiliar with the option. Billington wrote of her frustration at finding that her visits to Indian households were often 'expected', which meant people had dressed up for the occasion. She found Indian girls in frocks and bonnets, stripy stockings and German shoes, although she does not mention whether adult women ever deserted Indian styles on such occasions

---

22 According to the *dharmashastras* which emphasise high-caste orthodox Hindu ideals, a woman's garments should extend to her ankles (Leslie 1993: 201).

(Billington 1973 [1895]: 177). One woman who *did* temporarily cast aside her Indian dress was Swarup Rani, wife of Motilal Nehru, who adopted European dress when she accompanied him to Europe in 1905 (SWMN vol. 1: 61). She later changed back into a sari for her return to India. But maintaining more than one style of clothing was, till recently, relatively unusual for most Indian women. While it has become a well-established practice among cosmopolitan urban élites, it is only now beginning to emerge among women of the village élite. Its emergence coincides with and is an integral part of the changing expectations of women in contemporary Indian society.

Till recently, the lives of most rural women were confined to the house, the village or the farm. Though involving much hard labour, work in these spheres did not require women to step outside their caste role in the same way that male jobs often did. And since women were usually denied education, they were not introduced to many alternative role-models in the way that young boys were when they attended school. But recent attempts to encourage female education even among villagers is leading to a multiplication of roles for women and a new multiplication of clothing styles. As Leriben pointed out, she could not risk her reputation in the city by appearing at college in 'village dress'. She therefore needed an alternative set of clothes for going to Larabad. Her most traumatic time was waiting at the village bus stop, dressed in a *shalwar kamiz* and listening to the insults of other villagers. It was the age-old problem of what to wear in the border territory between one sphere and another, a problem familiar to many Indian men earlier in the twentieth century.

The question of when to change one's clothes is often, as we have seen, linked to the wider question of where to draw the boundary between public and private presentations of self. Till recently, North Indian married women experienced this dilemma differently from men, not only because they circulated less in social and geographic terms but also because they always wore some form of veil, which enabled them to draw the public/ private dichotomy around their own bodies. Being portable and obligatory, it provided the constant possibility of slipping into the private sphere at any given moment. Muslim women who wear the *shalwar kamiz* and *dupatta* (veil/scarf) maintain this same possibility of withdrawal. But a Hindu girl who wears a *shalwar kamiz* in a place like Jalia does so partly as a gesture of emancipation and an indication of her fashion-consciousness, and it is no longer considered appropriate for her to hide her face. Furthermore, the *dupatta* she wears is often little more than a thin decorative strip of cloth which acts more as a fashion accessory than as a means of concealment.

Some *Brahman* Dilemmas

Dressed thus, she has in effect lost both her means of protection and her right to it. She therefore remains both visible and exposed.

This had some grave consequences for Leriben. Having completed her schooling, she was all set to attend sewing classes in Larabad when one day a youth followed her in the city and tried to talk to her at the Larabad bus station. She threatened him with her sandal and he soon left her in peace. But there were young men from Jalia who had witnessed the event which, though totally unprovoked by Leriben, blemished her reputation. Had she been wearing a sari or half-sari, she might have been able to retreat into *laj*, but as it was she stood blatantly exposed to view and publicly humiliated. When she told her parents of the event, her father and brother decided that she must never take the bus or go to Larabad again unless accompanied by her brother. Her sewing classes were cancelled and from this time onwards she was confined largely to the house, only occasionally entering the village. This event shows how young women who abandon the veil take a considerable risk in a culture where female modesty is still so highly prized and female honour so intensely vulnerable. For the veil not only conceals women but it also acts as a shelter (cf. Papanek 1973) in a world where even comparatively modern women are taught that they should not be seen too much.

Echoes of a colonial heritage

To what extent can one compare the clothing dilemmas of the women in Sureshkaka's family to those of the male Indian élite earlier in the twentieth century? And to what extent are women's contemporary dilemmas related to the colonial heritage? At first sight there are some parallels. Though on a different scale, the silent but persistent struggles of the women of the household may be compared to the struggles of Indian nationalists who, subordinated by the British presence, chose dress as a means of non-violent but provocative rebellion. Furthermore in Hansaben's case the central focus of the dispute was a cardigan, a Western garment, suggesting that European dress is still a provocative issue in India today. But the parallels are not as self-evident, as they at first appear. It was not, for example, the Western aspect of Hansa's dress that was at issue. Her cardigan was perceived as being a *city* style rather than a *European* one, and much of the dispute revolved around questions of modesty and visibility more than style as such. Like the Gandhi cap, the symbolic value of the cardigan was cumulative, being constructed more through the actions and behaviour of those around it than through any stylistic features or properties of the garment itself.

The case of Leriben's dress presents a different problem. At first sight the question of whether she should wear a *shalwar kamiz* or some form of sari appears unrelated to colonial issues. Both garments are clearly Indian, suggesting that her problem of choice was purely an internal Indian affair – as indeed it was. However, the conflicting ideas of modesty and modernity that these different sartorial options embodied have their echoes in the colonial encounter. Cohn has discussed disputes in Travancore in South-West India in the mid-nineteenth century, when Protestant missionaries encouraged low-caste *Nadar* women, who had converted to Christianity, to cover their previously naked breasts. By covering their breasts these women, though conforming to European standards of decency, were breaking local hierarchical codes whereby they were expected to keep their breasts naked in front of *Brahmans* as a sign of respect (Cohn 1983a: 78–87). With the exception of the missionaries, the British made few direct attempts to interfere with Hindu women's dress, but British sartorial values were none the less invasive.

Although Leriben's problem of how to dress was entirely removed from direct contact with Europeans or Christians, it was, all the same, intimately bound up with the indirect historical consequences of both Muslim and British rule. The *shalwar kamiz* was perceived as controversial in Jalia, partly because it was considered 'Muslim dress' and partly because it was thought immodest for a mature girl to keep her head uncovered. The idea that it is liberal and advanced for women to expose their heads and faces is of course handed down from the British, who were shocked by veiling restrictions and the high-caste practice of female seclusion. Though not perceived in these terms, the dispute over how Leriben should dress was part of a long historical confrontation between opposing cultural values. To Leriben, the dispute was framed in terms of the conflict between 'traditional' village values as opposed to educated urban ones. But these educated urban values were, in turn, informed by the values of the cosmopolitan Indian élite who were the closest followers, though also the sharpest critics, of British attitudes and behaviour during the colonial period (cf. Srinivas 1968: 51). As Ashis Nandy has shown, colonial values were not only *in*vasive but also *per*vasive. Part of the very forcefulness of the colonial encounter was the infusion of alien cultural ideas in such a way that they can no longer be disentangled from Indian thought. They have become part of Indian society itself (cf. Nandy 1983). Leriben's clothing dilemma could be couched in terms of a number of different dichotomies: rural/urban, uneducated/educated, local fashion/national fashion, Hindu/Muslim, Indian/British. None of these taken individually quite covers the issues involved, yet each pair has contributed to the web of cultural meanings which the disputes about Leriben's dress seem to embody.

Some *Brahman* Dilemmas

As Saurasthran women become increasingly educated and take a more active role in the public sphere, it is likely that the problem of what to wear will become increasingly difficult for them, at least during the period of transition. For, as we have seen, circulating in different spheres often requires a change of clothes and a permanent change of clothes is frequently perceived as a threat to cultural values. It is likely that women will resort increasingly to the popular solution of changing their dress to suit the situation.[23] At present, however, this remains a problem confined largely to educated girls who, in Jalia, represent a small minority. Peasant women, whose lives revolve more around the village and the farm, do not confront such issues. Their clothing dilemmas are of a different nature.

23 In Southall, West London, for example, many Indian women change out of their saris and into Western styles just for work, returning to their saris before entering their homes at the end of the day. Their men are aware of the practice but do not prevent it. They recognise it as a valuable compromise which allows their women both to earn a living in the outside world and retain their cultural allegiance within the home where an Indian identity can be more easily sustained.

7 Some Peasant Dilemmas (*Kanbi* and *Kharak*)

The problem of Liliben's ghaghros (skirts)

Liliben is a *Kharak* girl of approximately fourteen years old. When I first met her she and her mother were busy sorting the winter crop of groundnut that had just been harvested from their fields. Liliben's mother, a woman in her late thirties, was dressed in a brightly coloured skirt (*ghaghro*) and bodice (*kapdu*), both of which she had embroidered herself with colourful stitching and inserts of mirror. Over these she wore a printed half-sari (*sadlo*). Liliben, by contrast, was dressed in a thin polyester petticoat, a plain blouse with buttons down the front and a synthetic floral *sadlo* in bright blues and greens. Despite her youth she had been married for four years, but was not due to join her husband's family for another three. Even so, she claimed to have stocked up clothes and ornaments for her future trousseau. When I asked if she would make embroidered *ghaghros* like her mother, she looked at me with serious disapproval and told me that she would *never* wear a *ghaghro*, and did not even know how to make them. The *ghaghro* was, she claimed, 'the stuff of the past' (*pelanu vastu*), and no one like her would be seen in such an old-fashioned thing. When her mother left the courtyard, Liliben added proudly that *she* was the sort of person who could mix with foreigners like me. Others in her caste would not even be able to talk with me, but she was modern. Her trousseau would contain not 'village things' (*gamnu vastu*) but saris from Larabad city. That embroidery was something of the past.

As winter gave way to summer and the arrival of hot windy days when agricultural activity more or less came to its annual halt, I returned more frequently to Liliben's house and was surprised to find her sitting with her cousins on a string bed in the open courtyard, embroidering a long strip of red cloth that was obviously meant for a *ghaghro*.

'Whom is that *ghaghro* for?' I asked.

'It's for me,' she replied, a little sheepishly. 'It's for my trousseau. But I won't ever wear it. I just have to make it to take with me to my in-laws' house, but I'll never put it on.'

Despite her negative attitude to the garment, Liliben was a serious and experienced embroiderer and it turned out that she had already stitched five

202

Some Peasant Dilemmas (*Kanbi* and *Kharak*)

ghaghros and that this was the sixth.

'Why do you embroider them if you think you will never wear them?' I asked simplistically.

'Because I have to display them at my *anu* ceremony. It is our custom. We have to show some *ghaghros* in our caste,' she replied.

Liliben lived in a large extended family. Two of her cousins (her father's brothers' daughters) were due to make their ceremonial departure to their in-laws' homes later that summer and were therefore in the midst of diligently preparing gifts and clothes for their trousseaux. Like Liliben, they were embroidering *ghaghro* cloths, and like Liliben, they too insisted that they would not wear their *ghaghros* unless absolutely forced. Vasantben, one of the cousins, asserted:

'You see, it depends on the mother-in-law. If my mother-in-law is kind and lenient, then I won't have to wear my *ghaghros* until I am an old woman of thirty or so. If she is strict and narrow-minded, then she could make me wear them at twenty or twenty-five.'

Asked if she would ever resist her mother-in-law's decision, she replied:

'How could I do that? If the mother-in-law insists, then I have to obey. But most mothers-in-law are good. They won't make us wear these *ghaghros* because they are no longer in fashion. They are for old women now. We don't even know how to put them on. Look at the *Kanbi* girls. They have advanced. They wear saris now.'

As the summer progressed and *anu* preparations reached a frenzied height, Vasantben's *ghaghro* embroidery was hanging up in the verandah, awaiting the finishing touches to be added by a tailor who had set up his equipment at her house (fig. 7.1). She had embroidered cloth for eleven *ghaghros* which she seemed to regard with a strange combination of pride and embarrassment – pride at the craftswomanship, but embarrassment at the prospect that she might one day have to wear the products of her labour.

This embarrassment did not prevent her from leaning over the tailor and supervising his stitching of the *ghaghro* borders. These machine-made borders seemed to excite her more than her own handiwork. And indeed they were more complex and intricate than those worn by older women. They consisted of extravagant quantities of different-coloured cloth strips, piled up in layers and one wider band of cloth, decorated with machine-embroidered motifs. Far from ousting hand-embroidery, machine-embroidery coexisted with it within the same garment, but whereas in older *ghaghros* the machine-sewn borders were narrow and fairly plain, in the new *ghaghros* they were two

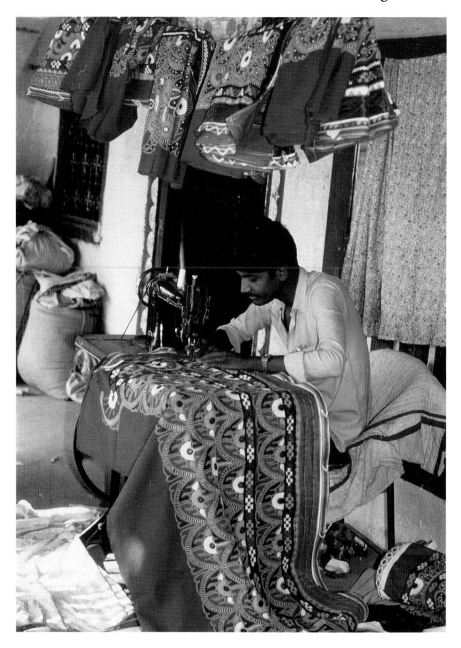

Fig. 7.1 A *Kharak* tailor stitches borders on to a girl's hand-embroidered *ghaghro* cloth in preparation for her trousseau, 1989. Her other trousseau *ghaghros* are seen hanging on the line above the tailor's head.

Some Peasant Dilemmas (*Kanbi* and *Kharak*)

or three times the previous width and complex in design.

Once the tailor had finished stitching the borders and had made up the embroidered cloths into complete skirts, Vasantben became quite proud of her *ghaghros*, but the idea of wearing them remained a sore point. Once I asked her to put one on and she had difficulty adjusting the garment and had to call for her mother's assistance. She and her companions soon fell about laughing and Vasantben complained that the skirt was too heavy and she could not walk with it on. Within a minute it was consigned to the bed. Vasantben's curious attitude seemed less an individual whim than part of a consensus shared among the new generation of *Kharak* women and girls, for whenever I visited *Kharak* families I invariably found girls preparing *ghaghros* but reluctant to wear them. A common complaint was that they were too *jada* (thick, heavy) or simply that the 'fashion had gone'. There was a strange disjunction between the extraordinary amount of time spent embroidering *ghaghros* and the adamant insistence that they would never be worn.

Pride in the *ghaghro* revealed itself not only in the act of embroidering when women and girls sat together discussing stitches and motifs, but also at the main *anu* ceremony when the entire trousseau[1] was displayed to relatives and friends. The *ghaghros* were usually either laid out on string beds or hung on a rope, but whatever the particular form of display they always occupied a prominent place, even though an additional twenty-odd saris were provided for the immediate wear of the new wife who nowadays was considered too young to wear a *ghaghro* immediately on reaching her conjugal home.[2]

1 Listed below are the contents of Vasantben's trousseau, which was fairly representative of those given to *Kharak* girls in Jalia in 1989:
   Clothes and household goods. 11 embroidered *ghaghros* (made by Vasantben), 21 saris with 21 matching blouses and petticoats, plastic bangles and bangle box, silver anklets, 70 steel vessels, 1 brass water pot, 1 quilt, 2 bed covers, 1 mattress, 1 wedding stool, 1 metal plaited dowry chest, 1 electric wall clock, 1 wooden display cabinet.
   Ornaments and decorations (made by her). Plastic beaded ornaments, crocheted cloth, embroidered door-curtain, hangings for above the door (1 embroidered, 1 sequined, 1 made from glass straws), 1 embroidered wedding canopy, 2 plastic straw mobiles, 4 sequined photograph frames, 2 plastic woven bags, 2 glass straw bags.
2 In the 1960s peasant girls were still wearing their embroidered *ghaghros* and *kapdus* as soon as they reached their conjugal home. Parmar, who has collected a number of folk songs in the area, records a song, sung by local women:
   Ghaghros, embroidered with flowers and fruits and lace on the head we have not yet worn, but will wear when we go to our in-law's home.
   Kapdus, embroidered with mirrors and beads, we have not yet worn, but will wear when we go to our in-laws' home.
   Chundadi from Navanagar, decorated with parrots and peacocks, we have not yet worn, but will wear when we go to our in-law's home (Parmar 1969: 13).

Embarrassment about *ghaghros*, on the other hand, revealed itself not only in women's reluctance to wear them but also in their attitude towards my embroidering a *ghaghro* myself. They laughed in disbelief when I expressed a willingness to learn, and Liliben's mother commented:

'You don't want to bother with such things. You know how to read and write. Why should you make *deshi* (local) embroidery? That is only for we people who know nothing. Liliben has not even studied one book.'[3]

Despite a certain reluctance, she began to teach me the process and soon became enthusiastic about my efforts. Other *Kharak* women would sometimes visit the house and I would visit their houses, and reactions to my embroidering seemed at once to fluctuate between pleasure, enthusiasm and thorough disapproval. Some women would tell me I was wasting my time and that embroidery would ruin my eyesight. Commonly I was told: 'Yoghurt will form in the brain.' Meanwhile men informed me that *deshi* embroidery was only for illiterates and that it would drive me *pagal* (mad) or that my mind would turn to water. But some women, both young and old, would be pleased that I was learning and would supervise my progress and criticise my stitches with interest. They seemed convinced that I was making the *ghaghro* for my own trousseau, although they found it difficult to believe that any woman in her mid-twenties would ever find a husband. One rather more sceptical woman informed her friends that I would cut it up and make it into handbags or *shalwar kamiz* decorations which I would sell in 'Foren' for a profit. She, like other women, was aware that embroidery had become high fashion in the cities and the cinema in recent years. Whereas in the 1970s her embroidered skirts were almost worthless in commercial terms, by 1989 they could fetch between 100 and 150 rupees each. But *Kharak* women rarely sold their *ghaghros*, unlike *Kanbi* women who would sell large quantities of embroidery to passing traders.[4]

3   The common local manner of ascertaining someone's standard of education was to ask them how many books they had studied. 'No books' meant total illiteracy whereas 'ten books' meant highly educated.

4   It has been suggested that for Greek peasant women the lace they made for their trousseaux performed the dual function of indicating status and acting as a form of currency that could be stored and used in times of economic distress (Schneider 1980). Similarly it has been shown that Gujarati women are sometimes forced to sell their embroidery in times of drought (Hitkari 1981; foreword, Nanavati *et al.* 1966). But farming women in Jalia disputed the idea that embroidery had ever been a useful form of wealth in the past, and argued that till recently nobody wanted to buy *deshi* embroidery which had backward connotations and was only village stuff. If peasant women needed money, it was valuable things like gold earrings which were pawned or sold, not embroidery. Nowadays, with the emergence of new ethnic fashions among the Indian élite, embroidered clothes and wall-hangings are recognised as valuable commodities. But despite this, women in Jalia, unlike those in some other parts of Gujarat, were not willing to embroider expressly for sale. They felt that the payment would be insufficient for the labour involved.

Some Peasant Dilemmas (*Kanbi* and *Kharak*)

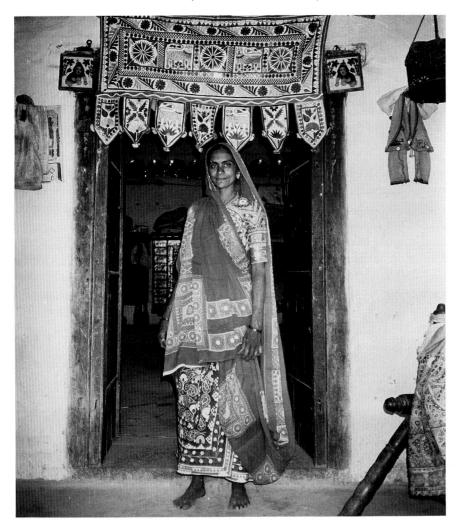

Fig. 7.2 A *Kharak* woman, wearing a hand-embroidered *ghaghro* and *kapdu*, standing in the doorway of her home which is decorated with an embroidered *toran* (door hanging), 1989. Wishing to look her best for the photograph (her first), she has changed into a new un-worn *ghaghro* which she has just taken out of her trousseau chest for the occasion. The faded *ghaghro* she was wearing a few minutes earlier is visible in the right-hand corner of the picture. Women usually wear their *ghaghros* until they are tatty and threadbare. They tend to keep two in use at any one time, storing the others for festival days and for the future.

Although in Jalia it is mostly *Kharak* women in their twenties, thirties and forties who wear embroidery today, embroidered clothes were never the exclusive preserve of the *Kharak* caste. In earlier times, wealthy élites had worn embroidered silks and till recently many other groups in the district were wearing embroidery (cf. Parmar 1969). Women of the *Kanbi, Karadiya Rajput, Pariwal Brahman* and *Koli* castes all wore a similar type of embroidered *ghaghro*, usually made from red *khadi* cloth and embroidered with silk threads and mirror inserts (*ibid.*). It was considered a practical garment since it was thick and durable and did not tear easily when they worked in the fields. In Jalia the two groups most renowned for such embroidery were the *Kanbis* and the *Kharaks*.

It is likely that historically *Kanbi* women were making embroidered *ghaghros* before *Kharak* women,[5] yet nowadays young *Kanbi* women no longer either make or wear them but instead purchase synthetic saris which they wear with plain blouses and petticoats, these being the only clothes they display in their trousseaux. Even some older-generation *Kanbi* women have ceased to wear embroidery[6] and are now disparaging about it, seeing it as a sign of backwardness. While a few elderly women still take pride in their embroidered heritage, others dismiss the *ghaghro* as 'Kharak dress' as if it has little to do with the *Kanbi* caste.

Why in recent years has the appearance of the two castes diverged so markedly, with *Kanbi* wives now wearing synthetic saris and *Kharak* wives modernised versions of the embroidered *ghaghro*, even if often reluctantly? What factors encouraged one group to modernise the *ghaghro* and the other to reject it? And why, in view of the reluctant attitude of young *Kharak* women, do the *Kharaks* continue to embroider *ghaghros* at all?

In order to explore these questions, it is necessary first to describe the clothing and adornment that *Kanbi* and *Kharak* women used to share, and to trace its evolution according to changes in technology and design since the 1940s. These changes are analysed in relation to parallel changes found in tattoos and in other hand-made items that women prepare for their trousseaux. The attitudes of these women both to their clothing and to

5 According to local geneologists, the *Kharaks* were originally a trading community who migrated from Rajasthan to Gujarat (cf. Seth 1980). Seth suggests that they probably learned both embroidery and agriculture from other farming groups, including the *Kanbis* (*ibid.*).

6 In the 1970s many *Kanbi* women bartered their embroidery for stainless steel vessels. These were hawked to villages by itinerant traders (*pheriyos*), who were gathering embroidery chiefly for the export market. Because women were not used to viewing their embroidery commercially, they often parted with large quantities for a mere steel bowl, and some even gave it away. For discussion of the process by which such embroidery entered the national and international market arena, see Tarlo, forthcoming.

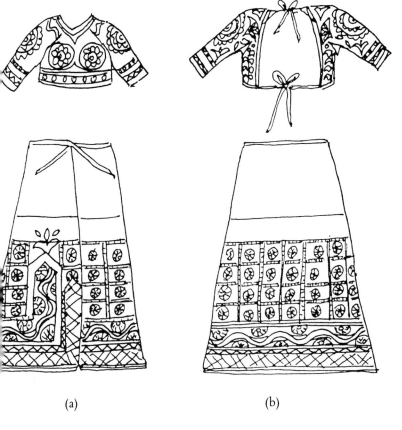

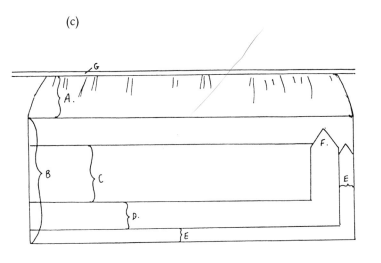

(a)

(b)

(c)

Fig. 7.3 Diagram showing the structure of the *ghaghro* and *kapdu*.

(a) Front view of a *ghaghro* and *kapdu*.

(b) Back view of a *ghaghro* and *kapdu*, showing the strings which tie round the neck and back, leaving the flesh of the back exposed to view.

(c) Diagram showing the structure of the *ghaghro*.

A = *chadavo*
B = *choliyu*
C = main hand-embroidered area
D = hand-embroidered border (*kor*)
E = machine-embroidered border
F = open flap (*vadkyu*)
G = string (*kaso*) which is tucked in rather than tied

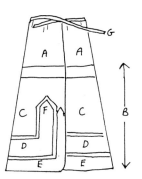

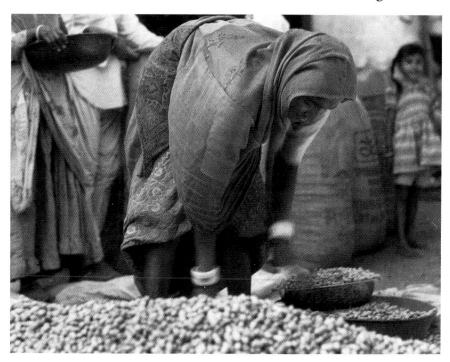

Fig. 7.4 A *kharak* woman sorting out ground-nut, 1989. To perform this task, she has folded back the hem of her *ghaghro*, thereby enabling ease of movement and the circulation of air. This also protects the embroidery which is folded back on itself.

their environment afford some insight into the reasons why the *Kanbis* and *Kharaks* have taken divergent sartorial paths.

Kanbi and Kharak dress (1940)[7]

A *Kanbi* or *Kharak* woman's outfit in Jalia in the 1940s consisted of *ghaghro* (wrapped skirt), *kapdu* (bodice), *sadlo* (veil), jewellery and tattoos.

The *ghaghro* was a wrap-around skirt, composed of two horizontal strips of red *khadi* cloth stitched together, the lower piece heavy and embroidered, the upper piece lighter and plain (see fig. 7.3).[8] The upper section was

---

7   This account refers specifically to the clothing and embroidery of the *Kanbi* and *Kharak* woman of Jalia. Their traditions are of course inserted within the wider context of regional clothing traditions. For a detailed account of the clothing and embroidery of Saurashtra people generally, see Parmar (1969). For a more specific account of the embroidery and decorative arts of the *Kharak* caste in Saurashtra, see Seth (1980). Both of these works are heavily illustrated and provide more extensive visual documentation than can be included here. I am grateful to both these scholars for our many fruitful discussions on embroidery.

8   Parmar (1969) and Seth (1980) use the term *ghaghro* to refer to a stitched skirt, reserving the word *chaniyo* for the type of wrap-around skirt described above. However, I have used the terminology favoured by women in Jalia.

slightly gathered at the top and given a string band. Embroidery always ran parallel to the width of the cloth, turning at a right angle at one end where it climbed vertically to form a triangular peak (*vadkyu*). A machine-made border ran parallel to the hand-made border along the bottom edge. The *ghaghro* was worn by being wrapped around the body so that the embroidered peak (*vadkyu*) fell at the front. The ties were then tucked into the body and the whole garment was hitched up an inch or two and tucked in at the waist. The weight of the garment prevented it from flapping wide open and the tightness of the tucking prevented it from falling down. While labouring in the fields or doing household chores, women usually folded back the hems of their skirts, which they tucked in at the waist (see fig. 7.4). This allowed them easy movement, but it also revealed most of the lower leg and was considered unrefined by high-caste groups. Nowadays young women who do not wish to wear a *ghaghro* claim that they are frightened of it falling down and that they do not know *how* to wear it.

The *ghaghro* was worn with a *kapdu*, a short bodice which covered a woman's front but was left entirely open at the back. It was held in place by two sets of strings, rather like a bikini top. These *kapdus* could be plain but were often wholly or partly embroidered and were generally made from satin or silk. While some young *Kharak* women still wear plain or embroidered *kapdus* today, young *Kanbi* women do not.

The *ghaghro* and *kapdu* were always accompanied by a *sadlo* (half-sari) wrapped once around the body and thrown over the head with the end piece falling forwards over the right shoulder. The *sadlos* worn by older farming women usually had blue and white floral and spotted patterns on a mud-red cotton background. Younger married women, however, wore a variety of brightly coloured *sadlos*.

A woman's outfit was never complete without her jewellery. In the 1940s this consisted of heavy silver ankle hoops, toe-rings, large white ivory bangles, a gold nose-ring and a variety of gold or silver earrings worn in the upper, lower and middle ear. Round their necks women wore threads, necklaces and pendants which varied according to their marital status. They never wore gold below their waists as this was considered an insult to Lakshmi, the goddess of wealth.

Tattoos (tajvus)
A woman's neck, lower arms, lower leg and part of her chest were usually covered in tattoos, the face bearing one spot on the cheek and one on the chin. Most of these tattoos consisted of small formations of dots in simple geometric forms or motifs, each with a name. According to most village

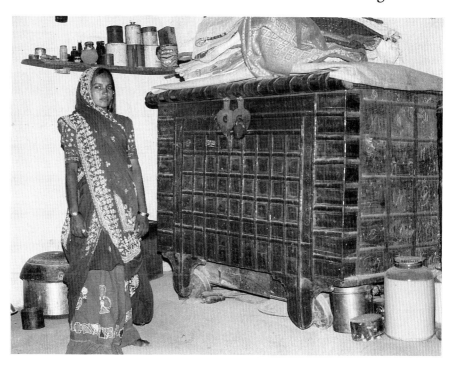

Fig. 7.5 A young *Kharak* girl beside her mother's dowry chest (*pataro*), 1989. She too has been given a similar chest which has been taken by truck to her in-laws' house after her *anu* ceremony earlier in the year. She wears a polyester petticoat, decorated with a few embroidered motifs, and a machine-embroidered half-sari. This is a fairly unusual outfit – most modern *Kharak* girls wear neither machine- nor hand-embroidery.

women today, these tattoos have always been purely decorative, although in the past there was considerable social pressure to have them. Without tattoos a woman used to attract rebukes like: 'Do your parents have so little grain that they don't even give you tattoos?' There was also the added fear that without tattoos she might be reborn as a camel. One woman suggested that the facial tattoo on the chin was important if a woman died since it prevented her from becoming naked and ensured that she would be identified as human rather than animal after death.[9] Some scholars have suggested that tattoos were also prophylactic marks, designed to protect a woman from the evil eye (*najar*) (Maloney 1976), but women themselves

9   Crooke recalls a similar belief that women are judged in the next life by whether they have tattoos. If not, they are told, they will never see their parents in the other world but be reborn as demons. He records a belief in the Central Provinces that women can sell the ornaments tattooed on their bodies in the next life and live off the proceeds (Crooke 1926: 298).

deny such explanations.[10] Unlike amulets or black threads, which are acknowledged to be protective, tattoos are today regarded as pure adornment. Even the belief in rebirth as a camel has attained the level of a saying without belief, at least in some cases. As one old lady put it:

'They *say* we will be reborn as a camel. But have you *seen* it? Have you ever seen anyone reborn as a camel? Have you? Have you? No? Well, then. That's what I was told when I was young but our young know better.'

Change in ghaghro design and motif (1940–1989)

Since embroidered clothing was the everyday wear of village women, there was no reason for them to preserve ancient pieces that might now provide historical insights into the origin of the tradition.[11] As we have seen, Jalia women were more interested in the demise of the craft than in its origins and this discussion is therefore confined to embroidery made in the past fifty years – which has made it possible to gain precise information on the embroidery made and worn by the different generations of villagers alive in the village today. Women of all generations were able to describe the contents of their own trousseaux and many still had examples of their trousseau embroidery stored in their dowry chests (see fig. 7.5). Thus recent

10 It is possible that the tattoo has undergone a process of secularisation over the years, having once had a protective function. According to the *Vishnu Purana* the custom of tattooing originated from the time when Lord Vishnu went to destroy a demon who was wreaking havoc in the three worlds (earth, nether world, heaven). His consort, Lakshmi, begged him not to leave her unprotected and to guard her against evils. Vishnu sketched on her body the figures of his weapons, the sun, the moon and the holy basil plant and ordained that any of his devotees who bore such marks would be free from danger and evil (Census of Gujarat 1961, vol. 5, pt. 6, no. 4: 18). Whether this story and the idea of protection did in the past influence women to have tattoos, it is difficult to assess. Writing in the 1920s, Crooke suggests that some tattoos are protective, some curative and others purely decorative (Crooke 1926: 196).

11 Despite the voluminous literature on the subject (cf. Nanavati *et al.* 1966, Dongerkery 1951, Irwin and Hall 1973, J. Jain 1982, Masselos n.d., Seth 1980, Parmar 1969, Gross and Fontana 1981, Dhamija 1964, 1988), little is known about the origins of embroidery in India. The *Rg. Veda* refers to embroidered garments (cf. Dhamija 1988) but existing samples do not predate the Moghul period. In Gujarat embroidery was clearly an established professional craft under the Moghuls and was taken up by Hindu men from the shoemaker caste (*Mochi*) who by the nineteenth century had established a distinctive style. This in turn is thought to have influenced and been influenced by the embroidery of rural women in Kutch and Saurashtra. Writing in 1838 without any of the modern nostalgia for rural life, Marianne Postans describes the appearance of Gujarati peasant women: 'Miserable and squalid, these time-worn crones yet retain the besetting vanity of womankind; and a love of personal adornment is betrayed by bodices interwoven with bits of looking-glass, and heavy bracelets of coloured ivory which, being worn in considerable number, rattle hideously together on their bare skinny arms' (Postans 1839 vol. 1: 195). I have been unable to find any early references to rural Saurashtran women's *ghaghros*.

Fig. 7.6 Diagram illustrating the stitches commonly found in hand-embroidered *ghaghro* borders.

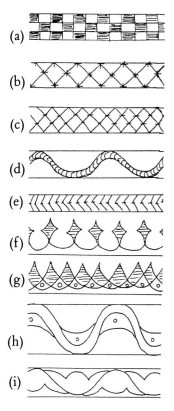

(a) *adadiya* (black gram)
(b) (c) *kanta* (thicket of thorns)
(d) *ardhakni* (half-closed eye)
(e) *jowla* (barley)
(f) *dodva* (buds)
(g) *dodva vel* (creeper of buds)
(h) *vijli vel* (wavering lightning)
(i) *kangsu* (comb)

changes in *ghaghro* design and motif could be discussed with the people who had actually embroidered them. While the structure of the *ghaghro* has remained stable over the fifty-year period, the motifs within that structure have undergone various changes. The following account describes *ghaghros* from the trousseaux of three generations of peasant women. The embroidery is dated according to the approximate time when the women first joined their husbands in Jalia, bringing their trousseaux with them.

Ghaghros in the 1940s and 1950s

In the 1940s and 1950s there was a fairly limited repertoire of *ghaghro* designs and motifs, with much repetition of certain basic stitching formations. Names were given not so much to individual stitches but to the eventual form that a combination of stitches resembled. Certain formations only appeared in the hand-stitched border while others tended to appear more on the main body of the embroidery. There was a strict system defining which colour of thread should be used for specific outlines or motifs. The framework of the border was always stitched in blue chain-stitch (*dori*) while other outlines were in yellow chain-stitch. Fig. 7.6 shows the types of stitch formation found in *ghaghros*' borders in the 1940s and 1950s. They bore the names *dana* (seeds), *dodva* (buds), *adadiya* (black gram), *jowla* (barley), *kanta* (thorns), *vijli vel* (wavering lightning), *ardhakhi* (half-closed eye) and *delo* (farmhouse door). These names referred mainly to aspects of the natural environment in which Jalia women lived. As agriculturalists, much of their year was spent weeding, harvesting and sorting the crops from their family farms, as well as grinding and preparing foodstuffs for the family's meals. The names of stitches appeared, then, to refer to the constituent elements of daily life: food, crops, plants, nature, the home.

Above the border, the main embroidered area was again decorated with a series of outlines, worked in yellow chain-stitch, often forming a square grid, always forming series of repeating patterns and motifs. Like the border area, the main area had its own grammar of stitches and forms which occurred repeatedly in different combinations (cf. Seth 1980). The most common motif was that of the *sikul* (circle or face), consisting of a small round mirror in the centre and a web of stitches flaring out from the mirror and forming a round. *Sikuls* were always yellow or white and were embroidered in cotton when all other threads were silk or imitation silk.

Besides *sikuls*, other common forms were largely taken from plants and animals. Where motifs were filled in, this was done in herringbone stitches in blue, green or pink silk thread. Colours were always alternated so that two never appeared consecutively. The overall effect of the embroidery

Some Peasant Dilemmas (*Kanbi* and *Kharak*)

was elaborate and highly colourful. Popular stitching configurations consisted largely of plant forms: *limbda* (neem leaf), *kevda* (fragrant flower), *dodva* (buds), *dana* (seeds), *badam* (almond), *keri* (mango), *bavaliya* (babul tree), and animal forms: *poput* (parrots), *mor* (peacock) and *dhel* (peahen), and *machli* (fish) (see fig. 7.7). A particular *ghaghro* was named according to the recurring central motif or composition of motifs on the main embroidered area. Fig. 7.8 shows four of the most popular *ghaghro* designs embroidered by wives who came to Jalia in the 1940s and 50s. The simple, fairly abstract motifs were first drawn on the lower cloth (*choliyu*) using a stick dipped in ink. This task was usually performed by a local woman, renowned for her skill in drawing. She would be paid a few annas or given some return service in exchange for marking the design. A woman would bring her own cloth to the specialist and would choose her own design from the local repertoire, which was learned from seeing other women's skirts. She would then embroider the outline in blue and yellow chain-stitch before filling in the motifs with bright blue, green and pink silk threads.

Women would start embroidering their first *ghaghro* cloth at the age of eight or nine, and many *Kanbi* and *Kharak* women who came to Jalia in the 1940s and '50s claimed to have completed more than fifteen embroidered *ghaghros* for their trousseaux. As the *anu* ceremony drew near, the bride's family would employ a tailor to do the finishing work. He would complete the *ghaghros* by attaching a strip of plain cloth and ties at the waist-band and by adding a simple machine-sewn border to the hem-line. Such borders were about the width of three fingers, consisting of a simple combination of layered, appliqué and stitched cloth arranged in a fixed format. The tailor would also stitch together pieces of embroidered cloth for the *kapdu* (bodice) and make other trousseau items such as quilts and borders for wall-hangings. Stitching charges were usually paid by the bride's in-laws.

After marriage, women would continue to embroider, particularly when they had daughters of their own who needed help in preparing their trousseaux. In the 1940s and '50s it was still possible to detect differences between the *ghaghros* worn by young wives and those worn by their mothers-in-law. Young wives wore the brightly coloured silk-embroidered ones, usually with green borders, whereas those of the mothers-in-law were simpler and embroidered mainly with cotton thread. The latter usually contained repeated patterns of interlacing stitch (*naka bharat*), with each *ghaghro* named according to its predominant stitch formation. Names of *naka ghaghros* were: *ladva* (sweet balls), *bavaliya* (babul tree), *panch phophal* (five betel nuts), *kankari phul* (spike and flower). Because they were embroidered in cotton and rarely contained inserts of mirror, these *ghaghros* were

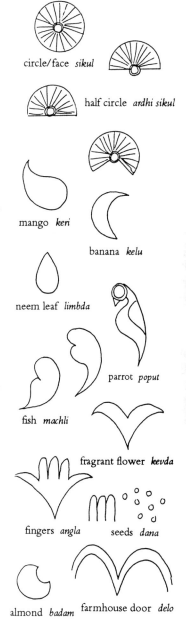

Fig. 7.7 Illustration of the motifs commonly found in the main embroidered area of the *ghaghro*. (1988)

circle/face *sikul*

half circle *ardhi sikul*

mango *keri*

banana *kelu*

neem leaf *limbda*

parrot *poput*

fish *machli*

fragrant flower *kevda*

fingers *angla*   seeds *dana*

almond *badam*   farmhouse door *delo*

215

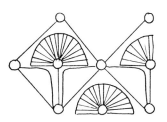

half flower garden *ardhi phulvadi*

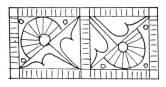

garden *bagicho*

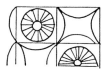
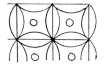

whole cotton pods *kala sakala*

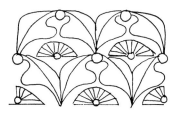

parrot creeper *poput vel*

considerably duller than those worn by younger women (see fig. 7.14a). Older women never wore green borders in their *ghaghros* or green *kapdus* since this colour was associated with youth and fertility. Those *kapdus* worn by old women today tend to be dark blue and pink, and are worn with plain red *khadi* waist-cloths and red and blue spotted *sadlos* (half-saris).

Ghaghros in the 1960s and 1970s
By the 1960s and '70s, the repertoire of *ghaghro* designs found in the trousseaux of new Jalia wives had both increased and diversified from the designs popular in the 1940s and '50s.[12] This did not involve rejection of the old designs and motifs, which continued to be embroidered. It was a case of adding to these rather than replacing them. Nor did it involve any radical departure from the structural framework of the embroidery or the stitching techniques. The grammar, as it were, remained the same. The change was in the increasing variety of new motifs that appeared within the old framework of the embroidery. These were no longer restricted to depictions of the natural environment (flowers, fruits, birds, lightning), and now included a number of mechanised objects such as radios, clocks, ceiling fans, aeroplanes, trains (fig. 7.9). Previously, the few man-made objects that had found their way into the *ghaghro* had been taken from the immediate life and environment of village women, such as a farmhouse door or a drinking bowl. But the new motifs which became increasingly popular in the 1960s and '70s depicted aspects of urban life with little relationship to the everyday lives of the embroiderers, for few farming families actually possessed radios, clocks and ceiling fans. These new motifs were not only incorporated within the familiar old structure of the *ghaghro* but were embroidered in exactly the same way as old motifs, using the same stitches and colour combinations. The popular *sikul* found new uses as a clock face, a wheel and a cup.

These changes in motif were related to changes in the technology of embroidery design. Many of the women who prepared their trousseaux in the 1960s, like their mothers before them, had visited the local specialist who had drawn the outlines of motifs by hand. By the 1970s, however, most women bringing their trousseaux to Jalia had visited a blockprinter's workshop in a local town or city before embroidering their *ghaghros*. These blockprinters, who were usually either of *Brahma Kshatriya* or Muslim origin, were scattered in towns throughout the district. They began to accumulate

12 Seth recorded as many as ninety-two different designs of *kharak* skirts in the 1970s, of which only twenty-six were described by women as 'old' (cf. Seth 1980).

Some Peasant Dilemmas (*Kanbi* and *Kharak*)

printed samples of most existing *ghaghro* designs and would print outlines for women to embroider. A woman would select her preferred motifs after looking through the available samples and would then pay the craftsman a small fee for printing the outlines on to her *ghaghro* cloths.[13]

While initially blockprinters were dependent on local women to supply them with existing designs, this dependence was soon reversed. Blockprinters were so quick and efficient that village embroiderers favoured them above local women artists. The demand for hand-drawn designs fell rapidly, with the result that very few women retained the skill of drawing.[14] Thus, instead of providing replicas of pre-existing designs, blockprinters gradually began to employ artists to create new designs which looked sufficiently familiar to village women but in fact incorporated new forms. By the early 1970s these apparently urban motifs began to appear regularly on the *ghaghros* of Jalia women.[15]

Whether a particular new motif originated in the village and was copied in the town or vice versa is difficult to fathom. But perhaps more relevant than the act of designing was that of naming motifs. For the names, it seems, rarely came from blockprinters, but usually originated with the embroiderers themselves. It is quite possible that the person who first drew the

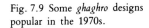

Fig. 7.9 Some *ghaghro* designs popular in the 1970s.

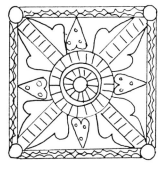

clock *ghadiyal*

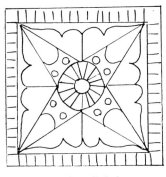

aeroplane '*balun*'

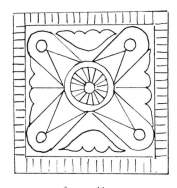

fan *pankho*

13 The idea of copying embroidery outlines from sample books is not new. Masselos shows how royal patrons would select motifs from pattern books provided by professional court embroiderers in Bhuj in the late nineteenth century. Ironically he admires the appealing freehand designs drawn by rural women, which he sees as less regular but also less 'sterile' and 'constrained' than the designs from sample books (Masselos n.d.: 44). But today the very women whom Masselos claimed 'escaped the constraints of the literal' now rely increasingly on the blockprinter and, if Jalia women are at all representative, are no longer capable of drawing their own designs.

14 Only one *Kanbi* woman in Jalia had retained the skill of drawing by hand but her services were rarely called for and her repertoire was limited to only a few designs. Most women had no comprehension of how to draw and regarded my ability to copy designs from their *ghaghros* with amazement. They assumed that I must have been taught each design beforehand and would not believe that I was simply transferring the image from the *ghaghros* to the page by copying.

15 Parmar suggests that European-style motifs of marigolds, garlands and dolls first began to appear in Saurashtran embroidery in the 1930s (1969: 24) but these were incorporated into the embroidery of the local élite, particularly those who received school education. They did not appear in farming women's skirts. Writing in 1895, Billington bemoaned the terrible effect of missionary influences on Indian embroidery, and named Kathiawad as one of the few places where 'the most interesting and uncontaminated indigenous needle-craft' could still be found (Billington 1973 [1895]: 192).

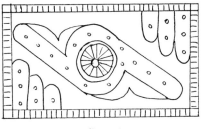

radio *redyo*

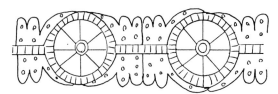

train *gadi*, or musical instrument *katra* (according to different opinions)

217

aeroplane (*balun*) motif did not think that the design resembled an aeroplane in any way. What is relevant, then, is that village women chose to interpret it as such and wished to incorporate it into their *ghaghros*. The most noticeable effect of the rise of blockprinting was that the printer's shop became a reservoir of designs which were now centralised in towns and became increasingly standardised throughout the district. Secondly, the skill of drawing by hand rapidly disappeared so that women were no longer in control of design, which was now in the hands of men who lived outside the village.[16]

Ghaghros, besides displaying an increasingly large range of motifs, showed other changes, including a more frequent use of cotton thread, rather than silk thread which was no longer easily available. The tailor's machine-sewn border also increased in size slightly at this time, although it remained fairly simple. There was no difference between the motifs on the *ghaghros* of *Kanbi* and *Kharak* women in the 1960s, although by the 1970s there was a marked increase in embroidery production by the *Kharaks* and a decrease by the *Kanbis*. While *Kharak* women were making between twenty-five and thirty-five *ghaghros* each for their trousseaux by the mid 1970s,[17] *Kanbi* women seem to have reduced the number to between ten and fifteen. The embroidered *kapdu* was already rare by the late 1970s and only some *Kharak* women continued to make and wear it. *Kanbi* women were choosing to adopt machine-sewn blouses (*polkas*), stitched by the tailor from plain polyester material. These blouses, unlike the older *kapdus*, covered a woman's back.

Ghaghros in the 1980s
By the 1980s most *Kanbi* women had stopped embroidering *ghaghros* altogether and were buying synthetic saris from the city which they wore over blouses and petticoats made from poplin, polyester or tericotton, stitched by local tailors. *Kharak* women, however, continued to embroider *ghaghros* for their trousseaux, and these displayed two major changes. First,

16 Not only do men play an increasingly important role in embroidery design, but they are also becoming increasingly involved in the craft of embroidery itself. As technological innovation increases, the craft is being gradually transformed from a predominantly female home-based domestic craft to a male-dominated commercial one (L.C. Jain 1986: 874). Most new machine embroidery is made exclusively by men.
17 Seth records *Kharak* women in the 1970s making between forty and fifty *ghaghros* for their trousseaux (Seth 1980), but I did not find a single woman in Jalia who claimed to have possessed this number, suggesting that such an estimate was either an exaggeration by the embroiderer or a reflection of regional differences.

Some Peasant Dilemmas (*Kanbi* and *Kharak*)

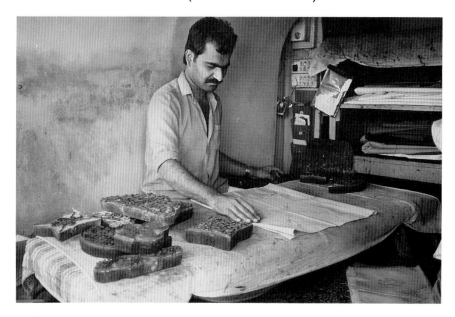

Fig. 7.10 *Above*: A blockprinter in Larabad city printing embroidery motifs for a *Kharak* girl from Jalia, 1989. With the cloth she will make herself an embroidered bag. *Below*: A selection of wooden and metal filigree blocks, designed specially for printing embroidery outlines for rural women's *ghaghros*.

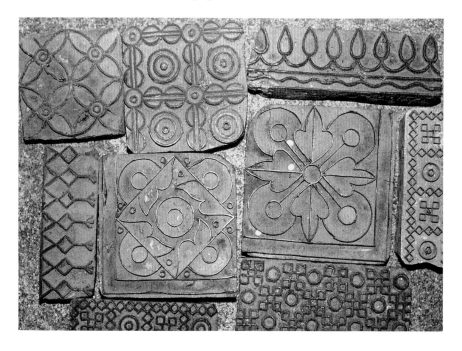

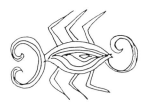

scorpion *vichi*

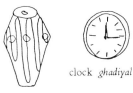

bicycle *'cycle'*

drum *dhol*

clock *ghadiyal*

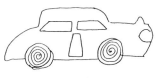

car *gadi*

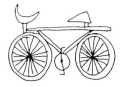

duck *batuk*

Fig. 7.11 Motifs taken from machine-embroidered borders on *Kharak* women's skirts, made in 1988 and 1989. They are more naturalistic than hand-embroidered motifs and are made by *Kharak* tailors who draw around cardboard cut-out shapes with a pen and then embroider the motifs.

larger and increasingly pictorial compositions of motifs were favoured. Whereas in the past the vast majority of motifs had been confined within some kind of grid, these new *ghaghros* were often without a grid and consisted of different motifs built on top of one another to form a large pattern that repeated itself only a few times within one garment (see fig. 7.16).

This tendency to favour more open designs was again facilitated by the changing techniques employed by blockprinters. Throughout the 1980s, they were gradually replacing their use of wooden and metal filigree blocks by the pricking and pouncing technique, a method which freed them from their dependence on block makers and enabled them to create their own designs. It has also changed the standard size of a unit of design. The old wooden blocks, being somewhat heavy and unwieldy, were rarely more than six inches square. But the perforated paper sheets on which new designs are prepared are commonly the standard A4 size, enabling large areas to be printed in a single operation. This appears to have encouraged the opening out and elaboration of the older, more rigid *ghaghro* designs.

The overall effect is that some modern *ghaghros* appear freer in design and less blatantly repetitive or constrained by geometric forms. The very designs that were most favoured in the early 1970s (radio, clock, aeroplane, fan) almost disappeared in the early 1980s since they did not conform to the new preference for open designs. However, the *objects* that these designs depicted re-emerged in a more literal, naturalistic form on the machine-stitched *ghaghro* borders.

It is the machine-sewn borders made by local tailors that form the most distinctive feature of the *ghaghros* made by Jalia women today. In the early 1940s these borders had occupied no more than 2 or 3 inches of space at the bottom of the *ghaghro*. Now they occupy anything from 5 to 7 inches and display an enormous range of technical skill and new motifs. The strips of coloured cloth that line the edge of the border have increased from three or four layers to as many as fifteen in some *ghaghros*. The borders themselves contain a variety of patterns which involve folding, layering and quilting pieces of cloth. Materials favoured are usually shiny, synthetic and bright, including fluorescent pinks and sometimes silver tinsel thread. And whereas in the past the tailor stitched wavy lines or a simple 'thorn' pattern, he now does machine-embroidered versions of flowers, animals,

Some Peasant Dilemmas (*Kanbi* and *Kharak*)

Fig. 7.12 Cross-section of three *ghaghros*, showing the increasing emphasis on machine-made borders and the comparative opening-out of designs. The machine-embroidered border displays plants, flowers, clocks, fish and cars. The appliqué layering (*guna*) has increased and the border occupies more space than in older *ghaghros*.

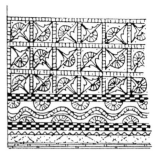

Made c. 1950. *Ghaghro* name: garden (*bagicho*). Border name: lightning creeper (*vijli vel*).

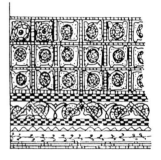

Made c. 1970. *Ghaghro* name: cup and saucer (*rukhabi*). Border name: parrot and electric fan (*pankho poput*).

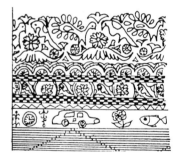

Made in 1988. *Ghaghro* name: five roots (*panch thad*). Border name: parrot and lotus (*poput gota*).

buildings, radios, clocks, cars and bicycles (see fig. 7.11). Fig. 7.12 shows a cross-section of three *ghaghros* made by three generations of *Kharak* women in one household. In the 1988 one, the machine-made border is large and pictorial, as opposed to the earlier ones where the borders are small and simple.

The highly complex machine-embroidered borders which *Kharak* women favour today are so technically demanding that none of the Jalia tailors from the *Darji* (tailor) caste could make them. Instead the *Kharaks* have a few tailors from their own caste scattered throughout various villages in the district (cf. Seth 1980) who specialise in these complex machine-embroidered *ghaghro* borders, making designs by drawing around cardboard cut-out shapes. These in turn have been taken from magazine images and picture books, and have entirely broken away from the original highly stylised forms. Instead they are naturalistic depictions, immediately recognisable by outsiders as well as by village women. Tailors make high charges for their services, and thus *ghaghros* are considerably more expensive than many of the ready-made saris and petticoats available in the shops.

Some problems of interpretation

Even after reviewing the evolution of the *ghaghro* over the past fifty years in both technology and design, the question remains how and indeed if these designs should be interpreted, and at what level. On the one hand there is clearly a definite grammar to *ghaghro* design. All have the peaked *vadkyu*, all have the set formation of two borders, and all have an established vocabulary of colours: outlines are yellow or blue; *sikuls* are yellow or white; *jowla* (barley) is blue and white; *dana* (seeds) are white and the filling in of motifs and forms is blue, green and pink. These rules present a framework which is rarely rejected or questioned by Jalia women, even today. When I began to embroider a *ghaghro* and once used yellow instead of blue for a border outline, it was quite simply 'wrong' and I was told to unpick it and start again. The structure of the *ghaghro* was therefore fundamentally fixed, but no one could ever suggest why this should be or what this represented. Nor, of course, did they consider it a reasonable question to ask. 'A *ghaghro* must be made like this because this is *how ghaghros are made*' was the closest I could get to an explanation.

221

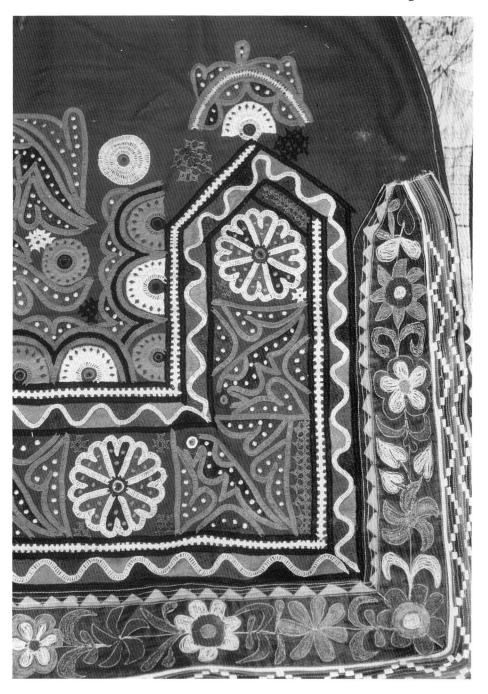

Fig. 7.13 Details of the end-flap (*vadkyu*) of two *ghaghros*, showing the intricacy of modern machine-made borders, including appliqué layering (*guna*), appliqué zig-zags

Some Peasant Dilemmas (*Kanbi* and *Kharak*)

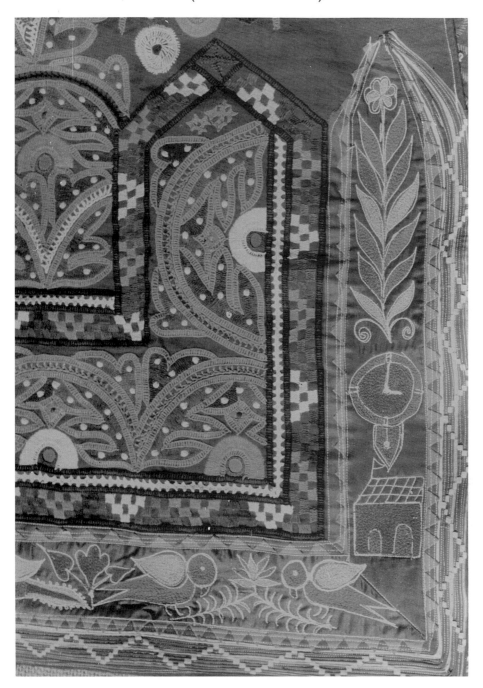

(*kangra*) and appliqué squares (*adadiya*). (a) *Left*: Potted plant. (b) *Above*: Plant, clock, temple, parrots and flowers. (1989)

There was also much ambiguity over the significance of the content or forms embroidered on *ghaghros*. Take, for example, the *sikul* form. Although *sikul* is a Gujarati word for face, the *sikul* form did not have the fixed meaning of face and was used more like an equivalent of the English word 'circle'. On some figurative embroidered wall-hangings the *sikul* did indeed act as a human or animal face. Yet on *ghaghros* it often represented a flower head, a tree or a cotton pod. And when *sikul* forms appeared in isolation, they were not intended to 'represent' a row of faces. They were seen simply as decorative round forms. Asking the meaning of *sikul* was, therefore, inappropriate for it was simply a round formation of stitches with a mirror in the centre which could be used to represent a variety of different things. Names of embroidery patterns often refer to what the patterns resemble rather than what they represent (Paine 1990: 17).

Similar ambiguity surrounded the names of other design elements. The checkerboard design found in most *ghaghros* was known as *adadiya*. Some women would insist that this did not refer to anything while others would say it was a reference to *adad*, a black pulse which they used for cooking.[18] The design itself, however, was an ancient one, found in early Jain manuscripts and paintings. Here each check represented a unit in a cosmological system of counting and dividing. The word for division into two parts is *addhadhun*, and it is possible that *adadiya* is a corruption of this and that over the years a system of counting and division has come to be interpreted as pulses owing to the similarity in the two linguistic terms. Certainly the local specialist in Gujarati art and folklore, Khodidasbhai Parmar, regarded the check design on women's *ghaghros* as representing a divine system of counting (interview). But no woman in Jalia ever came up with such an explanation. This raises the question as to whether women had once copied the design into their embroidery knowing its religious significance, or whether instead they had done so in ignorance or merely invented it for themselves. Perhaps, after all, such cosmological interpretations never existed at a village level or have been lost and transformed over time. Or perhaps it is simply inappropriate to seek verbal explanations of visual phenomena, which may take the very form that they do 'precisely because they cannot be explained away' and are 'not amenable to articulation in words' (Cardew 1978: 18).

The fact remains, however, that *ghaghros* are composed of set formations

---

18 Fischer and Shah, who found the same design in wall-paintings in the Saurashtran village of Ratadi, maintain that *adadiya* means 'small slices of sweets made from black *adad*-grains' (Fischer and Shah 1970: 63).

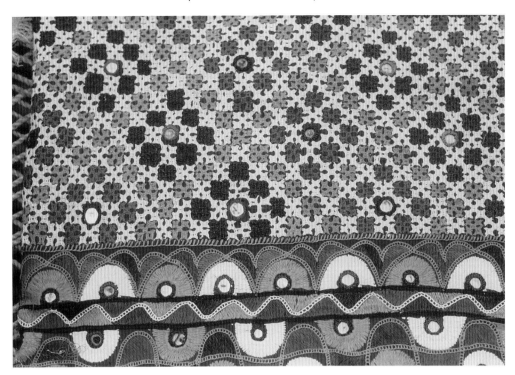

Fig. 7.14 Details of *ghaghro* embroidery popular in the 1940s and before. *Above*:
Bavaliya bharat or *naka bharat* (interlacing stitch, worn mainly by older women).
Below: *Ardhi phulvadi* (half-lower garden).

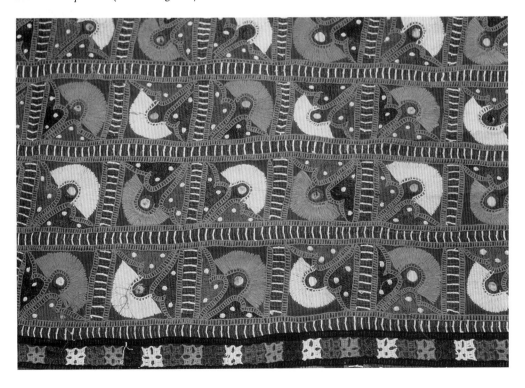

and stitches which take their name from natural phenomena and which, when joined together, refer to certain aspects of the local environment. Yet embroidery is not a form of graphic realism, for women are selective about the aspects of life that they choose to portray (Masselos n.d.: 41). Taking birds as an example, women embroider peacocks, peahens and parrots, which are the birds that appear in their farmsteads and fields. They are thought beautiful, auspicious and romantic and frequently appear in local songs; the dancing peacock in the early morning, they say, is the herald of the rains, the sign of a good monsoon in the coming months. And although such birds were common everyday sights, people never ceased to point them out to one another and appreciate their beauty. Yet other local birds, like crows and kingfishers, were never embroidered on *ghaghros* because these were considered inauspicious and to herald potential misfortune.

Similarly the fruits, nuts and flowers that appeared on early *ghaghros* were all considered auspicious – they were highly valued, desirable and worthy of offering to the gods – and the *ladva* (sweet balls) found on the *ghaghros* of older women were not merely sweets, which are themselves associated with auspiciousness, but were the specific sweets eaten and distributed at weddings, the most auspicious of all occasions. What these *ghaghros* designs portray, then, is an idealised picture of the pleasurable and auspicious things in life, the pleasant aspects of the local environment (cf. Masselos n.d.: 43).

Do the women of Jalia attribute anything more than this general auspiciousness to their *ghaghros*? From what women say, it seems not, yet around the border edges of the *ghaghro* other seemingly less desirable images appear, such as *kanta* (thorns) and *kangra* (spikes). Although women never explained these, it is possible that they originated as motifs of protection. Of the embroidery of the *Rabari* women of Kutch it has been written, 'The *kungri* design is found decorating and so protecting especially those elements of greatest importance in Rabari life' (Frater 1975: 53). Paine suggests a similar explanation of the zig-zag embroidery that edges Palestinian clothing and is locally known as *tishrifeh*, meaning 'to make good'. She illustrates how zig-zags and triangles are commonly found in the borders of embroidery in many parts of the world, and suggests that cuffs, skirt edges, necklines and other openings are particularly vulnerable to malevolent forces and are in need of heavy embroidery for protection (Paine 1990: 133–4). In Jalia the *kangra* design is also found in the borders of wall-hangings, in the tattoos on women's arms and sometimes on shepherd's faces. Again there is a discrepancy between local explanations, which focus on the decorative, and those of outsiders, which interpret tattoos as a form of diagrammatic protection against the evil eye (cf. Maloney 1976, Frater 1975). The

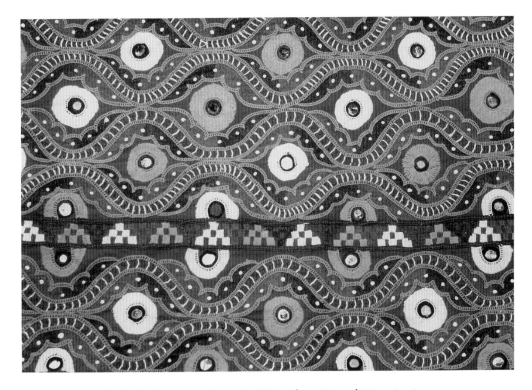

Fig. 7.15 Details of *ghaghro* designs popular in the 1970s. *Above*: *Nau nadi* (nine rivers). *Below*: 'Redyo' (radio).

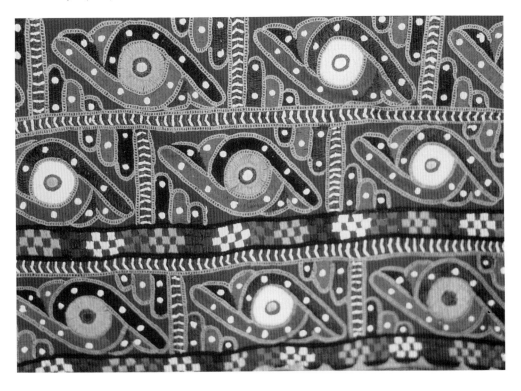

two explanations are not as incompatible as they first appear. What originates as a sign of protection may in time become one of beauty, since beauty is indicated by the suggestion that it is worthy of protection. Similarly, although women claimed to choose tattoos for aesthetic and social reasons, their fear of what might happen if they were not tattooed suggests that the tattoos may indeed have once been protective. Certainly the belief persists that desirable things should be protected from the evil eye. Hence a *Bharwad* (shepherd) woman binds her new ivory bangles with black threads, destroying their perfection so that 'the eye will not strike' (*najar na lagse*), and many women place a black mark on the foreheads of their babies for the same reason. But these are cases where the prophylactic qualities are acknowledged. It is possible that where protective designs have become incorporated into larger, more decorative designs, as in the case of embroidery, they become just another decorative element, and the once protective function dissolves over time.

What is clear is that local interpretations of the meaning of design elements can vary over both time and place (cf. J. Jain 1982). The scorpion motif presents another example of this. In Jalia I came across no scorpions embroidered by hand on women's *ghaghros*, but did occasionally find them in the machine-embroidered borders made by tailors. Women did not express any particular attitude to these embroidered scorpions, but regarded them as just one among many images of flowers, rabbits, drums, bicycles and cars. But according to Parmar the scorpion motif, which also appears in tattoos, is a sex symbol that was in the past commonly found at the top of the *vadkyu* of the *ghaghro*, at the top of the woman's thigh. These scorpions were not, it seems, merely decorative. They were potentially malevolent to anyone who should usurp a woman's *ghaghro* and, by implication, her husband's bed. Parmar recalls (1969: 57–8) a song which runs:

> *Manibai is having her bath, my beloved*
> *The scorpion has climbed her ghaghros,*
> *It climbed up and bit her, beloved.*

Here the scorpion in the song bit a woman's husband's lover. According to Parmar, dying women would often say: 'If my *ghaghros* are worn by my husband's second wife, she will be bitten by the scorpion.' Here the scorpion seems to be at once decorative, protective (of the wife's rights), malevolent (towards the impostor) and phallic. Yet in Jalia women have ceased to embroider it altogether and where it does appear, it no longer occupies a unique position against the woman's thigh, but is now incorporated along with other animals, plants and objects into the machine-

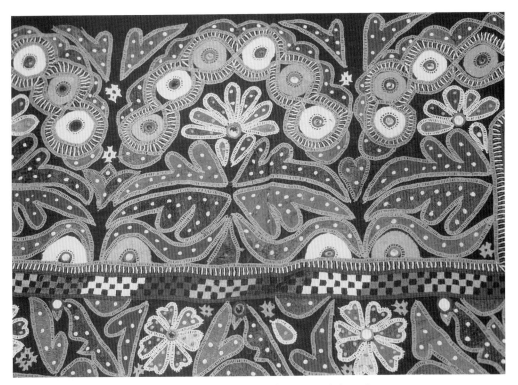

Fig. 7.16 Details of *ghaghro* designs popular in 1988–9. *Above*: *Suraj phul* (sunflower).
Below: *Naliyer* (coconut tree).

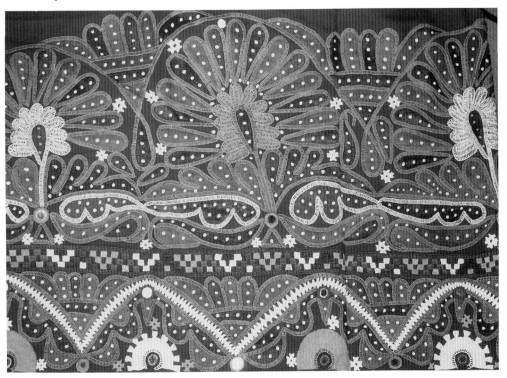

embroidered border where it is just another motif without specific value.

Yet although women in Jalia today do not make elaborate symbolic interpretations of their embroidery designs, they none the less select and favour certain motifs with great consistency. These motifs manifest themselves not merely in *ghaghros* but also in other embroidered items which women make for their trousseaux and in tattoos. To what extent do these represent a change in the value system or lifestyle of village women? To tackle this question, it is necessary first to examine the changes taking place in other popular arts besides embroidered clothing.

Changes in popular arts (1940–1989)

Tattoos. Fig. 7.17 illustrates new developments in tattoos between the 1940s and the 1970s. The 1980s have been omitted, since the art of tattooing had by then diminished. Few parents encourage their children to wear more than one or two facial marks today, but most older women still bear the marks they were given as children. Many are embarrassed by them as they feel tattoos mark them out as backward.

The early tattoos consisted mainly of a series of dots and simple shapes. Today many young women are unable to name their tattoo marks, but others recognise the forms of shrine, swastika, crescent, sun, flowers, seeds, bracelets, tree, scorpion and peacock. Like the images depicted in early *ghaghro* designs, these are stylised representations of the auspicious mixed with some more explicitly religious symbols such as the swastika and shrine. Yet by 1975 tattoos, like embroidery, had become increasingly naturalistic and were beginning to depict a new range of desirable objects. These included the watch motif, drawn on the wrist as a substitute for a real watch[19] (some well-to-do women now wear real watches over the tattooed image). They also included the radio motif, scissors, aeroplanes, household utensils, water-pumps and increasingly naturalistic depictions of flowers and peacocks.

Household arts. In household arts, a similar evolution was taking place. In the 1940's and 50's, farming women were embroidering not only their clothes, but also items for household decoration for their trousseaux. These consisted of wall-hangings, door-hangings, hangings to decorate shrines, wedding booth hangings and animal regalia for bullocks (fig. 7.18). Most

---

19   This might be compared to the recent custom in Greece of wearing T-shirts with depictions of seatbelts fastened across them (Brian Moeran, personal communication).

Some Peasant Dilemmas (*Kanbi* and *Kharak*)

Fig. 7.17 Diagram illustrating recent changes in tattoo designs. Like embroidery motifs, new tattoo motifs do not so much replace old ones as co-exist with them.

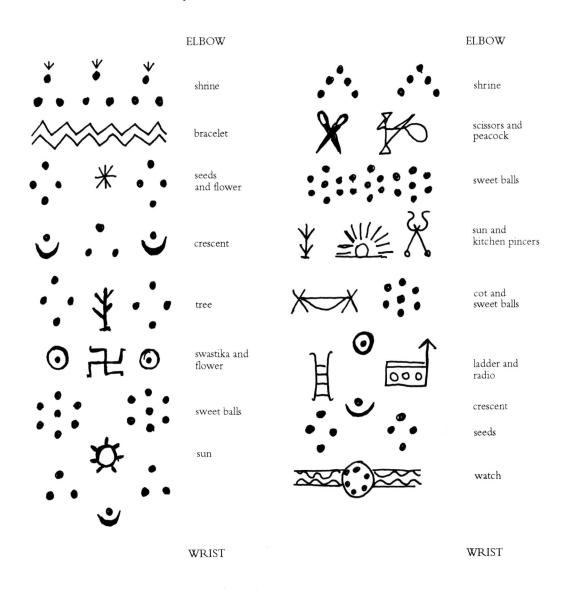

Designs on the arm of a woman now in her sixties, who was tattooed in the 1940s

Designs on the arm of a woman in her mid-twenties, tattooed in the late 1970s

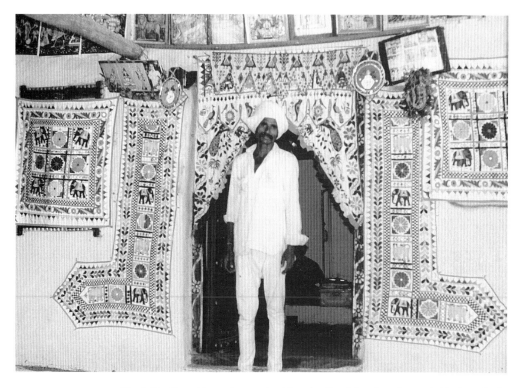

Fig. 7.18 *Above*: House decorated with embroidered hangings (*toran, chaklo, bar sakiya*), made c. 1980, using block-printed motifs. Earlier, designs were hand-drawn. Hanging in the doorway are the flaps of a *pardo*, showing the influence of foreign floral creepers. *Below*: Bullock, decorated with an embroidered blanket (*jhul*). (1989)

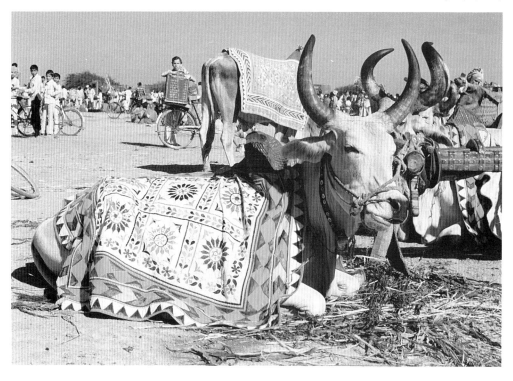

Some Peasant Dilemmas (*Kanbi* and *Kharak*)

of these were used as a form of display only on special occasions such as weddings when the plain mud walls of houses were temporarily transformed into a bright array of colourful embroidered cloth. Like *ghaghros* they were embroidered with a mixture of geometric forms, parrots, peacocks, flowers, buds and sometimes other animals such as lions and elephants. The only item of permanent display was the *toran* (door-hanging), hung in the doorway of every house to protect its entrance and welcome guests.[20] By the 1970s, some women were continuing to embroider wall-hangings and door-hangings, but a new embroidered item had become an obligatory part of the farming woman's trousseau. This was the *pardo* (curtain), a new style of door-hanging.[21] It was always embroidered on a white background with a new range of motifs easily obtainable from the blockprinter. These motifs consisted of animals (peacocks, parrots, deer, rabbits, lions), some of which had been popular in embroidery previously, but all of which now appeared in a new naturalistic style; gods (Laxmi, Ganesh, Hanuman, Krishna); flowers (flower pots, roses, creepers); other objects (bicycles, gramophone players, clocks); and, for the first time, written messages or slogans (such as *Jay bharat*, welcome, good luck etc.), usually embroidered in English lettering, sometimes in Gujarati.

The *pardo*, though another form of embroidery, represented a major break from local tradition for two main reasons. First, the motifs were no longer composed of the elementary embroidery forms such as *sikuls*, neem leaves, thorns and so on. Whereas in the past designs were produced by joining together these familiar embroidered forms, in the new *pardo* the local grammar of embroidery composition was ignored. Each motif was first and foremost a naturalistic drawing which, after being printed on to the *pardo* cloth by a blockprinter, could be embroidered using simple herringbone stitch, rather in the way that crayons or paints can be used to colour in designs. Secondly, the *pardo* was the first embroidered item

---

20 In some of the wealthiest households of the ruling families of Saurashtra, embroidery was on permanent or semi-permanent display in the late nineteenth century. Much of this embroidery was made by high-caste women or by professional male embroiderers from the *Mochi* caste. In particular the *Kathi* community, who ruled many of the central principalities, was renowned for its fine silk-embroidered house decorations. Much of this work now features in museum collections of Indian textiles (cf. the Calico Museum and the Shreyas Museum, Ahmedabad).

21 The Pardo is a door-hanging with two flaps which hang down on the inside of the door. It seems to have been inspired by the sight of European-style curtains, tied back in the windows of élite houses. Such *pardos* first came to Gujarat as early as the 1930s but it was not until the 1950s and '60s that some of the high castes in Jalia began to make them. Among the *Kanbis* and the *Kharaks* the *pardo* did not become popular until the early 1970s.

to include written inscriptions, which were to become increasingly popular among these illiterate farming women. By the 1980s such written messages had become common on cloth bags, tablecloths, *mandaps* (wedding canopies) and *torans* (door-hangings).

Trousseaux given in the 1970s were also beginning to include a number of other household arts, using new materials such as plastic beads, plastic wire, sequins and crochet. In particular the light-bulb flourished as a new form of decoration. This was before Jalia and the surrounding villages were to obtain a supply of electricity. The light-bulb, or 'globe' as it was known, was something that most women only saw when they visited the city. It was greeted with a mixture of wonder and in some cases fear, but redundant light-bulbs were rapidly to become a popular and desirable source of artistic expression. Sometimes they were simply strung together in rows and hung above doorways, performing the same role as the embroidered *toran*. More inventive women stuffed the interiors of bulbs with pieces of shiny coloured paper or rags to give the effect of a row of coloured lights. Yet others crocheted an elaborate covering for the bulbs using plastic wires (fig. 7.19), or covered them with a network of plastic beads and hung them from the beams of the verandah, where they looked like chandeliers. But there was no intention of using these bulbs as a form of lighting, nor would this have been possible since the plastic beads and wires would instantly have melted. These light-bulb arts flourished throughout the early and mid-1970s but went into a rapid decline in the 1980s, by which time most villages in the district had a supply of electricity and functioning electric light-bulbs replaced earlier decorative ones.

Although decorative light-bulbs still hang in some farmhouses, the artistic emphasis of the 1980s trousseau is on collections of beaded ornaments which are displayed in the popular new item of village furniture, the 'showcase' (see fig. 7.19). These items consist of small ornaments which women make from plastic beads, knitted together with plastic thread. Beaded items include animals (elephants, parrots, rabbits, scorpions, cockerels, fish, camels, deer, butterflies), often the same animals found in the embroidered *pardo*. They also include beaded images of Lord Ganesh, Shiva and Krishna's carriage. Among these usually crowded displays are miniature replicas of electric fans, radios, dolls in Western dress, bicycles, tables, aeroplanes and, the most popular item of all, the beaded sofa set. There is hardly a single girl in Jalia today who is not making a small beaded sofa with two accompanying chairs for her trousseau. These sofa sets are available in the shops in Larabad but women generally prefer to make them themselves. A girl from a reasonably wealthy family is usually given a small wooden showcase with

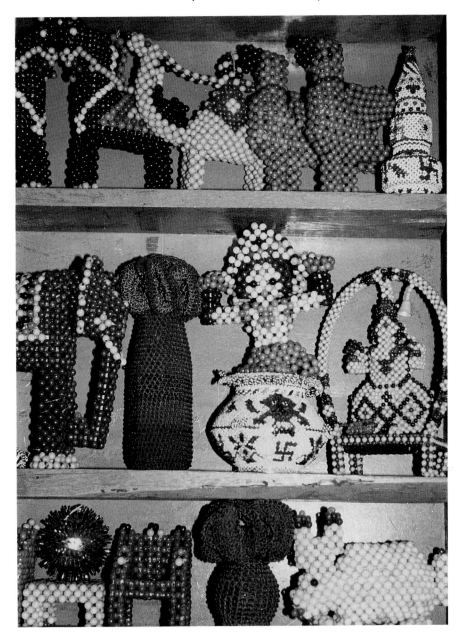

Fig. 7.19 Interior of a show-case (1989), containing (*top, left to right*): Plastic beaded horses, camels, parrots and glass beaded model of water pots. *Middle*: Elephant, plastic crochet around a glass bottle, pot, doll and beaded Ganesh. *Bottom*: Beaded table and gold sequin ball, beaded chair, crochet-covered light-bulb and beaded rabbit.

sliding glass doors in which to display all her beaded arts and ornaments in her new home.

Along with the increasingly popular plastic beadwork display, the more delicate glass beadwork is also popular in the village. Here tiny glass beads are knitted together (see fig. 7.20).[22] Usually, they do not form miniature models, but rather are knitted around actual objects. Some of these are auspicious objects used in rituals, such as decorated coconuts, betel nuts, rupee coins, water containers and *indhonis* (padded rings worn on the head to help balance a load). These items are used during the marriage ceremony, then returned to the showcase where they are kept on permanent display along with the plastic beaded items, crochet light-bulbs and other glass beaded objects such as biros (without ink), glass bottles, empty nail-varnish pots and toothbrushes. A single showcase usually contains a mixture of items from two or three different trousseau collections and therefore holds the arts of different generations simultaneously. The beaded arts are accompanied by an increasing emphasis on different techniques for decorating the house. *Torans* made from plastic straws, imitation flowers, paper roses, plastic beads, crochet, sequins and imitation leaves now adorn doorways. Women also make 'photo frames', consisting of elaborate sequined pictures of peacocks, gods and flowers that have a small blank area in the middle of which a family photograph can be inserted. Other items include plastic mobiles, sequined or embroidered pictures, and items such as bags decorated with embroidered writing and floral creepers. Designs are learned from borrowing and copying the ornaments and decorations of friends and neighbours.

Interpretation of changes in clothing and popular arts
The above survey of changes in embroidery, tattoos and household arts reveals certain consistent trends: first, a steady incorporation of new motifs which appear to take their inspiration from outside the village (electric fan, radio, car, aeroplane, light-bulb, sofa, chairs, watches, clocks and written inscriptions); secondly, a progressive movement away from stylisation towards naturalism; and thirdly, an increasing preference for new decorative media and techniques which are favoured above *deshi* embroidery (light-bulb

22 The knitting together of small glass beads is by no means a new craft in the area. It flourished in the latter half of the nineteenth century among the wealthiest families of Saurashtra (cf. Nanavati *et al.* 1966). They knitted together beaded wall-hangings, ritual objects and ornaments using imported Venetian beads. It was an art practised both by professionals and women in their own homes. It never flourished among the poorer agricultural castes, as beads were extremely costly. In Jalia the apparently new fashion for making beaded coconuts and ornaments is in fact a reworking of an older art tradition that declined among the Saurashtran élite earlier in the twentieth century. The beaded items made today are much less complex and intricate than earlier beadwork.

Some Peasant Dilemmas (*Kanbi* and *Kharak*)

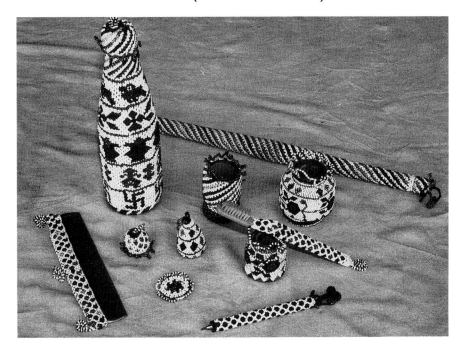

Fig. 7.20 Items decorated with small glass beads, including a toothbrush, comb, biro, rolling-pin, betel nut, bottle, rupee coin and two small pots used for carrying red powder. Some of these items are used in ritual performances. Although made in the 1980s, they replicate a style of beadwork popular in the late 19th century primarily among the local élite.

arts, crochet, plastic weaving, beadwork, machine embroidery on *ghaghro* borders). These various aspects of change are of course interrelated. To many lovers of folk art, they represent the gradual destruction and banalisation of 'traditional' skills. But what is their significance in local terms? What do they represent to the women of Jalia themselves? Taking the new motifs found in embroidery, beadwork and tattoos, it is clear they do not simply document changes in village life. They are more imaginative and inventive than descriptive. Images of radios and clocks appeared in embroidered *ghaghros* before the objects themselves appeared in farmhouses. Cars now appear on machine-made borders even though there is not a single family in the village that owns a car. Similarly, light-bulb arts preceded the installation of electricity and acted almost as the herald of electric lighting itself. Furthermore the current trend for making beaded sofa sets does not have anything to do with local furniture, since to my knowledge there is not a single farmer's house in Jalia that actually contains a sofa.

Yet many farming women, when asked to imagine their ideal home, would say it must be *pakka* (made from brick or concrete) and must contain ceiling fans, electric lighting, wall-clocks, a radio and a good showcase full of things. Ideally it should also have a water tap so that water can be obtained without going to the village well. And finally, 'everything should be up', meaning that it should have furniture so that people do not have to sit on the floor or cook at ground level. These were popular conceptions of a good life, derived from the idea of how 'well-off people' (*sarawalas*) and 'progressive people' (*sudharo manus*) live. Most such *sarawalas* were thought to live in the city, but some lived in the village. These were mainly *Vaniya* and *Brahman* families, some of whom had furniture and televisions in their homes. When asked where the fashion came from, people invariably gave one of two replies: 'It comes from the *Vaniyas*' or 'It comes from the city'. In fact many a *Kanbi* girl claimed to have learned beadwork from *Vaniya* girls. Both *Vaniya* houses and city houses seemed to represent wealth, comfort and success. While some farming women liked the idea of actually living in the city, others claimed that they preferred their village with its animals and fruit trees. They would describe the mangos and the custard apples which grew so big on their farms. But they too wanted the benefits that they saw in the city: the good shops, the tables, the chairs; the signs and proof that they too were 'forward, progressive people'.

Some of these modern aspirations have been fulfilled in the houses of farming women in Jalia, particularly among the *Kanbi* caste. Over the past twenty years, most *Kanbis* have built themselves *pakka* houses on the new 'plot'. These houses now have electricity and an increasing number have electric fans, radios, wall-clocks and occasional items of furniture, such as small tables, showcases, steel cupboards and metal-framed beds. *Kanbi* women no longer embroider clothes or hangings depicting these desirable objects, perhaps because they have the objects themselves. *Kharak* women too have ceased to make light-bulb decorations since the arrival of electricity in their houses. The only house in the village with a newly-made light-bulb *toran* was a small mud (*kacha*) house without electricity belonging to a poor *Vaghri* family. This suggests that the light-bulb arts act as a kind of precursor to electric lighting itself, perhaps even encouraging its advent in the minds of the artists.[23]

Such findings suggest that the new motifs that have appeared in embroi-

---

23   There is a custom in some Indian shrines of placing the image of a desired object at the shrine, along with an offering to the god or goddess. Worshippers make vows hoping that the gods will bring them the objects of their desire.

Some Peasant Dilemmas (*Kanbi* and *Kharak*)

dery, beadwork and tattoos since the early 1970s portray not merely the auspicious but also the desirable, the things that people want within their own homes. Far from rejecting modernisation, these creators of popular art portray their aspirations for an improved lifestyle in their house decorations and their clothes. Electronic goods such as fans, radios and electric light-bulbs are not in conflict with the older notion of the desirable, based on flowers, fruits, animals and birds. Rather, the two coexist simultaneously. And just as an electric fan appears beside a parrot in a *Kharak* woman's *ghaghro*, so a plastic beaded bicycle or toothbrush appears beside an image of Lord Shiva or a beaded scorpion in the showcase. Meanwhile Ganesh, that favourite of household gods, is often given the place of honour on top of the beaded sofa in the middle of the showcase or is placed, on a model sofa or chair, in a separate household shrine. And it is appropriate that he, the remover of obstacles, should have such fine surroundings, for it is he who might assist the people of the house to achieve one day a similar grandeur in their own lifestyle.

Once they are actually attained clocks and radios do not lose their desirability, but attention shifts away from images of the object and towards decorating or framing the object itself. Again a comparison may be drawn with the treatment of household gods, who are placed in shrines decorated with miniature *torans* and given suitable clothing and food. So, too, a valuable acquisition for the house should be well treated. Fig. 7.21a shows a small embroidered hanging, originally made to protect an embroidered image of Ganesh, now used to protect and frame a radio which was recently purchased from Bombay. This same family had hired a photographer from Larabad to come to the village and take photographs of different family members seated with the radio on their laps. Fig. 7.21b reveals a similar use of household arts to emphasise and frame a wall-clock that had recently arrived in a woman's trousseau. In this case, it is plastic-beaded images of flowers in their pots that flank the desirable object and ensure that it is noticed by anyone who comes to the house. Similarly, family photographs are given a place of honour in the middle of elaborate sequined pictures.

With the arrival of new motifs and the changing values attached to them, women have altered not only the subject-matter of their embroidery and arts, but also their attitude to certain embroidery styles, materials, forms and stitches. Certain forms have come to appear old-fashioned to village women, and to have a negative connotation through their association with illiteracy and backwardness. As described earlier, the embroidered *ghaghro* had its own grammar of stitches and forms which could be combined to

Fig. 7.21 *Above*: An embroidered hanging (1988) frames a much-prized radio from Bombay. Such hangings are usually hung above an embroidered image of Lord Ganesh. *Below*: Plastic beaded flowers frame a new wall-clock (1988).

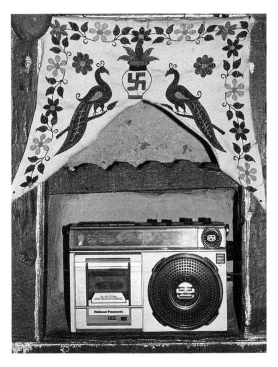

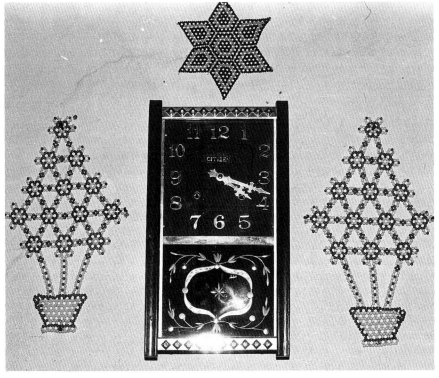

Some Peasant Dilemmas (*Kanbi* and *Kharak*)

achieve certain motifs. With the availability of blockprinted designs, traced from magazine images and photographs, a new emphasis on naturalistic depictions has encouraged young village women to scorn the older more abstract motifs as inaccurate and ridiculous. They are more impressed by a life-like peacock than by a *deshi* one that is sometimes scarcely recognisable as such. With the possibility of realism, the stylised forms found in their mothers' embroidery are seen as defective, as if representing an inability to portray things as they really are. Those *Kanbi* girls who make embroidered bags and bed-covers rarely combine the old stitches of barley, thorns, *sikul* and pulse. Rather they choose just one type of stitch at a time, such as interlacing stitch or the recently fashionable cross-stitch. Their emphasis is on neatness, simplicity, symmetry and realism. They embroider floral creepers, roses and baskets of fruit that are clearly of European inspiration.[24]

The increasing trend away from abstraction is in turn related to women's feelings about literacy and education. In the same way that realism is hierarchically opposed to abstraction, so is literacy to the old-fashioned *deshi* embroidery which seems to represent illiteracy in people's minds. Hence their embarrassment and confusion at my attempting to embroider a *ghaghro* myself. For a literate person, doing such embroidery was simply inappropriate. It represented a confusion of categories. When both men and women told me that my brain would curdle or my abilities would leave me if I spent time embroidering a *ghaghro*, it was as if they felt that the ignorance that such embroidery represented would somehow disrupt my educated mind. Embroidering a *ghaghro* was, as one woman put it, an activity for 'people who know nothing'.

The relationship between literacy and popular household arts was by no means straightforward. The act of embroidering a polyester shopping-bag or a sequined photo-frame of the new style was not considered degrading in the least. Nor was the act of knitting together plastic beads. In fact these

---

24 Billington described how educated Indian women were adopting European embroidery styles at the end of the nineteenth century. With the value judgements of a Victorian lady, certain in her opinions, she writes: 'In no branch of Indian art has British influence been so mischievously detrimental as in needlecraft. The native women are quick to seize upon a small novelty that can be passed on from one to another, and the vulgar showiness and easy accomplishment of our Western woolwork, in all the worst hideousness of Berlin cross-stitch and crewels, seems to have pleased some innate sentiment in them, for, unfortunately, they have adopted and perpetuated these in the vilest form. The mission schools are to be held responsible for most of the evil that has been wrought in this direction' (Billington 1973 [1895]: 189). One of the most popular styles of embroidering bags and cloth in Jalia today is cross-stitch using brightly coloured wool.

241

were regarded as high fashion, and as a sign of refinement and more generally progress. But these skills had spread from the town to the village rather than vice versa, and were the type of household arts that educated girls in the city learned at school. Similarly the idea of embroidering written messages such as 'welcome', 'sweet dreams' and 'good luck' came from outside the village and were not therefore defined as *deshi*. While these were usually written in English, none of the farming girls who were embroidering them or knitting them in their beaded *torans* were able to read what they said. And, with the exception of the word 'welcome', which has now been assimilated into Gujarati vocabulary, the messages were not only unreadable but also unrecognised when read aloud. When I asked women why they embroidered English writing, they often replied: 'It looks educated' (*bhunela lage*). Similarly their husbands and sons agreed that such messages were good as they made the people of the household look as if they had studied.

Written embroidered and beadwork messages seemed to encapsulate the predicament of village women. While few farming families showed much interest in educating their daughters, they were beginning to develop a sense of awareness and embarrassment about their lack of education. Some, particularly *Kanbi* parents, were sending their daughters to the village school in their early childhood. Here a basic knowledge of the rudiments of the Gujarati language was considered a very adequate education. But although farming women were on the whole far removed from literacy and especially from the English language, they were keen for their sons to study and felt that the greatest sign of advancement in the modern world was for a boy one day to become a bank official or at least have an office job. Some even suspected that my own willingness to go so far from home and study for so many years must have meant that I was seeking a qualification for a banking post.

Farming women were not by any means yearning for education, but they recognised it as something of value in the contemporary world and were often embarrassed and apologetic about their own lack of it. They appeared to want to 'appear' educated rather than 'be' educated. The ambivalence of their position is perhaps best expressed in the contorted misspellings that often occur when one illiterate woman copies another's writing. On the embroidered bags and *torans* of Jalia women, the following welcomes appear: 'Weccome', 'mellome', 'Wel Cowe', 'welccome', 'mflcowf', 'mellow' and other variations where all the letters are reversed as in a mirror image.

Writing embroidered messages and slogans was a clear case where the medium (embroidered writing) was more important than the message. As

Some Peasant Dilemmas (*Kanbi* and *Kharak*)

a medium, it was seen as bridging that uneasy gap between ignorance (the characteristic of *deshi* embroidery) and knowledge (the characteristic of literacy). Through the embroidered message, the ability to read and to embroider, two skills which were diametrically opposed in local thought, were temporarily, though precariously, fused.

The divergence of Kanbi and Kharak dress reconsidered

It has become clear that while *Kanbi* women no longer make embroidered *ghaghros*, *Kharak* women continue to embroider them. And while the former now wear synthetic saris, the latter still wear embroidered clothes even though the younger generation hope to avoid wearing them. These differences do not reveal a conflict between the values of the two castes, for members of both castes agree that the *ghaghro* is an old-fashioned *deshi* garment of the past – thick, clumsy and backward, marking its wearer as a villager and farmer. The self-conscious comments of Liliben and her cousins, and their reluctance to admit that they will one day wear their *ghaghros*, reveal that *Kharak* girls can be just as embarrassed by *deshi* embroidery as their *Kanbi* counterparts. So why do *Kharaks* continue to make and wear embroidery when the *Kanbis* no longer do so? And what has enabled the latter caste to rid itself of the 'backward' village label while the *Kharaks* continue to bear the village stamp? Any villager asked about these matters will invariably give a simple response along the following lines: 'The *Kanbis* are developed people [*sudharo manus*]. They are diamond cutters [*hirawalas*] and that is why they no longer wear embroidery. But the *Kharaks* are *deshi* people and only farmers [*khetiwalas*].' Such replies refer to the changing lifestyle and fortunes of the *Kanbi* caste and the relatively unchanging lifestyle of the *Kharaks*. Since independence the *Kanbis* (see chapter 5) have become increasingly involved in the diamond-cutting industry as a supplement to agriculture. This has brought them new wealth which they have invested in various ways that, in local terms, *prove* their progressiveness. Such proof is seen in their houses, their customs and their clothes. The new 'plot' area where they have built their *pakka* houses is considered the most prosperous part of the village. Apart from two sweeper families with small one-room houses, the plot is the exclusive home of members of the *Kanbi* caste and contains large and sturdy houses of concrete and brick that are considered far superior to previous mud constructions. These houses have been painted white or blue and people now consider it inappropriate to decorate them with *deshi* embroidery, which they say is suitable only for covering mud walls. Most *Kanbi* families have sold their old embroidered house decorations, either to passing traders in exchange for stainless steel or money, or to poorer people in the village such as members of the *Bharwad* (shepherd) caste. The latter still live in mud houses, but till recently had few embroidered house decorations since they could not afford the necessary materials.

Not only have the *Kanbis* improved their living conditions, they have also begun to adopt the customs more often associated with high castes in the village. For example, they have raised the age of marriage so that they no longer keep a gap of some years between marriage and the main *anu* ceremony. Like *Vaniya* and *Brahman* families, they now send the bride to join her husband immediately after marriage, and the custom of lavish ritual wailing at her time of departure has been curtailed since it is considered backward and excessive. Furthermore the *Kanbis* are switching increasingly from bride price towards dowry in their marriage payments. There is a new trend for the bride's parents to refuse bride price and to concentrate instead on giving an increasingly large and costly trousseau. Some *Kanbi* men now stress that it is a sin to accept money for the bride, as the *Kharaks* do. And although most brides today are still illiterate, the new generation of brides will be increasingly literate in Gujarati as many *Kanbi* parents now consider it necessary to send their children to the village school for at least a few years. All these factors are considered by other villagers to be proof that the *Kanbis* are now advanced and wealthy people.

This leads to the question of how and why these changes should have affected *Kanbi* women's clothes. Although on the whole the *Kanbis* live in superior housing conditions to those of the *Kharaks* and are generally more prosperous, the lives of *Kanbi* women have otherwise changed remarkably little. It is not as if the new money from diamond-cutting has made them exempt from working in the fields. On the contrary, while their husbands or sons cut and polish diamonds, they themselves continue to cook, clean and work on the family farm as before. Far from gaining more leisure, these women are labouring harder than ever since they lack the help of the new generation of young men and boys who now cut diamonds instead of farming. Why then, when their daily life has changed so little and they are clearly still 'farming people', have they ceased to wear their embroidered *ghaghros*?

This was best explained by a *Kanbi* woman herself who argued:

'It all started with the diamond business. First my husband's younger brother, then my son, went to learn the business in Surat. We have relatives there. There they stopped wearing *deshi* clothes because they felt ashamed and embarrassed. So they became fashionable and wore "bush shirt" and "pant". When they came back here they laughed at us and told us that we looked like village people.... Then I wanted to

Some Peasant Dilemmas (*Kanbi* and *Kharak*)

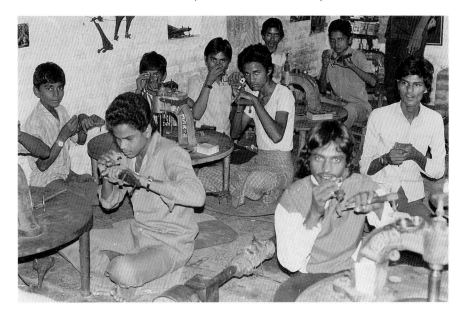

Fig. 7.22 A diamond-cutting workshop in Jalia. Most of the boys and young men employed here are from the *Kanbi* caste and wear Western styles of dress.

visit my second son. He rebuked me, saying "What will people think if they see my mother dressed like that in thick heavy cloth? They will all laugh and laugh." The first time I went to Surat I was wearing a *ghaghro*. But I felt *sharum* because all the women were wearing thin saris. I am old. For me it does not matter. Who cares what an old woman wears? But I would not want my daughters to look so backward. My eldest daughter married fifteen years ago. She took only two *ghaghros* to her in-laws' place. Now my two other daughters have married and they took only saris from Larabad in their trousseaux. They have never worn a *ghaghro*. My first daughter-in-law came here with fifteen *ghaghros* in her trousseaux, but some years back we sold them to some passing traders who came to the village and with the money we bought her saris. Now she wears only thin cloth [saris].'

Kanbi men did not have the same level of control over their women's clothes as the *Brahman* men discussed in the previous chapter, particularly since *Kanbi* women had till recently made their own clothes. But the young men of *Kanbi* families, through their travel and their new employment, developed a self-conscious and critical attitude to the clothes of their wives and mothers, and this attitude has gradually been assimilated by the women themselves. Although they continue to work in the fields, like their *Kharak* counterparts, *Kanbi* women no longer call themselves *khetiwalis* (farmers), but rather *hirawalis* (diamond people). This does not mean that the women themselves cut diamonds, but rather that, as the wives of diamond-cutters, they consider their status to be above that of farmers. And as diamond-cutters' wives it is no longer appropriate for them to dress in farmers' clothes.

This concept of appropriate behaviour was a strong influential factor in the question of how people should dress. It was readily agreed in the village that as wealthy people, living in *pakka* houses and no longer reliant on the land, it was appropriate for *Kanbi* women to dress in saris which were both the product and the proof of their advancement. This did not mean, however, that they could wear anything they liked. Asked why they did not wear the *shalwar kamiz*, a group of young *Kanbi* girls replied that people in the village would laugh and say things like: 'Look! They have become *"feshen-wala"* ', or 'They think they are *Vaniyas* now!', or 'Why do they dress like educated people when they have not studied more than one book?' For, although the *Kanbi* were recognised as *sudharo* (advanced, progressive), they were still not considered as *sudharo* as the more educated *Vaniyas* or some wealthy educated *Brahmans*. Similarly, married women dared not anger their husbands by wearing the 'Bengali' sari. As one girl put it, 'We must keep within our own customs. We can't just put shame on the roof. If I dressed in the Bengali sari, I would be cutting off my father's nose.' But while the Gujarati sari was considered acceptable and appropriate for *Kanbi* women, it was less acceptable for the *Kharaks*. Among them it was interpreted as trying to step out of their own caste and tradition. For the *Kharaks* were still defined as 'farming people' and their women were expected to dress accordingly. Many still lived in houses with mud-plastered walls, albeit large and prosperous ones, and even some of their men were still dressed in *deshi* clothes. Furthermore, owing to the exceptionally limited geographical distribution of their caste which barely extended outside the Larabad district, their marital ties and kinship links were almost entirely local. As a caste, *Kharak* identity was defined not merely in farming terms but also in local terms.

This helps to explain the ambivalence of *Kharak* attitudes towards the *ghaghro*. While they recognised a certain superiority in the saris of the *Kanbis* and other wealthy families in the village, they lacked the same intensity of urban contacts and the education and general level of caste 'improvement' considered appropriate to the sari-wearer. At a time when the *Kanbis* were beginning to reject embroidery (in the 1970s), the *Kharaks*, contenting themselves with the local idiom, chose to increase their embroidery production and

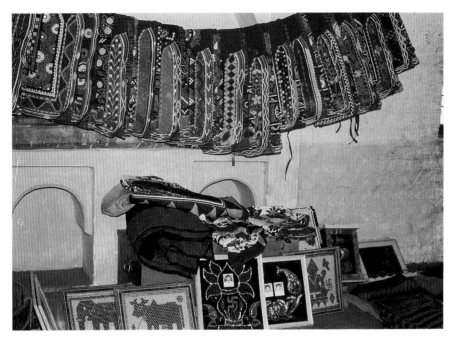

Fig. 7.23 Details of *Kanbi* and *Kharak* trousseau displays at the *anu* ceremony.
Above: Portion of a *Kharak* trousseau (1989), showing embroidered *ghaghros*, arranged
with the machine-made borders on display. In the foreground are beaded pictures,
sequined photo frames and an embroidered wedding canopy (folded). *Below*: Portion of
a *Kanbi* trousseau (1989), showing a wide variety of beaded items and plastic straw
chandeliers. The only embroidery is a woollen bag, a sequined *toran* and two floral
pictures, embroidered in cross-stitch. This trousseau contained saris rather than *ghaghros*.

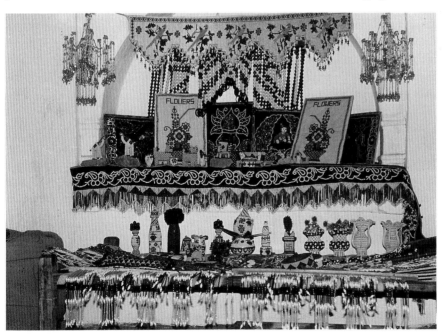

developed new styles of machine-embroidered borders which incorporated their modernising aspirations within the original structure of the *ghaghro* itself. While *Kanbi* families were installing electric fans and radios in their new *pakka* houses, *Kharak* women were embroidering images of fans and radios on their *ghaghros* and employing tailors to embroider images of cars, clocks and bicycles.

In the late 1970s and early 1980s, *Kharak* women exploited the potential of the *ghaghro* to its greatest degree (cf. Seth 1980). But now even they are beginning to reject it. What was once considered a fashionable new embroidered design has now fallen into the general category of 'old-fashioned', 'village-like' and 'backward'. For, as the *Kharaks* know, to most people outside the village and even to many within it there is no particular difference between an 'old' *ghaghro* and a 'modern' one. All are essentially hand-made *deshi ghaghros* which, by their very nature and origins, are old-fashioned. Even with sophisticated machine-made borders occupying an increasingly prominent space, nothing can hide the overall 'backwardness' associated with the garment.

The new generation, like Liliben and her cousins, are embarrassed that they are still making *ghaghros* and including them in their trousseaux. Like other girls in the village, they are more interested in making beaded sofa sets and decorative items for a showcase or for photo-frames, which they make alongside their *ghaghros*. They hope their mothers-in-law will be lenient and let them one day sell their *ghaghros* and wear saris in their marital homes. They look to the *Kanbis*' progress as a model for their own future when they too will be free to wear synthetic saris and rid themselves for ever of their ancestral embroidery. It seems that their hope will be fulfilled, for already *Kharak* girls are including saris with *ghaghros* in their trousseaux, and already they are not expected to wear *ghaghros* for the first few years in their marital homes. It is even possible that the very *ghaghros* that Liliben and her cousins were embroidering will never be worn by them, for by the time they are 'of age' to wear them the fashion may have advanced one further step away from the *deshi* embroidery. But the fact remains that *Kharak* girls are still illiterate and show little signs of going to school, and until they begin to replace their knowledge of embroidery with a knowledge of writing, they will perhaps be destined to continue embroidering *deshi ghaghros*, even if they never have to wear them.

It is often assumed that synthetic fabrics are replacing hand-woven and hand-embroidered dress in India simply because they are cheaper. Certainly price can be an important factor; many of the poorer communities in the village

Some Peasant Dilemmas (*Kanbi* and *Kharak*)

have adopted cheap synthetic or printed cotton and no longer wear locally produced cloth, because in the struggle to provide clothing and food for their families they often favour cheapness above other factors. But economic theories cannot adequately explain the complexity and variety of the different choices people make when they decide which type of dress to buy or wear (cf. Bayly 1986, Cousins 1984: 159). In the *Kanbi* and *Kharak* case, it was the wealthier of the two groups who adopted the cheap synthetic sari whereas the less wealthy group spent both more time and more money making *ghaghros*. In the same way that *khadi* was worn by nationalist sympathisers in the 1920s, despite being more expensive than machine-made cloth, so the *ghaghro* is still worn by *Kharak* women today despite being more expensive than the cheaper range of saris.

Here price is not the primary factor affecting people's choice, but aesthetic considerations are not paramount either. Just as *khadi*-wearing sometimes took the form of a moral obligation rather than an aesthetic preference, so *ghaghro*-wearing has become, for the *Kharaks*, a social expectation rather than a personal choice. These examples illustrate how people may be obliged – socially, culturally or politically – to remain in a particular type of dress despite the apparently easy availability of more desirable alternatives. In both these cases the obligation to remain within a certain category of clothing gave rise to an outburst of creativity as different individuals and groups exploited the full potential of the fabric without actually abandoning the category of clothing type. Thus many *khadi*-wearers chose to embroider, dye and tailor their *khadis* in order to beautify them, while the *Kharak* introduced new motifs and inserted increasingly large machine-made borders into their *ghaghros* in the attempt to update what had become an outmoded form of dress. Individual motivations no doubt varied from wishing to enjoy the full potential of a given medium to wishing actually to conceal the medium by embellishing it to such an extent that it was scarcely recognisable. Yet one important motivation in both cases was that people wished to escape the burden of the *deshi*, with the connotations of backwardness and lack of refinement that it implied.

In the same way that the *Kharak* retention of the embroidered *ghaghro* cannot be explained in economic terms, so the *Kanbis'* rejection of the *ghaghro* was not motivated primarily by economic factors. It was the social kudos attached to wearing the sari rather than its cost or cheapness that attracted the *Kanbis*. For them, being dressed in saris was a means of participating in a modern world that extended beyond the limited confines of the village. Cousins has shown how low-caste Rajasthani women describe those high-caste women who have adopted saris as 'coming from here, but taking on the manners of elsewhere' (Cousins 1984: 159). It was this outsider connotation that attracted the *Kanbis* and made them recognised as progressive in the village, but it was the same connotation that made it inappropriate for *Kharak* women, who lacked the same level of outsider connections, to wear the same dress. 'Consumption uses goods to make firm and visible a particular set of judgments in the fluid processes of classifying persons and events' (Douglas and Isherwood 1980: 67). For the *Kanbis*, adopting a sari was a means of moving one step closer to the social élite and one step further away from the category of local 'farmer'.

Examination of developments in the clothing of high- and middle-ranking groups in the village reveals the emergence of an overall progressive trend, led by the *Vaniyas*, followed closely by other groups including the *Brahmans*, *Kanbis* and *Kharaks*. Although different communities are at different stages within this progression, they are none the less moving in the same direction, away from more caste-specific Kathiawadi styles towards the sari, worn in the Gujarati style. And while young women are gradually expanding their regional sartorial borders, young men are busy escaping the confines of regional dress altogether by adopting Western styles which are now so common in India that they can no longer be described as foreign. Or can they?

8 Some Pastoralist (*Bharwad*) and *Harijan* Dilemmas

Bharwads: the traditionalists

Dilipbhai was unusual for a *Bharwad*. Unlike most men of his caste who had been brought up to keep goats, sheep and cattle, he had been educated at school and now, at the age of twenty-four, was studying for a qualification in medicine. For most of the year he lived and trained in the city of Baroda where, not surprisingly, he wore trousers and a shirt. But even during his lengthy sojourns in the village, he continued to wear Western styles, which made him conspicuous among his more traditionally dressed family and caste-fellows. It was therefore a surprise to see his family's photograph album with pictures of Dilipbhai's wedding in 1985, with Dilipbhai dressed as a conventional shepherd in a white cotton smock, baggy pantaloons, bright red and gold turban, and plentiful wedding jewellery.[1] Dressed in such clothes he looked much like any other *Bharwad* groom in Jalia. But the difference was that these other grooms both worked and dressed as shepherds in their daily lives whereas Dilipbhai claimed that he had never tended goats or sheep, or worn *deshi* clothes, either before his wedding or since. Noticing my surprise at his conventional appearance in the photographs, Dilipbhai explained that he had agreed to compromise his dress for the wedding day. It was a decision directly motivated by embarrassing events that had occurred some two years earlier at his cousin Kathabhai's wedding in Larabad. Below is a rendering of those events, based on Dilipbhai's eye-witness account.

The embarrassing case of the Bharwad groom in trousers

Dilipbhai's cousin Kathabhai had been brought up in the city of Larabad

---

1   It is often observed that people retain some form of 'traditional' clothing for religious or ritual occasions even when they have rejected such clothes in everyday life (Picton and Mack 1979, Kuper 1973). This is certainly true in some contexts in India, but it is by no means systematic. In most of the weddings I attended in Jalia those men who normally wore European styles continued to wear trousers, shirts or 'safari suits' for their own weddings. Some added a turban to these otherwise Western outfits, but there were other grooms who remained bare-headed throughout the ceremony. The educated village groom dressed in European styles may be contrasted to the educated upper-middle-class urban groom who nowadays favours a more 'traditional Indian' look: often a *kurta pyjama* with turban.

and, like Dilipbhai, was unusually well educated for a *Bharwad*.[2] His father continued to work in the milk trade, despite living in the city, but Katabhai never became a shepherd and was sent to school instead. As a schoolboy he dressed in shorts and later trousers and never wore the conventional *kediyun*, *chorni* and turban distinctive of his caste. When it came to his wedding day he felt awkward about wearing such clothes, especially since he was training to become a teacher. He thought it inappropriate for someone as educated as himself to be seen in *deshi* dress. So he decided to wear trousers and a shirt and even donned a tie for the occasion. His mother was upset to see him going to his own marriage in such dull 'foren' clothes but his father consented to Kathabhai's choice, being proud of the fact that his son had become an important and respected, educated boy.

Katabhai's wedding had been arranged since he was five years old. He was to marry a *Bharwad* girl whose family also lived in Larabad, where they kept cows and goats and sold milk products. She was eighteen and he twenty-two at the time finally fixed for their wedding, which had been delayed several times by Kathabhai's parents on the grounds that their son needed to complete his education first. On the appointed day for the marriage Kathabhai, mounted on a decorated horse, arrived at the bride's home with the *jan* (groom's party). But when his father-in-law saw him dressed in trousers and a shirt, he became angry, saying: 'How can you come to your own wedding dressed like that? Do you have no *sharum*?' He then turned to the *jan* and remonstrated:

> 'How can you allow the groom to dress in bushcot-pant? How can you do this to our caste? Are you real *Bharwads*, that you allow such a thing? Well, my daughter is a *Bharwad*. I have brought her up as a *Bharwad*. She does shepherd's work, wears shepherd's dress, and when she was still a baby I made arrangements for her future by finding her a good shepherd boy to marry. And now you bring me this. Do you call this pant-wearing boy a *Bharwad*? To give my daughter to him would be like throwing her out of the caste. To do such a thing is a sin. A *Bharwad* girl can only marry a *Bharwad* boy. I cannot give her to you. I shall find another groom, a real *Bharwad* for my own daughter who has lived till now as a shepherd and knows only the shepherd's way of life.'[3]

2   According to an educated *Bharwad* in Larabad, the literacy rate among the caste in Gujarat as a whole is only 1 per cent, with women almost entirely uneducated. This calculation may be exaggerated, but it is certainly true that as a group the *Bharwads* have shown very little interest in education.

3   These are the father-in-law's words as recounted by Dilipbhai, who translated them into English, using the words '*Bharwad*' and 'shepherd' more or less interchangeably.

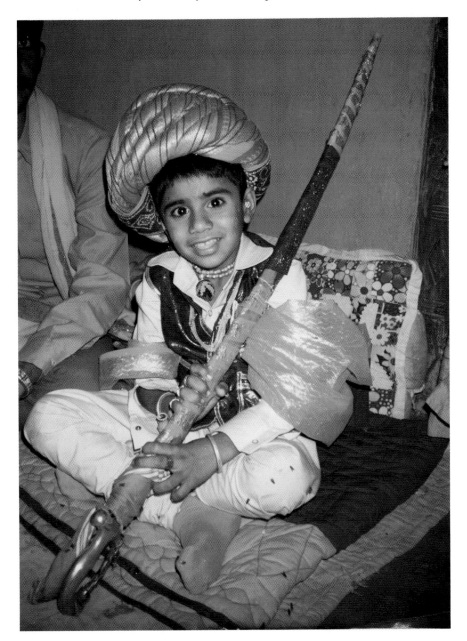

Fig. 8.1 A young *Bharwad* groom (aged seven) dressed for the marriage ceremony, 1989. He wears a *chorni* with a shirt and waistcoat and large brocaded turban. Around the turban is a sequined turban band (*bokani*) and around his neck a pompom (*mala*). Both are worn only on festive occasions.

Kathabhai remained silent throughout this tirade – he was young and it was inappropriate for him to address his elders in front of the crowd – but the *jan* were in an uproar. They felt insulted. They were not even allowed entry into the courtyard – Kathabhai's father-in-law had shut the gate in their faces and refused to admit anyone to his house. So they stood in the street and began to argue back. Some tried to argue that Kathabhai was educated, that he had progressed and he had never worn a *kediyun* and *chorni*. Any normal father-in-law would be pleased that his daughter was marrying such an important man. It would be impossible to find another such groom in their caste. But the bride's father was deaf to all entreaties. He was furious with the senior men of the *jan* for even allowing this to happen. He cancelled the marriage there and then and declared the engagement void.

The whole *jan* were left in the street, humiliated and insulted. What should they do? How could they cancel this marriage after all the preparations had been made and the time was astrologically right? Many senior men of the *jan* were themselves unhappy about Kathabhai's dress and suggested that he should change his clothes. Although angry and insulted, everyone wanted the marriage to take place, and after much squabbling a solution was agreed upon. Katabhai was led to a relative's house and given a clean *kediyun* and *chorni* to wear, and a large red and gold brocaded turban with an embroidered turban band (*bokani*). They put a silver chain (*kandoro*) around his waist, and a large silver anklet (*toda*) on his ankle and he remounted the horse, arriving at the bride's home richly adorned as a conventional *Bharwad* groom. This time his father-in-law opened the door and welcomed him and the marriage took place.

Dilipbhai was in the groom's party and witnessed the entire scene. It was, he claimed, a very bad day for the caste. Marriage was meant to be the most auspicious time of one's life. The groom was meant to be king – he was meant to be welcomed with admiration and respect – but his cousin had been gravely humiliated in front of everybody. Dilipbhai interpreted this as a sign of the great backwardness of people in his caste who felt that failure to wear a *kediyun* and *chorni* meant deserting the caste itself.

When it came to Dilipbhai's own marriage time, his father approached him anxiously and asked him what he would wear for the wedding. He told Dilipbhai:

'It is your choice. I cannot tell you what to wear. But you remember the wedding of your cousin and all the trouble and humiliation of that day. As your father, I beg you to wear *Bharwad* dress, just for your wedding. You see that even Kathabhai's father-in-law accepts that Kathabhai

Some Pastoralist (*Bharwad*) and *Harijan* Dilemmas

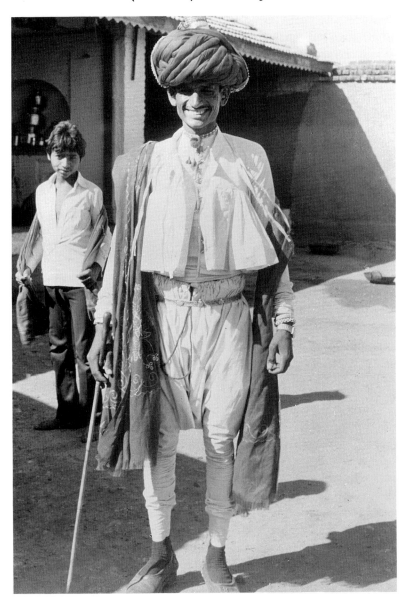

Fig. 8.2 A *Bharwad* man dressed to attend a wedding, 1989. He wears a large red twisted turban and a white *kediyun* and *chorni*. The festive nature of his dress is revealed by the additional features of socks, shoes, turban-band and jewellery. Over his shoulders he wears the pink wool and acrylic shawl now so popular among members of this caste. In the background is a boy wearing trousers and a shirt. He too wears a pink embroidered shawl, thereby marking himself out as a *Bharwad*.

wears bushcot and pant every day. But for his marriage it was different. If you have love for your parents you will do this thing. You will wear *kediyun* and *chorni* like a shepherd just for one day in your life, and then you will be free to dress as you like.'

Dilipbhai, unable to resist these persuasions, agreed to his father's request. He said his parents had provided everything for him and allowed him to be educated, which was unusual in his caste. How could he deny them this one thing and upset them in front of the community? So he told his father that he would wear full *Bharwad* dress for his wedding without making any fuss. This he did, as the photograph album bears witness.

But Dilipbhai's album required careful scrutiny. For, tucked behind a picture of Dilipbhai and his wife at the marriage ceremony, there was an *extra* photograph that Dilipbhai was only prepared to show me when his mother had left the courtyard. Drawing this second photograph from behind the first, he announced with a smile:

> 'This is the *secret photograph*! Nobody knows it is here except my sisters and my wife. If my mother saw it she would throw me out of the house and never speak with me again. But she would never think of looking under here. She does not know how the photos are attached to the page and would never try to move them.'

The secrets of the secret photograph
The secret photograph showed Dilipbhai and his wife standing in a cornfield, with corn up to their waists. They were arm in arm and both were smiling broadly. Dilipbhai looked much the same as ever in his fawn-coloured trousers and white synthetic shirt, but his wife was almost completely unrecognisable from the timid woman I had seen earlier, sheltering beneath her *sadlo* (half-sari), dressed in the typical waist-cloth (*jimi*) and *kapdu* worn by the women of her caste. Not only was she wearing a bright red synthetic sari in the photo, but she had it flung back from her head to reveal her hair and her bold and smiling face. Dilipbhai explained:

> 'This is how my wife would look if I had the choice. But I cannot control it. Her parents would refuse to send her to me if she changed her clothes and my parents would have refused to accept her as their daughter-in-law. Even if she came to live with me in Baroda, she would have to wear *kapdu* and *jimi*. For what if my parents came to visit without warning? They would see her in a sari and we would be thrown out of the caste. I am controlled by my parents. They are controlled by the caste association. *Bharwad* people are very backward-looking, especially the

women. They say "If you change your clothes, then you change your nature." My mother especially thinks this.'

The 'secret photo' had been taken by Dilipbhai's friend from Larabad, who had borrowed a camera for the day and had also provided one of his wife's saris for Shantaben (Dilipbhai's wife) to wear. The actual taking of the photo was planned a week in advance and on the morning of the event Dilipbhai and his friend set off 'to visit a temple' in the hills. Shantaben and her sister-in-law followed soon afterwards. They were supposed to be taking bread (*rotlo*) and buttermilk (*chas*) to some men in the fields. But they made a quick diversion and met up with Dilipbhai and his friend. There in the long grass, Shantaben took off her *sadlo* and exchanged it for the red sari. Then she and her husband posed for the shot. Only one pose was taken, since this friend had obtained the camera to take photos of his own family. But Dilipbhai was very pleased with the result. As he said, 'It could be from a movie, don't you think?'

The picture might have had less impact had it not been hidden immediately beneath a photograph in which Shantaben was completely concealed beneath her marriage veil (*gharcholu*). She was doing *akhi laj* seated opposite Dilipbhai, who was dressed in his *kediyun*, *chorni* and turban. The two were linked by a cotton thread. Just as Dilipbhai's desired image of a modern couple was suppressed in everyday life, so the illicit photograph was concealed behind the overtly conventional *deshi* image. When I spoke with Shantaben about it, she laughed and said that it would be impossible for her to wear a sari in everyday life. She said: 'if you wear a sari then you can no longer be called a *Bharwad*. That is the way it is among our caste. Better to die than to change your clothes.'

Although the *Bharwads* were the only group in the village to show such sartorial conservatism regarding both men and women, there were other shepherd communities in the area, such as the *Rabaris*, who shared a similar style of dress and a similar reluctance to accept change. Even as far away as Ahmedabad city, they tended to cling tenaciously to their traditions. In Ahmedabad it is common to see prosperous *Rabari* men delivering milk on expensive Honda motorbikes but still dressed in *kediyun*, *dhoti* and turban, despite living in a large industrial city. Like Kathabhai, they met with considerable resistance if they tried to cast off such conventional attire. One example of such resistance took place in 1985 when a reluctant *Rabari* wife threatened to reject her husband on account of his clothes.

The tale of the reluctant Rabari *wife*
This tale was recounted by a professor in a university department in

Ahmedabad. In one of his classes he had a bright young student from the *Rabari* community, who apparently suffered from bad body odour because he always wore the same dirty trousers and shirt. One day the professor asked the student why he never changed his clothes and received the following reply:

> 'Sahib, I am a *Rabari*. We people keep goats and sell milk. I too must do this work even though I am studying. When I come home from college I deliver milk on my bicycle. But I have a problem. At home I am expected to dress in *kediyun* and *dhoti* like the rest of my caste. Most of them are still dealing in milk and are very backward-looking. When I came here to college I could not wear *kediyun* and *dhoti* for people would have laughed and said: 'Look! A shepherd in college!' So I purchased one pair of trousers and this shirt that you see me wearing. But it became very difficult for me at home. My wife despised me in these clothes and refused to allow me to come to her. She said that she had married a *Rabari* man and she could only sleep with a *Rabari*. She said that if she saw me in trousers and shirt again then she would never again share the same bed. So you see, I don't let her see me in my college dress. I leave the house each morning in a *kediyun* and *dhoti*. Then I visit my friend's house where I keep these college-going clothes. I change into trousers and shirt for college and then, in the evening, change back into *deshi* [dress] before returning home. Because of this I only have one shirt and one trouser and so I never wash them. And certainly I cannot ask my wife to wash them. She would refuse.'

Before discussing some of the reasons for the sartorial conservativism of pastoral groups it is worth recounting two further examples, this time taken from Kavakshibhai Barot's collection of *Bharwad* folk tales from the villages of Saurashtra (cf. Barot 1977).[4] From these it is clear that even when clothing traditions were questioned and criticised by members of the herding communities, this seldom resulted in the outright rejection of a custom. Rather, the retention of a custom such as a particular style of dress often acted as a barrier to other forms of social change. The first story concerns women's inability to give up the custom of wearing *boloya* (ivory bangles) and the second the difficult relationship between clothing and education. Together with the clothing incidents from Jalia and Ahmedabad, they help to provide some overall view of the attitudes of shepherds to their dress.

4 The tales have been summarised here and should not be taken as literal translations.

Some Pastoralist (*Bharwad*) and *Harijan* Dilemmas

The tale of the boloya (ivory bangles)

Boloya are the thick white ivory bangles given to a young wife by her in-laws. As we have seen, it was customary for members of all castes in the village to give at least one pair of ivory bangles to a new wife. The term *boloya* refers only to the heavy bands of undecorated ivory worn by *Kanbi, Kharak, Bharwad, Koli* and those low-caste women who could afford them;[5] these bangles were usually given to the bride a few weeks before the *anu* ceremony and were one of the symbols of marital bliss (*saubhagya*). Today *boloya* are very costly, particularly because of increased restrictions in the ivory trade.[6] They are also notorious for the pain they cause when they are first squeezed on to the wrists, which have to be bound and greased for the purpose. Most communities have given up the custom of wearing *boloya* and have replaced them with gold or plastic bangles. Among the *Kharaks*, those women who wear *ghaghros* usually continue to wear *boloya* but young women are reluctant to do so and, like the *Kanbis*, now regard them as clumsy and old-fashioned. The *Bharwads*, however, still value them highly and give them to new young wives. The tale of the *boloya* runs as follows.

There was a *Bharwad* girl still living at her parents' house but married into a poor family who had fallen on difficult times. Because of their desperate poverty, the girl's in-laws did not send her *boloya*. According to custom, the girl's mother refused to send her daughter to her in-laws' house until she had received the *boloya* which were her due. Three times the groom's relatives arrived to fetch the bride and each time the girl's mother refused to allow her daughter to leave, saying that she would never join her husband until she had received her *boloya*. On the fourth occasion, the mother relented and agreed to send her daughter on the condition that the daughter should receive *boloya* within one week. The groom's family, despite their poverty, agreed. When the girl arrived at her in-laws, the wife of her husband's elder brother was jealous and annoyed. She was

---

5   The origin of the custom of giving ivory bangles to married women is unknown. Parmar suggests that before they adopted ivory women wore conch shell bangles (interview). Certainly in Bengal the latter are worn by married women (Fruzzetti 1982). According to a census report on ivory manufacture in Saurashtra, it was only wealthy married women who wore ivory bangles 'in early times' but the practice gradually spread down the social hierarchy. The original *boloya* worn by peasant women were apparently made from wood which was dipped in oil to give the bangles a deep maroon colour. Once ivory bangles were adopted they were often dipped in dye to obtain the same deep red colour (*Census of India 1961*, vol. V, part VII–A, no. 4: 3–5).

6   Recent attempts to protect the elephant have resulted in a prohibition on the export of raw ivory from Africa and a restriction on ivory production in India. This has reduced the stock of ivory available and sent prices soaring.

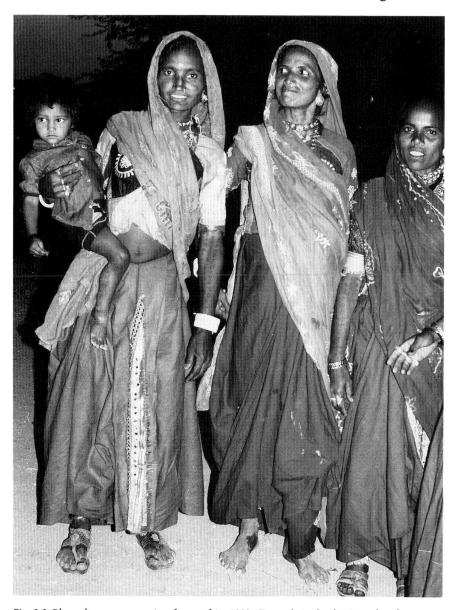

Fig. 8.3 *Bharwad* women returning from a fair, 1989. From their chunky ivory bangles (*boloya*) and their heavy gold earrings (*porkhani*) it is possible to tell at a glance that the two women in the left of the photograph are married and now reside chiefly at their in-laws' home. They wear the *jimi* (waist-cloth), machine-embroidered *kapdu* and veil which is typical of fairly young *Bharwad* wives.

Some Pastoralist (*Bharwad*) and *Harijan* Dilemmas

older than this newcomer and still had not received *boloya*, owing to the family's financial problems.

Within a week of the girl's arrival at her in-laws', the women of the household set out for town to visit the ivory shop. They were given the choice of real or false ivory and said they could only accept real. The shopkeeper asked for 1,800 rupees, and accepted 1,400 rupees after bargaining. The women said that the *boloya* must be tightly fitted. They celebrated the purchase by eating chick pea snacks and sweets. Then, at an auspicious moment, the new wife's arms and wrists were greased with butter and her fingers and thumbs bound together. The girl screamed in agony but the women held her down and the shopkeeper forced the *boloya* on, scraping and bruising her hands. She cried and screamed and said that she no longer even wanted *boloya*. Finally, she fainted with the pain and, when she came round, felt so frightened and ashamed that she wet herself and had to ask for clean clothes. Meanwhile, many city people gathered around to see what all the commotion was about. They looked at the *Bharwads* with disgust and told them they must give up this bad social custom. Why didn't they invest in gold or silver instead?

When the girl returned home, her wrists and hands became septic and swollen. She could not work and her hands smelt bad and the family wasted a lot of money on ointment and medicine. Finally, they had to break each *boloya* off into three parts. When, after three months, she had recovered, they re-fixed them, but this time using metal joins so that they looked ugly. Seeing all this, the women began to wonder if they really should wear *boloya*, but they felt they must because they feared what might happen if they broke this old tradition.

The tale of the Bharwad's dislike of education
A *Bharwad* boy called Lakshman went to school. But it was against *Bharwad* custom to sit still in one place. His own people scolded him and accused him of no longer mixing with the rest of the caste. One day he went down with fever and they called the exorcist (*bhuva*), who said that he had been affected by the evil eye (*najar*). The *bhuva* was given a coconut and tied a thread around the boy's wrists to protect him. His family refused to allow him back to school. Three days after the fever, he was ambling along when a bullock raised its tail and knocked him over. The women exclaimed: 'It is because he is reading that he did not see the tail. It has made his eyes weak.'

Some time later, Lakshman went to his teacher's house and was impressed by the cleanliness and order. The teacher encouraged him to continue his studies and not to bother about what people said. He put Lakshman in school lodgings. Lakshman's father wanted him to study but was worried about *najar*. The teacher told the parents that they could not see their son for six months, and agreed to pay all his expenses himself.

Lakshman's mother disapproved. She said, 'People will talk', 'He will be different from the others' and 'He will be affected by the evil eye'. She cried and cried, and finally after four months she begged the teacher's permission to see her son. But Lakshman's mother did not recognise him because his skin was so pale, he was no longer wearing a *dhoti*, earrings and bangles, and his hair was all one length. She was frightened by his whiteness, which made it look as if his blood had turned to water. She thought that without his silver bangles he looked like a widow. If her mother-in-law saw him now, she would surely object. She was frightened also because his tuft of uncut hair (*chotli*) had been removed. This was a pledge that should only be removed by the *bhuva*; now that he was without it, the mother goddess might become upset.

The head teacher explained that all the other pupils would have laughed at Lakshman if he had kept his *chotli*, and with his earrings and bangles he might have injured himself when playing sports. The teacher returned the jewellery to Lakshman's mother, but she did not believe his explanations. She thought her son's skin had turned white from disease. Lakshman said he was better off at school than at home but his mother would believe none of it. She returned home and told people that her son had turned as white as buttermilk (*chas*). She would never allow him back to school.

At Diwali, Lakshman came home on holiday, dressed in neat clean clothes and wearing shoes and socks. People were impressed by this but they did not like the way he had turned so white. At the end of the Diwali holiday, Lakshman prepared to return to school but his family did not allow it.

Being a Bharwad

Bharwad attitudes to clothing and identity, of which these stories give a general impression, may be summarised as follows. To fulfil the expectations of the *Bharwad* community, a *Bharwad* had to be clothed in something that conformed to the idea of '*Bharwad* dress'. The mere fact of being born of *Bharwad* parents was not enough to convey the full requirements of *Bharwad* identity. Rather, such identity needed to be reconfirmed by a willingness to look like a *Bharwad* and to be seen to be one. Failure to achieve this was not merely considered a threat to the caste but was interpreted as a visible sign of unwillingness to be a *Bharwad*, and was therefore perceived as a *desertion* of caste. This was summed up in the two common phrases: 'If

Some Pastoralist (*Bharwad*) and *Harijan* Dilemmas

you change your clothes, then you change your nature' and 'Better to die than to leave your clothes'. In other words, embodied within a person's clothes was part of the *Bharwad* way of being, some kind of contribution to a more general *Bharwad*ness which included all manner of *Bharwad* customs.

Thus rejection of *Bharwad* dress meant rejection (voluntary or involuntary) by the *Bharwad* community at large. Like the *Rabari* wife who refused to sleep with her husband if he wore 'foren' (non-*Rabari*) apparel, so Kathabhai's father-in-law refused to marry his daughter to a man dressed in non-*Bharwad* clothes. Implicit in these disputes were the two ideas of caste exclusiveness and endogamy. These ideas were major concerns of the caste associations which, according to Dilipbhai, sought to keep *Bharwads* in line. He claimed that all decisions concerning the caste were taken through these exclusive *Bharwad* meetings and that caste matters rarely, if ever, went to court. At times of difficulty important members of the caste came together and elected their own jury. Minor decisions were made by local groups, composed of members of a few neighbouring villages, while major ones were discussed in larger assemblies, containing *Bharwad* representatives from a wider geographic area.

The local association in which Jalia men participated did not have any fixed policy concerning dress but members were opposed to the introduction of 'too many "foren" elements', especially on such occasions as marriage. They felt it better to reject a groom and his clothes rather than marry a *deshi* girl to a 'foren'-looking boy and so risk mixing unlike categories and diluting the *Bharwad* community. In some stricter associations unmarried men were apparently made to swear to keep *Bharwad* customs for the rest of their lives before they were allowed to marry. Failure to do so could result in excommunication from the caste. Many told me of an incident in a neighbouring district where a groom had announced his intention to wear trousers at his wedding. An emergency caste meeting was held in which a jury voted not only to boycott the proposed wedding but also to kidnap the groom's mother. This was rationalised on the grounds that the groom's mother should remain within the community even if her wayward son was willing to desert it by wearing trousers.

Thus in the same way that wearing foreign clothes was perceived by Gandhi and his followers as an act of disloyalty at the national level, so it was perceived as such by the *Bharwad* at the local level. And in the same way that Indian women earlier in the twentieth century remained faithful to Indian clothes even when their husbands deserted them, so *Bharwad* women were even less willing to desert caste dress than their menfolk were. There were fewer disputes about women's dress than men's among the

Bharwads because women were conformists; until their husbands changed their own sartorial image more radically, the women were unlikely to 'step out of caste'. One of the few incidents where women's dress was at the centre of a controversy concerned female modesty rather than caste loyalty. It took place at a wedding in Larabad during which an educated *Bharwad* man announced that it was backward for the bride to be fully veiled. The bride's maternal uncle, upset by this insult, apparently lifted back the veil to expose the young girl's face. Horrified at seeing the bride, the older generation turned their backs on the wedding ceremony, saying that if the bride would not keep *laj*, then they, the old men and women of the community, would have to keep *laj* themselves. Such, they argued, was the perversion caused by people deserting the *Bharwad* tradition and losing all sense of shame.

Marriage, being an important and auspicious occasion when members of the community created and reaffirmed their social bonds, was, as we have seen, a particularly sensitive time for sartorial disputes. Sisters or female cousins from the same village were often married on the same day to grooms who came from other villages, each one bringing his own wedding party (*jan*). Such group marriages brought large crowds of *Bharwads* together, a factor which heightened the likelihood of disagreement, particularly when the uneducated majority met with the small minority of educated *Bharwad* men. Furthermore, the practice of direct exchange marriage and the ideology of equality associated with it reinforced the idea that clothing traditions should not be changed. In a discussion about village fashion, one *Bharwad* man attributed the impossibility of *Bharwad* women wearing saris to the principle of exchange marriage itself:

> 'If I dressed my daughter in a sari, then she would never be able to marry. For in our caste we give our daughters *hame hame* [opposite opposite = exchange] and when we arrange their engagements they are just small children. Now suppose it came to *anu* time and one girl was wearing a sari and the other wearing *jimi* and *kapdu*, how could it be said that they were equal? They would not be the same, and one or the other family would feel cheated. So the marriage, arranged for so many years, would have to be cancelled.'

Similarly, fear of *najar* (the evil eye) served to reinforce the idea that all *Bharwads* should look alike, for any peculiarity in dress or manners risked attracting the envious and destructive glance of others. Beliefs associated with *najar* therefore served to constrain individual interests in favour of group ones, for the eye struck hardest among those of the same caste who

Some Pastoralist (*Bharwad*) and *Harijan* Dilemmas

should in theory be equal but are not quite so (Pocock 1973: 39). Pocock sees *najar* as 'symptomatic of a whole dimension of village life ... particularly expressive of a conflict between the desire to do and be well and the fear of appearing superior' (*ibid.*: 2). In the last *Bharwad* story above, Lakshman's somewhat brief school career was cut short because his parents feared he would attract *najar*. Wearing shoes and socks and other clothes associated with education seemed to imply a sense of superiority which risked inviting the envy of other *Bharwads*. As Pocock shows, *najar* is linked to the dual feelings of envy and guilt which, taken together, serve to discourage blatant displays of individualism within a caste.

In Lakshman's case it was his altered appearance and the suspicion it caused that made his parents remove him from the school. In the case of some Jalia women, it was the fact that being educated would *necessitate* a change of dress that was often put forward as a reason for their lack of education. As one woman put it, 'How can we go to college when we wear the *kapdu*? It is totally open [at the back]. People would laugh at us and call us backward.' Yet, asked why she and her relatives did not wear blouses like the women of other castes, she reversed her argument:

> 'How could we do that? Those things are for educated people. They are for progressive people. We have not studied at all. How can we dress like *bhunelawala* [educated people] when we are not educated? Our people would say we were stepping over the limits of our caste and trying to look more important than we actually are.'

Thus in the same way that women could not go to school because they could not change their dress, so they could not change their dress because they had not been to school. Such reasoning was caught in a vicious circle, with each custom being justified simply by the fact of its existence. So even when the women recognised the physical discomfort and financial burden caused by their custom of wearing *boloya*, they could not reject it because they feared what would happen if they did. According to *Bharwad* reasoning, the *Bharwads* could not leave their clothes because if they did so 'they would no longer be *Bharwads*'. A favourite saying among women was 'You can change your *desh* [locality] but not your *vesh* [clothes].'

Defining Bharwad dress

So we can see that among the *Bharwads* dress plays a vital role in creating and maintaining caste identity. The fact that failure to wear *Bharwad* dress is treated as an act of desertion suggests that for the *Bharwads* clothing does not merely symbolise social identity but also 'transforms' it (cf. Bayly 1986).

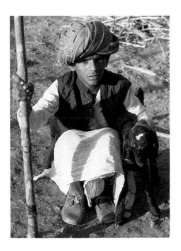

Fig. 8.4 A young *Bharwad* boy, on returning home after a day of goat-herding, 1989. He asked to be photographed with one of his father's goats. Unlike most boys from other castes, he wears *deshi* (local) styles.

According to Bayly, the distinctive feature of pre-colonial Indian ideas about cloth lay in this transformative aspect. By this he means that cloth, being porous to purity and pollution, did not merely mark out the status of its wearers, but also altered their physical and moral properties. In other words cloth was capable of actually transforming the bio-moral substance of the individuals who wore it (*ibid*.: 287). According to such reasoning, a person dressed in silk was considered not merely wealthier than someone dressed in cotton, but morally and physically superior through contact with the cloth.

Of all the people in Jalia, the *Bharwads* would appear to believe more strongly than most in the transformative aspects of cloth. But what is the precise nature of this transformation? For although clothes help to define caste identity, they are not considered sufficient in themselves actually to confer caste identity, any more than eating the appropriate foods can transform a *Harijan* into a *Vaniya*. Obviously, a *Brahman* dressing as a *Bharwad* would never be a *Bharwad*, even if looking the part to perfection. Yet a *Bharwad* without *Bharwad* dress was somehow 'not a *Bharwad*', in view of the fact that he or she was not dressed in the appropriate way. This raises various questions regarding definition. First, what exactly is *Bharwad* dress and to what extent has it remained constant over time? And secondly, are there any specific criteria of *Bharwad* dress which enable us to see which types of changes are permissible before a single garment crosses the boundary between the *Bharwad* and the non-*Bharwad*? Is it the specific type of fabric, the clothing style, the colours, the designs, the mode of production, the geographic origin, or a mixture of some or all of these factors, that makes *Bharwad* dress into *Bharwad* dress? Or is it, as Bayly might suggest, the bio-moral properties of the cloth which actually serve to transform the wearer's physical and moral being?

The accompanying table summarises the various changes that have occurred in the production of different articles of *Bharwad* woman's dress since the early twentieth century. While it may be artificial to carve up the different aspects of an item of clothing in this way, it is, however, helpful in trying to locate precisely what is meant by *Bharwad* dress. These changes may be summarised as follows. There has been a radical change in the raw materials used to make *Bharwad* women's clothes, with synthetic fibres often replacing natural ones. This fits well with Bayly's hypothesis that there is a cultural preference in India for fine fabric, which has been easily satisfied by the ready availability of machine-manufactured cloth (Bayly 1986: 308). For among the *Bharwads* each garment worn in the early twentieth century seems to have been replaced by a new finer machine-

Some Pastoralist (*Bharwad*) and *Harijan* Dilemmas

manufactured version. However, *Bharwad* women were pragmatic about this change. Not only were the machine-produced goods finer and lighter to wear, but they were also cheaper, especially bearing in mind that women could sell the wool they once used for their veils at a much higher price than they now paid for new synthetic materials. Most *Bharwad* families were relatively poor and for them cost was an important factor in their choice of fabric type. While *Kanbi* and *Kharak* women favoured synthetic fabrics because they wanted to boost their social image and escape being classified as backward or uneducated, *Bharwad* women seemed to favour them for predominantly financial reasons and were not concerned with whether or not other castes regarded them as backward. This was clear because they made no attempt to adopt the sari and were on the whole proud of retaining a *deshi* look.

BHARWAD WOMEN'S DRESS (1900–1989)

	Early 20th century	1989
LOWER GARMENT		
Garment style	*Jimi* (waist-cloth)	No change
Raw materials	Wool[7]	Polyester or cotton
Producers	Woven by *Harijans*, Spun by *Bharwads*	Factory
Mode of production	Hand-woven	Machine-woven
UPPER GARMENT		
Garment style	*Kapdu*	No change
Raw materials	Cotton or satin cloth, silk threads, mirror	Polyester, synthetics and sequins
Producers	*Bharwad* women and local tailor	Factory
Mode of production	Hand-woven[8] and embroidered	Machine-woven and stitched
HEAD COVERING		
Garment type	Veil-cloth	No change
Raw materials	Wool	Polyester, cotton or wool
Producers	Spun by *Bharwads*, woven by *Harijans*	Factory (if polyester or cotton)
Mode of production	Hand-woven	machine-woven (if polyester or cotton)

7 Some women claim that it was only *Motabhai Bharwads* who wore woollen *jimis* in the past while *nanabhai Bharwads* wore cotton ones. Unfortunately I was unable to find visual records which might have clarified the situation.

8 It is likely that some *kapdus* were made with machine-woven cloth by the twentieth century. These would have been hand-embroidered by *Bharwad* women, who probably employed a tailor to stitch together the pieces of cloth into *kapdus*.

Changes in material were, of course, related to changes in the mode of production and in the identity of the producers of *Bharwad* clothes. Whereas in the past women embroidered their own *kapdus* by hand, they were now buying ready-made polyester versions of the *kapdu* which were machine-embroidered with coloured thread and which often contained inserts of fake gold brocades and shimmering synthetic materials. Similarly, they were no longer spinning their own wool for their veils, which were now largely factory-produced and machine-printed with new patterns.[9] These changes suggest that it was not necessary for *Bharwad* clothes to be hand-made, or for them to be made by the *Bharwads* themselves in order for them to fulfil the criteria of *Bharwad*ness. City merchants were quick to recognise this and in Larabad there were a number of shops which specialised in ready-made versions of shepherd's clothes.[10] From the readiness with which *Bharwad* women accepted these innovations we can conclude that it is not in the act of creation that *Bharwad* clothes gain their particular *Bharwad*ness. Nor is it in the texture of the fabrics employed, since these fabrics seemed easily replaceable.

When it comes to decorative elements, the situation becomes more complicated. Although patterns and motifs have undergone many changes, these can best be described as transmutations rather than innovations. The *jimi* (waist-cloth), seems to have changed little. It is still plain-except on special occasions when it is worn with a decorative border. Young women wear red *jimis* and older women black ones, a distinction which apparently existed in earlier times. *Kapdu* decorations have perhaps changed more noticeably. Whereas in the past women relied on silk threads and mirror inserts to make their bodices lavish, today they rely mainly on shimmering synthetics to make their best *kapdus* glow. Those modern *kapdus* that are still embroidered are decorated with simple machine-stitched flowers and symetrical patterns. They are commonly embroidered in only one colour (often gold or white), since this enables the man operating the sewing machine to continue sewing without having to change the thread too often. Machine embroidery has also become the most popular decoration for young girls' veils on festive occasions. Whereas in the past embroidery on

9 Many older women still wore woollen veils, particularly when travelling outside the village. These were still hand-woven and could be purchased from specialist shops in Larabad.
10 In Ahmedabad there are equivalent shops which cater to the *Rabaris* of the city and neighbouring area. These *Rabaris*, unlike those in Larabad, used to embroider their own skirts and wore a strip of embroidery on their veils. Nowadays many of them have their skirts decorated by machine embroidery which they order through the city merchants. Unlike Larabad, Ahmedabad attracts tourists from India and abroad. To tourists these specialist shops appear exotic and the merchants now cater to a mixture of *Rabari* and tourist demands.

Some Pastoralist (*Bharwad*) and *Harijan* Dilemmas

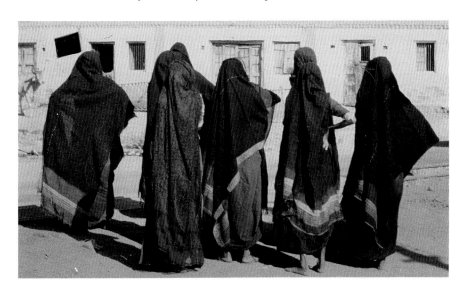

Fig. 8.5 Some *Bharwad* women going to town, 1989. Most such 'old women' wear thick woollen tie-dyed blankets which are black with red dots and red decorative borders. Here one woman (*second left*) wears a red and black printed cotton veil, a design which loosely imitates the woollen blankets worn by the other women. Such cotton veils are considerably cheaper than their woollen equivalents and are increasingly popular.

Bharwad veils was sparse or non-existent, since women had little time or money to embroider, nowadays embroidery often covers the veil-cloth, creating a rich and colourful effect. Yet again, the modern patterns are often transformations of those of the past. The tie-dyed spotted patterns formerly worn by married women were often replaced by machine-printed imitations of tie-dyed patterns or simple floral ones. The black woollen veils (*dhablos*) of old women which were decorated with red tie-dyed spots are sometimes replaced by black cotton veils with a red floral print, which from a distance resemble the old *dhablo* in its overall colour and effect. Thus although it cannot be said that the *Bharwad* have insisted on retaining certain patterns, they do retain a preference for patterns and colours that resemble those worn by past generations.

The most constant factor that *Bharwad* women have retained since the beginning of the century is the garment style and to some extent its colour, and altering these elements would inevitably be perceived as a threat to caste identity. While there was some flexibility in the styles worn by young girls, there was none in the styles worn by women once they were married and living in their conjugal homes. A veil could not be replaced by a sari, or a *kapdu*, though it could be machine-made, by a blouse. And this was one of the reasons why Dilipbhai and his wife were so secretive about their illicit photograph. It showed not only that they had sneaked out of the house together, but also that Shantaben, dressed in a sari and with an uncovered head, was willing to question the necessity of wearing *Bharwad* dress.[11]

While women have remained consistent in their choice of clothing style, men have been less so. Despite their insistence on the importance of preserving '*Bharwad* dress', it remains difficult to define just what this dress actually is for it seems to embody a number of different alternatives. Enthoven described it in 1920 as follows: 'The true *Bharwad* dress for men is three woollen blankets of undyed wool, one wound in broad bands around the head, a second tied around the waist reaching the knee, and a third thrown across the shoulder' (Enthoven 1920, vol. 1: 119). That Enthoven spoke of 'true *Bharwad* dress' suggests that already by 1920 there were some *Bharwads* who did not wear this type of dress. Certainly photographs of *Bharwad* men in the early 1930s show that many were wearing cotton *dhotis* rather than woollen wraps. And today in Jalia *Bharwad* men wear mainly white cotton or white poplin, and no longer restrict themselves to simple unstitched cloth. On their upper bodies they wear either the smock (*kediyun*) with a vest (*gunji*) or sleeveless shirt (*bundi*) underneath, or a long shirt which is sometimes worn with a green waistcoat. On their lower bodies they wear either pantaloons (*chorni*) or *dhotis*. On ritual occasions the *kediyun* and *chorni* combination is the favourite, although some men appear in *dhotis* or wear shirts with their pantaloons. On such occasions men often add other items of adornment such as socks, watches and additional jewellery (silver waist-bands, silver button ornaments and woollen pompoms round the neck). Young men wear red turbans and old men white turbans, wrapped in a variety of styles which, though fairly uniform on ritual occasions, often appear haphazard in daily life. Since the mid-1980s young *Bharwad* men have taken to wearing a new shoulder-cloth which is usually bright pink (occasionally bright red), made from a mixture of wool and acrylic and embroidered by machine in coloured threads (see fig. 8.6). This has largely replaced the thick hand-woven woollen blankets that *Bharwad* men wore in the past. The new garment acts not only as a shawl, but also as a scarf that can be draped around the neck or over the shoulders or even wrapped around the head instead of or on top of

11 Her wearing a sari would not have mattered much if she had been in a photographer's studio where dressing up for photographs is common practice. But to dress up in a field, a public place where women should take care to safeguard their reputations, was a disgrace to the community and a betrayal of the caste.

Some Pastoralist (*Bharwad*) and *Harijan* Dilemmas

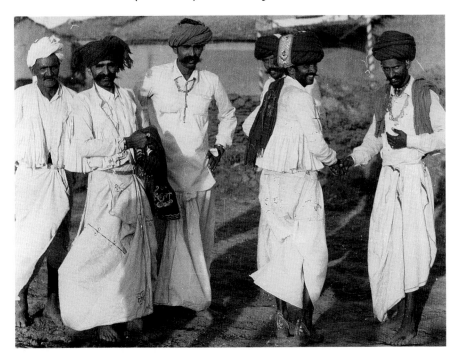

Fig. 8.6 A group of *Bharwad* men at a fair, 1989, wearing *dhotis* with either *kediyuns* or long-sleeved shirts. Note the variety of ways in which they wrap their turbans. The men shaking hands (*far right*) have draped their fashionable pink/red embroidered shawls over their shoulders. Two other men have used similar shawls to bind around their heads in the absence of a fuller turban. *Far left*, a man reveals his seniority by wearing a white turban rather than a pink or red one.

a turban. Although Jalia *Bharwads* have only been buying and wearing these 'shocking pink' cloths during the past few years, they have none the less incorporated them into their image to the extent that few young men are seen without them. At social gatherings and marriages when large groups of *Bharwads* get together, there are inevitably some youths in Western dress, but even they don one of these distinctive pink shawls to show their allegiance to the caste. Indeed this new machine-made acrylic and woollen pink shawl is, in a sense, the single most recognised symbol of *Bharwad* dress, even though it is also the most recent.

Two points emerge from an examination of the features of *Bharwad* men's dress. First, the *kediyun* and *chorni*, which so many *Bharwads* wear on ritual occasions, may, if Enthoven's description is to be believed, be a relatively recent form of dress for *Bharwads*. And secondly, although the *Bharwads* have a strong sense of the need to preserve *Bharwad* dress, the actual features of this dress vary considerably in both material and style and have incorporated some very recent elements. In the same way that their conservativism has not prevented *Bharwads* from adopting modern methods of organising their milk production, so it has not prevented them from adopting new types of dress. Yet, despite the variety of clothes now worn by male pastoralists, it remains easy to recognise them; and perhaps this is the most important feature of *Bharwad* dress – that it should be distinctive. The precise materials employed, the properties of the weave and even the styles chosen were perhaps less significant than this one element of group distinctiveness. And if *Bharwad* men in Jalia today are free to choose from a wider range of styles than ever before, this is perhaps partly because the farming men of the village and region are in the process of rejecting such styles which they now perceive as embarrassingly *deshi*.

The importance of group distinctiveness to the Bharwads
One question remains unanswered, and is worthy of further research: why should pastoral groups like the *Bharwads* show such a strong determination to resist the pressures of mainstream fashion? This resistance applies not merely to dress, but also to education, Western medicine and the *Bharwad* refusal to change certain customs which other castes now regard as humiliating or backward. In Jalia the *Bharwads* are probably the only group who still arrange marriages between young children, and some even claim that in neighbouring areas *pet chandla* (marriage of children while in the womb) is still practised. Quite apart from this, the *Bharwads* hold a complex network of beliefs concerning *najar*, exorcists and diviners which seem to play a more prominent role in the lives of shepherds than for other social groups.

The answer to these differences lies perhaps in that aspect of the pastoralist lifestyle that differs from the lifestyles of other groups in the area. Whereas most communities are fully settled, and travel only for work, shopping or visiting relatives, the shepherd groups have always maintained a semi-itinerant existence, moving if necessary in search of suitable pasture during the driest months of the year. And although today the *Bharwads* of Jalia are largely settled, there seems little doubt that their identity has long been forged on the notion that they are by definition people on the move.

It might be argued that an itinerant lifestyle would put pastoralists in touch with many outside influences, all of which might combine to make their dress less regionally specific than that of other groups. Yet it should be recalled that the continuity and persistence of itinerant groups, the members of which are often forced to separate for months at a time, relies and is indeed dependent upon a strong sense of group solidarity and shared

Some Pastoralist (*Bharwad*) and *Harijan* Dilemmas

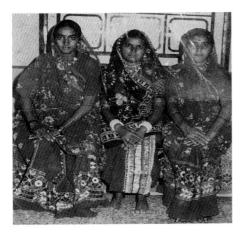

Fig. 8.7 A photograph of three *Bharwad* girls, taken in 1988 by a professional photographer in Larabad. The central figure wears the decorative *jimi* and *kapdu* typically worn by married *Bharwad* women on festive occasions. But her companions wear embroidered *ghaghros* similar to those worn by *Kharak* women in Jalia. Such play with dress is restricted either to secret venues or to the photographer's studio where fantasies can be enacted. It would not be possible for *Bharwad* girls to wear such clothes in everyday life as this would be considered a desertion of caste.

values. Such groups have to preserve their distinctiveness in relation to the outside world literally in order to survive, and the shepherds of Gujarat appear to have done just that.[12] Dress, along with other customs, was one of the means by which men and women reconfirmed their allegiance to the caste and expressed their loyalty to the group. The women's saying, 'We can leave our *desh* [locality], but not our *vesh* [clothes]' was not merely metaphorical; it described the code of conduct and indeed the very lifestyle on which the *Bharwad* community was built. It was therefore vital to the future of the caste's wellbeing that educated men like Kathabhai and Dilipbhai, rather than emphasising their difference through wearing trousers, should express their continued allegiance to the group at least during their own marriages – marriage being a time when the potential future of the community was forged through new alliances.

The sense of solidarity promoted by a shared sartorial image was not merely psychologically important, but also had practical importance to the *Bharwads*. Travelling in search of pasture, they often passed through 'foren' villages where they required hospitality from strangers. The *Bharwads* had a unique custom of providing food or hospitality to any other *Bharwad*, without first inquiring about the stranger's village or name. Here it was the clothes and tattoos of the stranger that provided the key to recognition and subsequent welcome. I was told that earlier in the twentieth century all *Bharwad* men had a tattooed image of Lord Hanuman (the monkey god) on their upper arm and of Lord Krishna on their lower arm, and that these would be inspected by other *Bharwads* if there was any doubt over a person's

12 Gypsies are, of course, the clearest example of this process at work. Scattered throughout the globe, they have retained some form of recognisable dress that distinguishes them from the settled populations around them.

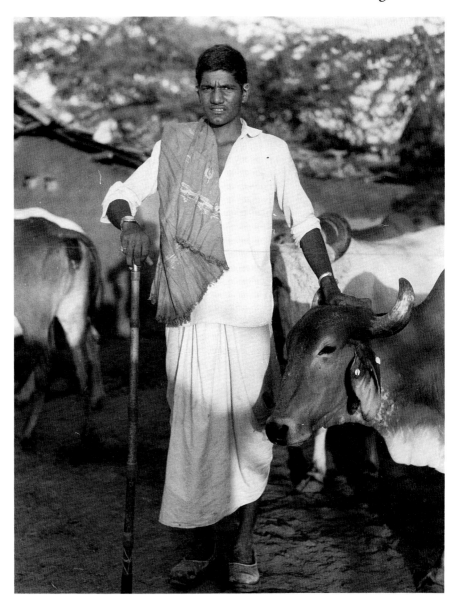

Fig. 8.8 A *Bharwad* youth with his family's cattle, 1989. Relaxing at home, he wears his pink embroidered shawl over his shoulder, having just removed it from his head. This is his first experience of posing before a camera and he has borrowed his father's wristwatch for the occasion. The cattle were included in the photograph at his request.

identity. Examining the groom's tattoos had even been an integral part of the marriage ceremony, for people apparently reasoned that while anyone could dress as a *Bharwad* for the day and so abscond with the bride, no one but a *Bharwad* would ever bear these markings on his arms. The tattoos seem to have acted literally as a guarantee of *Bharwad*ness.

While to shepherd groups the fact of caste distinctiveness and the ability to be recognised were probably the most important aspects of their appearance, there were other groups in Jalia whose concern was to underplay differences and escape the burden of recognition. We turn finally[13] to the *Harijans*, whose progressive attitude to dress provided a stark contrast to *Bharwad* conservatism.

Harijans, the modernists

Bharwads, like other 'caste Hindus' in Jalia, never entered the *Harijan vas* (settlement) for fear of being polluted. If they had, however, they might have been surprised, as I was, by the neat *pakka* houses, freshly painted in blue and white, decorated with posters and ornaments and altogether more prosperous-looking than the small and simple mud houses of the *Bharwads*. Tucked outside the original village boundaries and surrounded by a mud wall, the *Harijan vas* was well secluded so that once inside it one felt that it might have been a different village altogether. But despite its seclusion, it was clear that some 'caste Hindus' had an idea of its appearance; they made comments like '*Harijans* live like kings', or 'The *Harijans* are the only people who can live well these days', or 'Nowadays unless you are a *Harijan* you don't stand a chance of getting a good job'.[14]

13 The term 'finally' is appropriate, because the *Harijans* were, as mentioned earlier, the last group with whom I worked in the village. I was in fact unable to visit the *Harijan* settlement till late in my stay owing to objections from other people in the village with whom I was working. Although all castes considered the *Harijans* as potentially polluting, their precise attitudes varied considerably. No one in the village seemed prepared to accept water from *Harijans* or allow them to share the village well and enter the main temple, but for some (usually high-caste) people, overt prejudice ended there. It was largely among the middle-ranking and low-caste people that discrimination against *Harijans*, and fear of them, was strongest. A *Kharak* woman, with whom I was very friendly, told me that if I ever entered the *Harijan* area I could never visit her house again. The *Brahman* family with whom I lived were more tolerant about my visiting *Harijans*, although they would never do so themselves. As one member of the family put it, 'On paper they are equal to us, but everyone knows there is a difference between what we say and what we do. You know what I mean? As *Brahmans* we are higher. How can we mix with the lower? We would not be performing our duty to our own caste.'

14 I had left India by the time that the then prime minister, V. P. Singh, proposed increasing the quota system for backward and scheduled classes. This proposal, which resulted in rioting in much of northern India, has no doubt increased the resentment that high castes feel towards low castes in Jalia, as elsewhere.

When I had from time to time asked people how it was possible to recognise a *Harijan* in the street, they would usually reply with some derogatory but vague comment like, 'Oh, you can tell from the way they walk, slouching and lolloping', or 'They are dirty', or 'They are always drunk and swaying about'. But sometimes I got other replies such as 'They have a branch [*jaklu*] tied around their waists', or 'They wear a spitoon [*thukdani*] around their necks', or 'They have a whole roll of cloth tied about their heads so you can see that they are untouchable and avoid them'. When I suggested that these customs must surely have been in the distant past and that one never saw such sights today, I was told 'No, not today, but when I was young it was like that', or 'No, but in my mother's time these customs were still there. And she told them to me.' Only one of the people to whom I spoke on this subject actually claimed to have *seen* such practices herself. She gave a lengthy description of the spitoons worn by the *Harijans* in her natal village, saying they were made from earthenware if the people were poor and brass if they were wealthier. Her description sounded convincing.

When I entered the *Harijan vas* what I actually saw were rather modern and fashionable-looking people. There were young women dressed in *shalwar kamizes* and even adolescent girls wearing skirts and blouses, with their calves exposed, such as I had rarely seen before in the village. Married women were dressed mainly in neat saris, tied in the Gujarati style, and men almost without exception wore trousers and shirts. Some of the older generation had a more *deshi* appearance; two old women wore black *jimis*, black and red veils and *boloya* on their wrists, and might have been *Bharwads* apart from the fact that they had rejected the *kapdu* in favour of a blouse, which they claimed was more modern. One woman explained her *Bharwad*-like appearance:

'You see, sister, in the past we had nothing, I mean nothing. We wore what we could get. My father was a weaver and used to weave veils for the *Bharwads*, and in exchange they would give us something to wear, like a *jimi*, a *kapdu* or veil. So after that we looked like them. And now I am old. People would laugh if I started to wear a sari now. They would say, look at her with her white hair and fancying herself young.'

Another woman looked more like a *Kanbi* or *Kharak* and wore the plain red waist-cloth used by the older women of those castes. She explained that years ago she had worked for a *Kanbi* family, doing small jobs. She had been very poor and used to beg for clothes. The *Kanbi* family sometimes gave her a *ghaghro* or a *kapdu* – sometimes both – and for a while she went

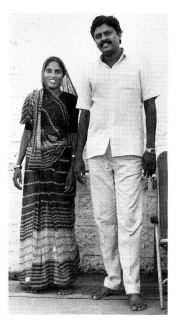

Fig. 8.9 A *Harijan* couple wearing comparatively anonymous styles of dress not associated with any particular caste, 1989. The wife wears a sari in the Gujarati fashion while her husband wears plain trousers and a shirt.

Some Pastoralist (*Bharwad*) and *Harijan* Dilemmas

about in embroidery like them. She had no time to embroider herself and accepted whatever she could get. Nowadays, *Harijan* women had large trousseaux with saris and fine clothes, but in her day, she claimed, she had not received a single item of clothing because her family was too poor.

Asked if they ever had any caste-specific clothing of their own, these women laughed and said they were too poor to care what they wore. They just wore whatever they could get, whatever it might be. The men, too, seemed to have worn a hotchpotch of clothing in the past. Some, if they could afford it, wore a *kediyun* and *chorni* with a small untwisted turban. Others wore a *dhoti* or *langoti* (loincloth). They agreed that they had no real clothing of their own. So I put it to them: 'If you go into the village and see some *Bharwads*, you know that they are *Bharwads* from their clothes. But how do people know when they see a *Harijan*?' One man gave the following reply:

'Nowadays, they don't know. We look like anyone else. We are developed people. Our sons can read and write and even our daughters. We are more educated than any *Kharak* or *Bharwad* of this village. But people used to know us because we had to wear special signs to show them who we were. This we did by tying a whole roll of cotton cloth around our heads like a huge untwisted turban. We called it *talfad*. When they saw *talfad* from a distance, then they knew a *Harijan* was approaching and would avoid us if we did not first step out of the way. Otherwise, if we wore *kediyun* and *chorni* with silver bracelets [*kudla*], people could not tell us apart from other castes. Then there were other things. We wore spitoons of earthenware round our necks so that our spit never touched the ground and polluted the path. Then we tied a branch round our waists so that it hung behind sweeping the ground after us to purify the place where we had trodden. So when people saw these things, they knew that we were *Harijans*. But all this is past now.'

He went on to tell me how these symbols of stigmatisation had come to an end:

'There was a king, a great king who wanted to build a lake in Patan. He constructed a huge ditch but it was empty and he did not know how to find water. He was told that he must sacrifice a boy who was virtuous in thirty-two different ways, and only then would water come. But it was difficult to find a virtuous boy and no father wished to sacrifice his own son. Finally one *Harijan* man came forward and sold his son to the king. The boy, who was named Mayo, agreed to be sacrificed only on condition that the wearing of symbols by the *Dhed*[15] (*thukdani, jaklu, talphad*) should be ended. The king agreed and the worship (*puja*) began. But at the last moment Mayo changed his mind, telling the king that it was wrong to sacrifice someone from his own kingdom. He tried to run away but he slipped and fell into the empty lake, cutting his foot. From the blood, water sprung and filled the lake. So we worship this boy. We call him Malapal. He was so truthful that no one swears falsely on his name.'

When asked when these events were thought to have taken place, he said that it was before independence, in his grandfather's day. He claimed that his grandfather, a weaver, had worn all these signs. But when I discussed the story with some *Brahmans*, they agreed on all the details except for the date. They argued that the king in the story was Sidh Raj (1094–1143). It was therefore impossible for anyone in the village to have seen any of the signs of untouchability, and they merely *claimed* to have seen them.

The *Brahman* interpretation of the story as a legend from the distant past seemed more valid than the popular perceptions of other villagers, for surely if such customs had persisted into the twentieth century they would have gained more exposure from politicians like Ambedkar and Gandhi who took up the *Harijan* cause. Yet, to my knowledge, neither had publicised these humiliating customs. The story of Mayo is, however, recorded (in slightly different versions) in the district *Gazetteer* (1884 vol. 8: 157) and in Enthoven (1920 vol. 1: 322–3), where again it is attributed to the reign of Sidh Raj. Certainly by the beginning of the nineteenth century these stigmatising articles of apparel must have entirely disappeared, for the Rev. A. Taylor, writing in the late eighteenth century, recalls:

> *Dhedas* used to drag thorns after them, and till lately *dhedas* were not allowed to tuck up the *dhoti* but had to trail their dress along the ground. Though traces of this practice have disappeared, an abusive term *kuladi* or *kodivala* or spittoon-men, shows that at one time the *dhedas* had to hang spittoons round their necks (in Enthoven 1920 vol. 1: 322).

Leaving aside the absence of education and the concurrent lack of historical accuracy among most older-generation villagers, the time-lag between the *Brahman* and other more popular interpretations of the *Harijans'* plight could not be ignored. Had·villagers claimed that these symbols of untouch-

---

15 *Dhed*: a weaving caste, later known by many as *Vankars* and later still as *Harijans*. The more politicised term 'dalit' was not used in Jalia.

Some Pastoralist (*Bharwad*) and *Harijan* Dilemmas

ability were simply the habits of *pelana varus* (years gone by), then there would have been no discrepancy, since this multi-purpose category of time stretched back anything from a few years to infinity. But the fact was that almost everyone I spoke to on the subject (mainly *Harijans*, *Bharwads*, *Kanbis* and *Kharaks*) claimed that either their parents or their grandparents had witnessed these things 'with their own eyes'. The result of this telescoping of history, this insistent recounting of a story as though it had happened in the immediate past, was that the idea of the untouchability of the *Harijans* remained ever-present in the minds of the new generation. And what remained present for all except the *Harijans*, it seemed, was not the tale of how these symbols came to be abolished, but rather the details of what they were and why they existed in the first place. For many uneducated women in the village, the story provided a means of convincing their children of the polluting nature of *Harijans*. It was a means of saying that although *Harijans* no longer look different today, they *are* different and must be avoided accordingly. Indeed they are *so* different and *so* polluting that they even used to have to wear special items of clothing to warn people of their coming and purify the ground on which they trod. It might be imagined that while many villagers attribute these symbols to the immediate past, for the *Harijans* themselves they belong to a more distant past, since they must surely find the association with these traditions humiliating. But, on the contrary, *Harijan* men and women of the older generation did themselves attribute the symbols of untouchability to their recent past, recalling how their parents and grandparents used to have to wear these visible statements of their own impurity.

To understand this attitude, it is necessary to recall briefly some popular ideas about the *Harijans'* impurity which were shared not merely by other groups in the village but by the *Harijans* themselves. Untouchability, as practised in Gujarat, encompassed the belief that *Harijans* were so impure that the mere sight of them was potentially polluting. They were therefore forced to live on the outskirts of villages and were barred from entry to the village centre, to shops, temples, wells and the houses of other villagers. They were denied the services of the barber (where contact with a *Harijan*'s skin and hair would have been particularly polluting), and even at times access to local transport facilities for fear that they would pollute other passengers. The polluting qualities of the *Harijans* could be transmitted not merely through touching them, but also through contact with objects which they had touched.[16] Thus most people refused to take money that was in a

---

16 Among the objects which could be polluted by a *Harijan*'s touch was, of course, cloth. But was cloth any more permeable to pollution than other objects? It is difficult to gain any clear

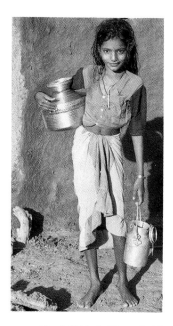

Fig. 8.10(a) A *Bharwad* girl wearing a full-length *ghaghri* tucked up at the waist for ease of movement, 1989. In a couple of years she will learn to cover her head with a veil cloth.

Harijan's hand without purifying it with water. Acceptance of these restrictions by *Harijans* themselves rested not merely on fear of reprisals (usually beatings) from other castes, but also on their own belief that through polluting other castes they were committing a sin which affected their own chances of rebirth at a higher, more desirable level of society in the next life. According to this internalised ideology, it was in the interests of the *Harijans* themselves to avoid polluting other castes.[17]

It is difficult to assess whether or not the outer symbols of untouchability mentioned by villagers actually existed in concrete terms. Yet perhaps the question of their existence is less significant than the fact that they have been retained in modern memory as if they did exist, and as if their demise were only recent. For *Harijans* as much as for members of other castes, the story of the symbols of untouchability has reminded them of their lowly position and their need to distance themselves from other groups. At the same time the story of Mayo, the untouchable boy who was virtuous in thirty-two different ways and who became a god, acted as a hope for the future, suggesting that good deeds were worthy of reward.

But the implications of these stories are changing over time. For young, and even middle-aged *Harijans*, the outward symbols of untouchability seem to be retreating into history and myth. As discrimination lessens[18] and *Harijan* education increases, the story becomes important as an indicator of just how badly treated their ancestors were in the past and of how they themselves must strive for a better future. Knowledge of their past humilia-

---

historical insight into this question, owing to lack of concise data, but I. P. Desai's study of untouchability in rural Gujarat (1976) provides detailed statistics of contemporary attitudes and practice. By the 1970s cloth ranked fairly low in its permeability to pollution as compared to other substances such as food and water. In two-thirds of the villages studied, tailors were willing to mend a *Harijan's* clothes (I. P. Desai 1976:132), and tailoring itself was an increasingly popular occupation among *Harijans*, who had clients from various castes (Desai 1976: 155).

17 The *Harijan* practice of stepping aside in the road to avoid meeting a person from another caste was still widely practised in the 1970s (I. P. Desai 1976: 205–6).

18 It is important to distinguish here between those whom villagers classify as *Harijans* (ex-weavers previously known as *Vankars* or *Dheds*) and those whom they refer to as '*Bhungis*' (sweepers who are not locally accepted as *Harijans*). The latter live separately from the former in comparatively poor conditions and remain the recipients of taunts and prejudice from other groups, including *Harijans*. In Jalia there were *Bhungi* children who had stopped attending school because of the bullying they received from other pupils who refused to sit near them. Such families continued to pursue their traditional occupations of sweeping and preparing the dead for the funeral pyre, polluting tasks which reinforced local prejudice against them. In general, it would seem that ex-weavers have been able to benefit more easily from government assistance in education and employment than the more stigmatised '*Bhungis*'. It is surprising, however, that it was the *Dheds* or *Varkars*, and not the sweepers, who in the past were required to wear visible indications of their own untouchability. Were the latter perhaps too ill-clad and poor to require further distinguishing features? I can offer no answer to this.

Some Pastoralist (*Bharwad*) and *Harijan* Dilemmas

tion is supplemented by school and college education and the knowledge that Gandhi declared himself a *Harijan* and was not ashamed to live and eat among them. Furthermore, access to government-backed education and jobs in government institutions has made *Harijans* less dependent on the village for their livelihood and reputation. Many have either left the village altogether or commute to other cities or towns for their work. They are more concerned with education and earning a decent living than with the attitudes of less educated villagers whose prejudices they cannot radically change.

Over dress the *Harijans* present an interesting case. They never had any caste-specific clothing of their own and it was precisely because of this lack of an immediately recognisable identity that they were forced to wear signs which marked out their status to other castes. These marks should not be regarded as '*Harijan* dress', for, by all accounts, if they existed at all they were never worn within the *Harijan* settlement but only when *Harijans* went into the public domain where they needed to be recognised and avoided.

The absence of a coherent caste dress in the past, combined with the relatively high levels of education and urban employment among *Harijans* today, gives them more freedom in their choice of dress than many other villagers, for they have neither a caste tradition to protect nor a good reputation to preserve in the eyes of others who do not respect them anyway. The future of the *Harijans* lies not in the maintenance of tradition but in breaking with it and trying to forge a new, more acceptable identity independent of the hierarchical foundations of caste. They are therefore free to adopt synthetic saris and *shalwar kamizes* which enable them to participate in progressive, mainstream fashion, and they have no desire to compete in the caste-bound hierarchy of dress within the village itself where prejudice against *Harijans* continues to abound.

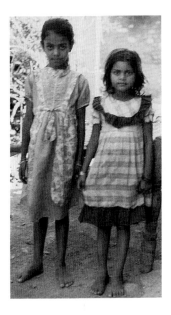

Fig. 8.10(b) Two *Harijan* girls wearing Western-style 'frocks' which link them more to city fashion than to *deshi* styles, 1989. Unlike the Bharwad girl, the latter attend school.

The *Bharwads* and the *Harijans* provide two examples of contrasting attitudes to dress. While *Bharwad* identity is based on the notion of preserving group distinctiveness through time, *Harijan* identity is built on the principle of building a new, more anonymous identity in the future. It is worth comparing the situations of the two groups in more detail. The *Bharwads*, though poor, never had the stigma of untouchability attached to them. Rather, they were defined by other groups as outsiders, as 'jungle people' who spent too much time in the forests and were rough and uncouth. This outsider status in fact contributed to the strength of the *Bharwad* community, which had its own rules and traditions and deliberately reinforced its own distinctiveness in relation to other groups. Clothes were an important means of both preserving social distance and reinforcing the group's own sense of solidarity. Dressing in a *Bharwad* way (however defined) has not only helped modern *Bharwads* to resist certain changes, but has also been a device that has prevented change: dressed in the *deshi* style; a person's environment is immediately restricted. Lacking the geographical boundaries which keep individuals in the village from stepping above their station, the *Bharwads* have created their own sartorial boundaries which play a similarly restricting role in preventing individuals from stepping out of line.

There are certain parallels between Gandhi's choice of a *deshi* image and the *Bharwads'* veneration of the *deshi*. In both cases, the fact of choosing a *deshi* mode of expression was also linked with the fact of distance from the *desh* (locality). It was through spending years in England and South Africa that Gandhi came to appreciate the Indian way (defined in terms of an idealised past). And, similarly, it is through leading a semi-itinerant existence and seeing a variety of alternatives that the *Bharwads* have come to appreciate the benefits of the local Kathiawadi style and to venerate the *deshi* above the new. It is somewhat ironical that the only group in Jalia which actively favours *deshi* dress and attributes positive values to it is the only group which never had a well-defined *desh* (place) in which to live. Those whose lifestyles are fixed within the boundaries of the village itself are more inclined to favour 'foren' clothes which carry the appeal of exoticism and imply sophistication.

While the *Bharwads* needed to create boundaries in order to survive, the *Harijans* have had the opposite problem. They needed to change their image and reformulate their social identity to escape the closely-knit and oppressive social and spatial boundaries that limited their actions in the past. They have, not surprisingly, rejected the *deshi* idiom which to them represents poverty and oppression. It is no coincidence that while Gandhi, who came from the *Vaniya* caste, chose to represent the *Harijans* by dressing as a poor man in the *deshi* style, Ambedkar, himself a *Harijan*, chose to represent them by wearing a full set of European clothes. Coming from a *Harijan* background, and having felt the full weight of social prejudice, he needed to break with tradition and had no nostalgia for the *deshi* past which summed up centuries of poverty and degradation. Having said this, there are of course some old *Harijan* men in the Larabad district who wear *khadi* and the Gandhi cap, but their sons and daughters usually do not choose to share this image. In Jalia, as we have seen, *Harijan* women seem freer in their choice of dress than *Brahman*, *Kanbi* and *Kharak* women who rely on what 'people of the village think and say'. In fact the *Harijans* (at the bottom of the social system) and the *Vaniyas* (considered by many to be at the top of it) are the two groups least concerned with village attitudes and least constrained in their choice of what to wear. While confronted with financial and aesthetic considerations like anyone else, they are the least hampered by the pressure of local opinion.

Viewed in a broad perspective, Jalia is but one village among thousands participating in what is undoubtedly a national trend: the dissolving of narrowly defined social and regional sartorial boundaries in favour of broader, more encompassing definitions. Yet, as we have seen, villagers are by no means swept up blindly or unwillingly by industrialisation. Many feel constrained by the limitations of previous regional traditions and actively *seek* variety and change. Even the *Bharwads*, despite their veneration of the *deshi*, have introduced an increasing range of styles and fabrics within their definition of *Bharwad* dress. And who would deny them the choice?

As an outsider, equally bound by the perceptions and limitations of my own consumer-oriented society, I inevitably liked many of the hand-made clothes that villagers were rejecting. And while I was trying to understand their changing tastes, they too were trying to understand mine. When I finally left the village, the family with whom I was staying gave me a gift of clothing which, this time, I received without hesitation. And I was touched by their choice. No longer were they trying to dress me in shiny synthetic rayons, but instead presented me with a *shalwar kamiz* of pure cotton. In the front they had inserted a large panel of local embroidery which, they said, 'they will like in Foren!' I shared their sense of irony at the fact that I, the foreigner, could wear the fabrics from which local peasants were trying to escape. But there was more irony to come. And much more Gujarati embroidery. I found them both in Delhi.

9   Fashion Fables of an Urban Village

Prologue: through 'ethnic chic' eyes, 1989

As *Vaniya* and *Harijan* women lead the women of Jalia into synthetic saris
and *shalwar kamizes*, as *Kanbi* and *Kharak* women throw aside their hand-
embroidered skirts and bodices in favour of button-down polyester blouses,
as the wilful *Brahman* Hansaben struggles for the right to wear a cardigan
and a bra, I enter another village where 'traditional' arts are respected and
admired, villagers are proud of a *deshi* look, and even some men seem to
enjoy wearing Indian styles. I see before me a young man clad in white
khadi and wearing delicately embroidered Rajasthani shoes. On his forehead
is a mark of henna paste. Beside him, his friend tosses a shimmering silk-
embroidered shawl over his shoulders so that it hangs, half obscuring his
loose cotton *kurta pyjama*. Women, glowing with embroidery and mirror
work, dressed in the very *ghaghros* and *kapdus* that Jalia women spurn,
flit before my eyes. Clad in hand-dyed fabrics and bulky silver jewellery,
these are clearly women proud of their 'traditional' clothes and proud
of their village.

As I walk from house to house among the buffaloes and the mud (it
is November but there has been a freak rainstorm and the earth is sodden),
I see none of the plastic beaded sofa sets, stainless steel vessels, metal cupboards and crude calendar pin-ups that are common sights today in the
houses of Jalia. Instead I see 'An Indian Story', for among the 'cane and
wicker' are embroidered wall-hangings of 'ethnic splendour', delicately
hand-carved wooden furniture and pillars, carefully patterned mud-covered
walls, hand-painted scenes from Hindu mythology, brightly decorated pup-
pets and masks, earthenware jars, old brass oil lamps – in short, a feast of
'beautiful designs from a rich past'.[1] I thought of Coomaraswamy and his
disillusionment with the modern India he knew, how he had implored people to recognise 'the luxurious simplicity of Indian culture' (Coomaraswamy
1908: 33) and told his readers:

> Look about you at the vulgarisation of modern India. . . . our use of
> kerosene tins for water jars and galvanised zinc for tiles – our caricature

---

1   These are quotations from shop hoardings and publicity cards.

of European dress – our homes furnished and ornamented in the style proverbial of old seaside lodging houses (Coomaraswamy 1911: 3).

Would he not have been content to stand where I was standing, in the heart of a 'genuine' village 'where art is tradition' (publicity card)? Or would he have felt confused? After all, where is this village? Those embroidered hangings that adorn the walls suggest I am still in Gujarat. Yes, it must be Gujarat with those carved wooden doors and pillars, although I have rarely seen such ancient craftsmanship in such good condition. Had I chosen the wrong village when I went to Jalia? Were there *really* still villages where craftsmanship was so highly valued and preserved? But wait, those hand-painted murals, beautiful though they are, are not in the Gujarati style. They remind me strangely of Bihar. But then that 'cane and wicker' has a distinctly southern flavour, while those woollen hats look positively Himalayan. I could think myself in a National Crafts Emporium if it were not for the buffaloes and the mud and the small winding streets with a tea-stall at the corner.

I follow the distant sound of music. I am back at the entrance to the village where musicians are sitting cross-legged on the ground with their colourful tie-dyed turbans gleaming under the spotlights (it must be Rajasthani village! But spotlights?). The crowd has thickened since I first arrived and my eyes feast on the brightest and most lavish 'village belles' I have ever beheld. They are moving around the Gujarati pillars, which stand strangely aloof, without any houses to support. But there seems to be a division in the crowd. All around the pillars are women dressed in 'genuine' Indian clothes. But just across the road, out of the glare of the spotlights, stands a bunch of people miserably clad in greys and browns: women in rayon *shalwar kamizes* with plain shawls flung around their heads and shoulders; men in jeans and tight-fitting trousers and shirts. Who are these people infiltrating this beautiful 'traditional village scene'? How dare they spoil the aesthetic bliss with their fake, Western look? No wonder there are two security guards to protect the *real* villagers from this urban onslaught, lurking like a shadow on the dark side of the street. Who are these intruders?

Then the show begins. A young villager gets up on stage. She is dressed in a beautiful raw silk *khadi lehnga* (full gathered skirt), her hair loose about her shoulders. She offers flowers to a woman in the crowd and there is clapping and cheering. Who is that woman wearing a red and black tie-dyed scarf over her shoulders, the very scarf that *Bharwad* women wear as a veil? 'The film-star, Jaya Bacchan', I hear people mumble as they strain their necks to see. The dark intruders on the outskirts of the village are pushing forward, excitedly. The security guard is holding them back. The Rajasthani music gets louder, the lights get brighter and on the stage. . . .

Not 'luscious *lehngas*' and 'ethnic splendours' but, for a moment, models clad in the stark, sleek tailored clothes of Shahab Durazi, an Indian fashion designer, trained in New York (see fig. 9.1). More models appear dressed mainly in black and white, in pin-striped jackets and pleated trousers, tailored skirts above the knee. They prance self-consciously between the Gujarati pillars to the incongruous beat of the *tabla* (drum). However, they are soon followed by a stream of models in *lehngas, ghaghras* (Hindi for *ghaghros*) and even *kapdus*, made from a variety of village cottons, expensive silks and mirrored embroidery. Many have bare feet or simple embroidered shoes. Some wear veils over their heads, which they toss and swirl, peering seductively from underneath, flashing their painted eyelids and pouting their shining lips. Others wear more modern styles such as skintight *shalwar kamizes* or miniskirts containing patches of Gujarati or Sindhi mirror work.

The village is Hauz Khas, tucked away in what was a strangely quiet corner of South Delhi. In 1989 it was fast becoming one of the trendiest and most expensive shopping centres for designer clothes in the capital. The event was Delhi's first fashion show ever to be staged outdoors in a village setting. It was the celebration of the opening of Ogaan, the latest in the recent range of designer stalls. The crowd around the stage was composed of film-stars, fashion designers, boutique-owners and industrialists from some of India's leading families. Most of the women in the crowd were wearing so-called 'ethnic' clothes and jewellery. Some were dressed convincingly like Gujarati or Rajasthani peasants, although their make-up and hair-styles betrayed their urban roots. Their men were mainly in Western dress though a few had donned *khadi kurtas*, silk pyjamas and embroidered shawls. And as for the other crowd held back by the security guard, they were the people who actually lived in Hauz Khas village. They had come to watch the Indian glitterati, dressed as glamorised villagers in styles of clothing that no actual inhabitant of Hauz Khas would consider fashionable enough to wear. As the village headman put it, 'Previously people were looking down on us because we were wearing *dhotis* and looking like farmers. But now they actually come to the village and dress in our old clothes.'

His assessment of the situation was all too accurate. For Bina Ramani, a high-society fashion designer and one of the key inspirations behind this village revival, had told me earlier that evening as she was preparing to attend the show, 'I think I shall go as a village peasant tonight.' Selecting a flared cotton *lehnga* from the rails of her own boutique, she added:

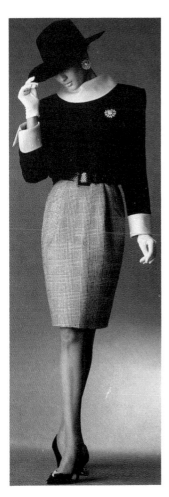

Fig. 9.1 An outfit designed by Shahab Durazi whose collection was modelled in the fashion show at Hauz Khas. Reproduced from *Glad Rags*, 1989, vol. 2, no. 2.

Fashion Fables of an Urban Village

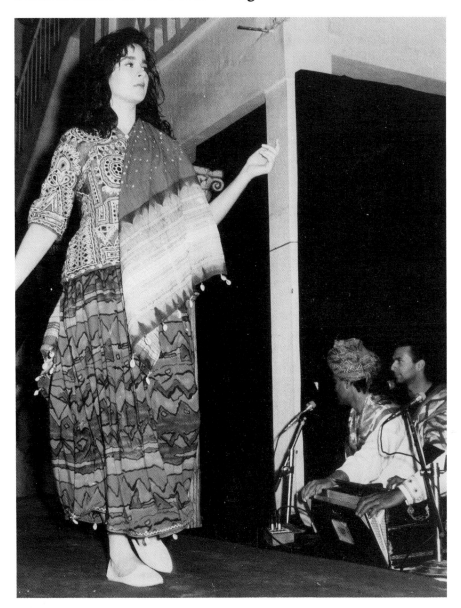

Fig. 9.2 The fashion show at Hauz Khas, 1989. Here a model takes the stage wearing an 'ethnic' skirt, embroidered *kapdu* and tie-dyed shawl. To the right a musician clad in a stereotyped version of Rajasthani dress plays music to accompany the show. Behind him is a fashion designer who wears a black *kurta pyjama* with a *phulkari* (embroidered cloth from the Punjab) draped over his shoulders. Courtesy of Kavita Bhartia.

'You see, this is a *real* peasant skirt. The village women come to me and sell their stuff. Village women wear such fabulous clothes. Really, I think they know how to dress like nobody else. . . . Villages are beautiful. They are the *real India*.'

Hauz Khas – the village and its environment
Hauz Khas village takes its name from the great (*khas*) water reservoir (*hauz*) built by *Ala-ud-Din-Khilji* at the end of the thirteenth century. In the fourteenth century Emperor Firoz Shah Tughlaq repaired the damaged tank and built alongside it a series of buildings commonly identified as a *madrasa* (college or seminary). These vast stone constructions had led to the displacement of a small village of Muslims, *Jats*[2] and sweepers. Some years after the fall of the Sultanate, these original inhabitants returned to the site of their former village and set up homes within the abandoned buildings, filling up the open spaces between pillars with a mixture of stones and mud and cow dung paste.[3] Over the centuries, the condition of the buildings declined but the residents remained. By the early twentieth century there were approximately 100 families (of which two-thirds were Muslim) living in these patched-up ancient monuments and earning their livelihood by farming the surrounding land. This was the situation when in 1913 the Archaeological Survey of India, then under British authority, declared the monuments worthy of protection and forced the inhabitants to move outside the original walls. With gold guineas as compensation the locals built themselves a new village just beyond the protected archaeological zone. It is this comparatively modern construction that is known today as Hauz Khas village.

The village's somewhat brutal history continued with Partition when many of the wealthy Muslim families fled to Pakistan, leaving most of the land and property in the hands of *Jat* farmers. But even the position of these farmers was insecure, for by the late 1950s and '60s the Delhi administration was buying up vast tracts of land in and around the city in order to cater to the massive influx of refugees. Having already seen their homes transformed into an archaeological site, the villagers of Hauz Khas now witnessed their farmland transformed into a public park and picnic area, a so-called 'green lung' for the expanding capital. Ironically, it was this 400-acre green lung which protected Hauz Khas from the property

2 *Jats*: a caste of agriculturalists found mainly in North India.
3 The historical details recorded here were collected from elderly villagers. That villagers were previously living inside the monument walls is confirmed by an account by Carr Steevan (1876).

developers, who soon pounced on other urban villages,[4] incorporating them into the densely populated urban mass. While the outer and inner ring roads ran either side of the green zone, the absence of a through road prevented the village from attracting traffic. It therefore remained both architecturally and economically aloof from the city around it. In 1986 it housed a small population of 1,500 inhabitants, spread among 160 houses, of which well over half were *kacha* or semi-*kacha*.[5] Non-residential commercial activities were restricted to a printing press, a small manufacturing unit for washing-machines, two export garment units and a marble go-down. Local commerce was limited to tea-stalls, two small grocery shops, *pan*-sellers, a flour-mill and a washerman's stand (cf. Narendra 1989). This low level of economic development made Hauz Khas village an unusual and forgotten feature of the capital.

Population and residence

The village, as it stood in the early 1980s, was divided into two main residential sections: the *pakka* area which branched off to the right as you entered the village and the semi-*pakka* and *kacha* area which branched off to the left. The former consisted mainly of large, narrow houses, built of brick, stone and lime with wooden beams and roof-tops. These were usually of one or two storeys[6] and built around inner courtyards. Floors were either of stone slabs or plastered with mud and cow dung paste. Interiors were generally simple, with the typical North Indian features of decorative metal *jalis* (filigree ventilation holes) and small niches for storing goods and for placing the household gods for worship. Wooden pegs for hanging clothes and oil lamps were still common features of the houses, even though the necessity for them had been largely eliminated by the arrival of steel cupboards and electricity. Buffaloes and cows were generally kept within the house compound and at either side of the open courtyards.[7] This

---

4 There were 111 'urban villages' recognised in the Master Plan of Delhi in 1962. The land surrounding them was purchased by the government in the period 1958–76 at the rate of 50 paise per square yard. Villagers were given the opportunity to buy land elsewhere at a special rate, but many did not take up the option since they were attached to their villages and did not want land in another area.

5 These figures are taken from R. Narendra, 'Hauz Khas Village, Delhi, an approach towards redevelopment', unpublished thesis, School of Planning and Architecture, Delhi, 1989, and I am extremely grateful to Rachna Narendra not only for making her thesis available but also for returning to Hauz Khas with me six months after her study was completed, thus enabling us to compare notes about the development of the village over the previous twelve months.

6 I am counting the ground floor as the first storey.

7 For further details and architect's drawings of village houses, see Narendra 1989.

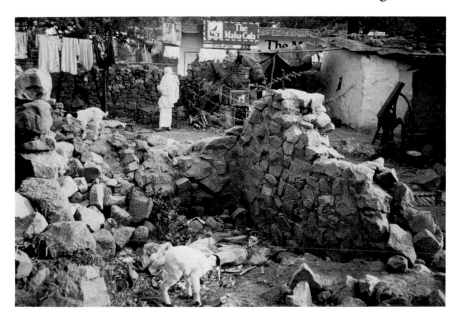

Fig. 9.3 Views of Hauz Khas village in the winter of 1989. *Above*: The poorer side of the village where bill-boards advertise Maha Cola and Thumbs Up. *Below*: The pakka section of the village where hoardings advertise fashionable boutiques. A Rajasthani musician has been hired for the day to lend an 'authentic' village atmosphere.

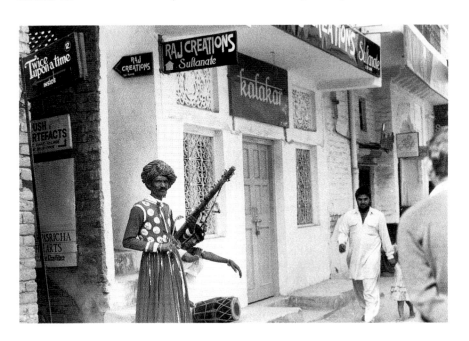

Fashion Fables of an Urban Village

pakka section of the village was inhabited mainly by *Jats*. Since losing their land in the 1960s, they had found alternative employment in a variety of occupations, usually outside the village. Many supplemented their incomes by keeping cattle and selling the milk. A few of these men were highly educated and had professional jobs in the city.

In the poorer half of the village, housing conditions were shabby and varied. Some people had built concrete houses. Others lived in mud or brick constructions or entirely makeshift patchwork houses, made from scraps of whatever material was available. Most of the inhabitants were poor Muslims and *Harijans*, who earned their livelihood mainly from casual labour such as building, carpentry, plumbing and vending. Women of these families were often employed as home helps or sometimes as sweepers in Delhi. In the 1950s the eminent writer and activist Mulk Raj Anand had bought a plot on the outskirts of the village and tried to set up pottery and weaving workshops for *Harijans* under the auspices of the social welfare organisation, Lokayata. But his attempts failed and have left little trace on the evolution of the village.

Apart from *Jats, Harijans* and Muslims, who can be considered the indigenous inhabitants of the village, there were some more recent arrivals. In the higher-income group, these consisted of a few educated families, mainly Punjabi, who had built their homes in the village in the 1980s. They were professionals who had found that Hauz Khas offered easily affordable accommodation as well as proximity to their work. Their choice of location had been considered extraordinary by most professional Delhiites at that time, who regarded the village as too 'primitive' and ill-equipped for modern living. In the lower-income group were individuals and families who could not afford urban rents, but who rented rooms at village-type rates in the houses of the *Jats*. These families often lived in cramped conditions, sometimes with as many as ten people to a single room.

A new style of tenant

From 1987 onwards, a new category of tenants was rapidly emerging. These were fashion designers and boutique-owners from some of Delhi's wealthiest and most fashionable families. They had started renting rooms in the smarter quarter of the village, where they were establishing exclusive boutiques selling expensive designer clothes, art and furnishings, most of which were sold under the classification of 'ethnic' or 'antique' goods. In February 1989 there were twelve such boutiques in the village. By December the number had more than tripled to thirty-eight, with over half specialising in ethnic clothes. Unlike the Punjabi tenants, the boutique-owners

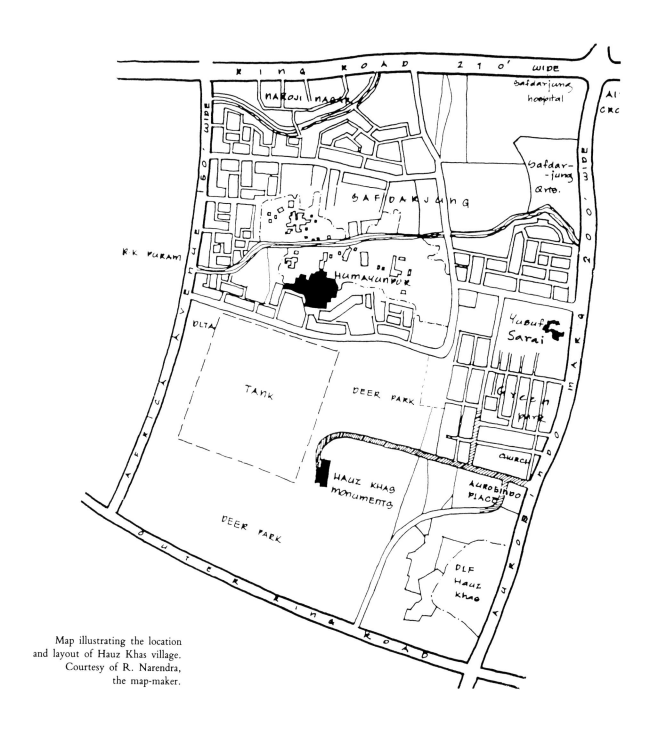

Map illustrating the location
and layout of Hauz Khas village.
Courtesy of R. Narendra,
the map-maker.

Fashion Fables of an Urban Village

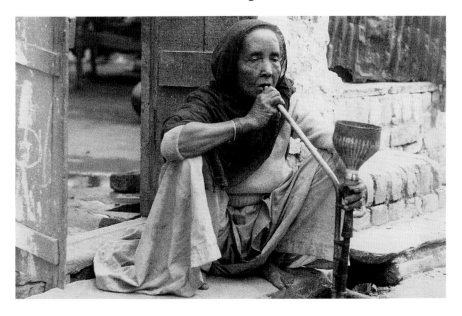

Fig. 9.4 An old *Harijan* woman sitting in the doorway of her home, 1989. She still dresses in a flared skirt. Conscious of what constitutes a 'genuine village scene', she insisted on bringing out her hookah for the photograph.

formed a relatively cohesive group to the extent that they tried to establish shared objectives. They had recently formed the Creative Arts Village Association (CAVA), through which they hoped to articulate their plans and work towards the general 'improvement' of the village as an ethnic shopping centre with an 'exclusive village flavour'. CAVA met jointly with a council of village elders to seek resolutions to the differing desires and expectations of the resident landlords and their new tenants, but despite these attempts at diplomacy there were mounting tensions between the two groups over ideas of progress in the village. These stemmed from the differing values and expectations of the village landlords and their glamorous tenants, both of whom harboured idealised perceptions of the other's lifestyle. Hitherto tensions had remained dormant because of the mutual satisfaction gained from financial profit, but there was a growing feeling on both sides that conflict was imminent. This was because the village was rocking precariously on the brink of an unstable paradox.

The composition of Hauz Khas village has been described in some detail because it helps to explain and support the nature of the fashion that was developing there. When a woman bought a garment from Hauz Khas, she was buying not only an outfit but a slab of carefully marketed village life.

It was through exploiting the exclusive appeal of this 'village life' that boutique-owners were able to sell their clothes at inordinate prices. This is not to say that 'ethnic' fashions were unique to Hauz Khas. On the contrary, the 1980s had seen an 'ethnic boom' throughout India, with 'ethnic' clothes selling in every major city, whether in street markets, state emporiums or exclusive boutiques.[8] But Hauz Khas was unique in selling 'ethnic' clothes in a 'genuine village setting', and as such was an ideal environment in which to explore the significance of the 'ethnic fashion revival'.[9] It also gave an opportunity for analysing the relationship between village fashion and élite urban fashion, for here the two coexisted in a state of uneasy harmony as old villagers and new village tenants observed each other's clothing with amazement, amusement and at times disgust.

Village fashion

The fashions favoured by the inhabitants of Hauz Khas in 1989 expressed their social, economic and aesthetic choices within the framework of recent cultural and historical changes in the area. Before independence, Muslim women were wearing *shalwar kamizes*, while *Jat* and *Harijan* women wore full gathered skirts (*lehngas*), blouses (*angis*), veils (*odhnis*) and large quantities of jewellery. Their dress was not unlike that worn by many Rajasthani peasant and tribal women today. For daily use most women wore cotton, but on special occasions those who could afford it wore *lehngas* of rich silk. The greater the quantity of cloth, the greater the swirl of the skirt and some skirts contained as much as 30 metres of material. Hindu men dressed largely in white *dhotis*, turbans and optional shirts while Muslim men generally favoured the *kurta*, worn with either a *pyjama* or a *lungi*. The clothes of the villagers of Hauz Khas were in fact very similar to those worn by a variety of different groups throughout Northwest India.

After independence the rapid expansion of the city of Delhi brought Hauz Khas within easy access to urban goods and finally incorporated the village within the urban structure itself. Although the village maintained

---

8 For a more general account of the different strands that have led to the emeregence of ethnic fashion, and for an understanding of how this fashion operates at the level of the street trade, see Tarlo, forthcoming.

9 The idea of an ethnic shopping village was not of course unique. The village of Suraj Kund was constructed near Delhi in 1987 with the express purpose of housing an annual craft fair. Unlike Hauz Khas, it was purpose-built and therefore contained no resident villagers who might have interfered with authorities' attempts to construct an idealised portrait of Indian village life. Similarly the village houses constructed in the grounds of the Crafts Museum (Delhi) and at Vishala ethnic restaurant (Ahmedabad) do not have any villagers inside them. They therefore fulfil the aesthetic expectations of visitors more easily than Hauz Khas, where real villagers hamper the élite's appreciation of the aesthetics of 'village life'.

Fashion Fables of an Urban Village

its geographic and architectural particularity, this was not through any concerted effort by the villagers themselves. On the contrary, most villagers were interested in the opportunities for change and both men and women began to alter their dress accordingly. Many men took to trousers and shirts, keeping their *dhotis* only for relaxation and home use, and many Hindu women, impressed by shiny synthetic materials which resembled silk, first had their skirts made from synthetic rayons and finally rejected them altogether, following the increasingly popular urban fashion of wearing the *shalwar kamiz*. Like *Kanbi* and *Kharak* women in Jalia, they felt that their village skirts marked them out as backward and uneducated, but unlike the fashionable women of the city, the *Jat* and *Harijan* women of Hauz Khas retained the idea that their heads should be kept covered once they were married. They resolved this problem of how to look both modern and modest by following the Muslim women of the area in wearing large veil-sized *dupattas*. This enabled them to continue with the practice of veiling (*ghunghut*).

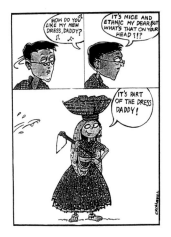

Fig. 9.5 Cartoon by Crowquill (1989).

In 1989 most village women were wearing shiny synthetic *shalwar kamizes* in baggy styles with large *dupattas*. Many had adopted accessories such as bras, socks and high-heeled shoes, and woollen pullovers or cardigans were often worn in the winter under their shawls. A few old *Harijan* women retained their cotton skirts and silver anklets, but they were becoming a diminishing minority. Many women had in fact sold their old skirts or used them for stuffing quilts or as household rags. With the exception of the older generation, the men of the village dressed almost exclusively in Western styles.

The only women in the village (with the exception of some boutique-owners) who wore what might be termed 'traditional village dress' were the semi-migrant Rajasthani labourers who worked as bricklayers and camped in the dry reservoir basin. They wore flared Rajasthani skirts, bodices and veils, and elaborate bangles up their arms. Despite being alien to the village, they represented to outsiders the very 'romance of village life' that gave Hauz Khas its charm. And although impoverished, overworked and homeless, these women found themselves unconsciously at the height of a new fashion trend. The irony of the situation is expressed in fig. 9.5.

This trend of wealthy urbanites dressing up like villagers emerged in the early to mid-1980s. Journalists were quick to identify it as 'ethnic chic', but remained largely puzzled about how to interpret the phenomenon. What was it, they wondered, that was leading the sophisticates of Delhi, Bombay, Ahmedabad and other major cities back to the village in search of 'things ethnic'?

Hauz Khas: an ethnic transformation

The transformation of Hauz Khas village into an exclusive fashion centre was engineered primarily by the fashion designer, Bina Ramani. Her autobiography to some extent mirrors the development of 'ethnic chic' itself. Although Indian-born, she had spent twenty-five years of her life in London, San Francisco and New York, working with top designers including Christian Dior and Givenchy, and latterly supplying such major London department stores as Harvey Nichols and Liberty with her 'classic designs'. In the earlier days of her career she was both designing and wearing Western-style clothes, but on her periodic visits to India she became interested in Indian dress. In an interview in 1989 she recalled:

> 'Coming back to India I realised the richness of India's traditional heritage. I travelled around a bit and saw the whole place with foreign eyes. Foreigners have always appreciated our wonderful fabrics and our village traditions, but Indians always neglected them. . . . I saw for the first time those rural women in their fabulous colourful garments. I thought, why not combine these wonderful rural costumes to suit our city women? So I developed my own style, quite unique, of using old saris, embroideries, brocades, whatever, and incorporating them into my own designs. The newspapers here call it 'ethnic chic'. In the States they tend to call it 'the Raja Look'. . . . Most of my early customers were foreign women. I introduced them to a new fashionable and exclusive Indian look. I have always felt it important to market the Indian image abroad. Now women come from Bombay specially to visit my boutique and the fashion is taking off in India too. . . . But I am not concerned to capture the ordinary Indian woman who is mediocre and conventional in her sari. She is not interested in my stuff and, quite frankly, I have no interest in her. The clothes I sell are for people like me, people who lead international lives.'

Bina Ramani opened her first boutique in Delhi in 1986, before her 'discovery' of Hauz Khas. She called it 'Once Upon a Time' because she saw her clothes 'as a story'. Chapter 1 of this fairy tale began with her 'discovery' of beautifully clad rural Indian women. Describing them to the magazine *India Worldwide*, she commented:

> 'They are the only ones who I find still dress *authentically*. The rest of us wear saris or Western clothes. The costumes of centuries ago were so varied and so glorious. It is such a joy to see these women wearing them on a daily basis' (*India Worldwide*, August 1989: 60, emphasis added).

Fashion Fables of an Urban Village

Chapter 2 was her realisation that old abandoned cloth could be resuscitated: 'It's the old sari that was put away in a trunk and discarded which I took out and gave new life to...creating new wearable garments' (*ibid*.). Employing refugee tailors and destitute women, she set about using the dejected members of society to revitalise neglected cloth, concluding: 'It's just an experiment which is a very happy one' (*ibid*.). It was indeed a happy experiment for Bina Ramani, particularly when she hit upon the idea of selling her clothes in Hauz Khas village. When she first visited the village, she had no intention of setting up another shop, but was simply looking for a cheap place in which to house her workshop. She told me:

'I instantly fell in love with the place. There was the beautiful old monument, the countryside and of course the wonderful people. I adore peasants, villagers, ethnic and rustic things. Peasants and tribals are really the best people. In fact they are the only real authentic people of India.'

In an interview with *Society* magazine, she recalled:

'When I first walked in here [the village] in 1986, I knew instantly that there was going to be a wonderful romance between the villagers and me. The people came running out to see me, touching and pulling my clothes as if I was some creature from outer space' (*Society*, October 1989: 90).

But despite her enthusiasm she did not open a boutique in the village: 'The idea was unthinkable. Many of my friends thought me totally mad even having my workshop there.' However, defying such conventions, she rented two rooms for a minimal rent in the house of one of the *Jat* families and set up her workshop of Afghani refugee tailors. That was in 1986. One year later she took the plunge and opened a boutique in the village itself, calling it 'Twice Upon a Time'. She explained her decision thus:

'Most of my original customers came from abroad, either visiting India as tourists, or businessmen's wives or embassy people, that kind of thing. . . . Sometimes I invited them to the village to visit my workshop or to have some alterations done, and they simply went berserk about the place. You see, they had spent their time in five-star hotels or in comfortable parts of South Delhi and they had never seen an Indian village before. They loved everything: the people, the buffaloes, the winding streets and of course the monument and the countryside around. They found it so picturesque. So I thought, why not open my second boutique here in the village itself? . . . Of course, the idea caused quite a stir. My Indian friends thought I was completely mad. They had a horror of villages and talked of the dirt and the backward people. One told me "Oh Bina, you and your mud and flies and peasants! You are crazy!" But I managed to persuade a few other designers and art collectors to join me here. They were sceptical at first, but they decided to give it a try and rented out rooms from the villagers. And from then on the whole idea took shape and people just love it. . . . At first it was mainly diplomats and foreigners who came, international people. Delhi women have never been creators. They simply follow the ideas of the international élite. Now it is Indian film-stars, celebrities, the high society people from Delhi and Bombay who come. It has become *the* fashionable place to go. In fact, it's a wonderful opportunity to see a real Indian village and to buy at the same time. Everyone enjoys the novelty, and each shop has its own unique atmosphere of village life.'

To create her own unique atmosphere of village life, Bina Ramani furnished her boutique in a simple style with woven wicker panels on the walls, wooden carvings from Gujarat, and an Indian rug on the floor. Her clothes, many of which were selling in the 2,000 to 5,000 rupees range, were hung on railings, with a few choice garments displayed on wooden frames with heads made from hand-painted Orissan masks.

Bina Ramani's story seemed a pre-eminent success. In May 1989 she opened a boutique in New York, staging a charity fashion show in Washington one month later, where her clothes were modelled by the wives of American politicians. The event was widely covered by the Indian press which delighted in images of US Congressmen's wives parading around the Indian embassy in Washington, dressed in Indian outfits and sporting red spangles on their foreheads. Bina herself wore a 'genuine peasant skirt' for the occasion which she sported with one of her elaborate silk tops and elegant shoes.

What is striking about Bina Ramani's return to an Indian identity is that it appears to have been stimulated at all stages by her sense of foreignness. First, there was her perception of her own foreignness when she returned to India and saw it 'with foreign eyes'. Secondly, there was her awareness of those aspects of India that appeal to foreigners – not the modern streamlined boutiques of South Delhi, but the 'rustic' village with its 'peasants and buffaloes' and 'authentic Indian people'. And finally, there was her realisation of how to market this appeal of 'Village India' in such a way that foreigners would buy it, exclusively gift-wrapped in a new aesthetic form.

The question arises whether the path to Indian ethnicity commonly takes such a convoluted route,[10] or whether Ramani's story with its 'international people' and 'foreign' perceptions was unusual in the village. Certainly she moved in the wealthiest and most jetsetting circle of new tenants. But further interviews with other boutique-owners and fashion designers (often the very same people) revealed that such an outsider perception of 'Village India' was integral to the development of this 'ethnic' enclave. A large proportion of the designers had trained abroad, others had visited foreign countries, and even those who had not travelled were aware of the exotic appeal that India had abroad and its backlash effect in India. One designer who specialised in selling Gujarati peasant embroidered *ghaghros*, *kapdus* and adaptations of both concluded:

'I think ethnic stuff really took off in India because of the Festival of India abroad. It got so much publicity, and suddenly we began to think: "If foreigners are buying and wearing our stuff, why can't we begin to like it?" Then when one person starts to wear ethnic clothes and be noticed, others start following suit and the fashion takes off.'

This theory of the spread of ethnic chic was widely accepted, among both sellers and buyers of ethnic clothing and furniture. The magazine and television coverage of the Festival of India in England, Japan, France, the United States and Russia dwelt much on the foreign appreciation of Indian things and clearly had a profound effect on encouraging Indians to buy Indian.[11] While some boutique-owners were stimulated by this collective foreign appreciation, others had more individual motivations for selling Indian things, as one woman explained:

'The idea came to me through travelling. My husband is in the merchant navy and I worked in the airlines for twelve years, so we travelled a lot. I sometimes used to wear something Indian, just a small thing like a ring or a scarf, and I got so many compliments from foreigners that after a while I began to dress in deliberately ethnic things – flared *ghaghra* or *lehngas* or *shalwar*-type trousers. . . . I got the idea of opening a shop from my experience of making gifts to foreigners. Because we travelled so much, we were always having to give presents to people. I started off giving Western things as presents because I thought that was what

10   Certainly, many important historical figures such as Mahatma Gandhi, Jawaharlal Nehru and Ananda Coomaraswamy all discovered India through leaving it.
11   Other influential factors have been the Hindi film industry and the craft revival movement which can be traced from pioneering figures such as Ananda Coomaraswamy and Mahatma Gandhi through to the establishment of national and state handicraft boards.

people would want. But I soon realised that what they wanted was the traditional hand-made Indian stuff. So I began offering skirts, scarves, *khadi* shirts, etc. and people loved it. That was when I got the idea of trying to sell Indian stuff in Delhi.'

A man who occupied one of the prime spots of the village, setting up his boutique for antique Indian textiles in the front of the village *chaupal* (traditionally the central meeting place), commented:

'About ten years ago, only foreigners were interested in traditional textiles and antiques. Now my Indian customers get upset because they realise that years back they threw out this type of thing [he points to a Paisley shawl]. Now these, for example, are worth a lot of money and people have started to appreciate them and are wanting their old things back again.'

The attitude of the boutique-owners generally was perhaps best summarised by the secretary of CAVA, who was fully aware of the paradox:

'Basically, in India people are reluctant to acknowledge anything that has not been appreciated by foreigners first. They still seek validation from the West in everything. I started off selling to foreigners and now sell mainly to Indians, but I still get a few Indians walking into the shop and saying "Oh, this is just for foreigners" and marching out without even taking a look.'

But although the inspiration behind the establishment of boutiques in Hauz Khas village had a distinctly Western flavour, many of the boutique-owners were genuinely attracted towards the village precisely because of its non-Western feel – this was not a case merely of urban Indians following foreign trends but also of their experiencing the village as foreigners themselves. Some of them had never visited an Indian village before and enjoyed the exoticism and sense of adventure in much the same way that a tourist does.[12] They also experienced the same type of weeding-out

---

12 In trying to expose the dominant ethos of the boutique-owners, I would like to stress that not all of them shared this ethos. In particular the people involved in the craft development organisation, Dastkar, had extensive experience of working in rural areas and did not share this naive approach to villages and villagers. The Dastkar boutique was, however, an exception. It was established at the time when Bina Ramani had already opened her workshop in Hauz Khas but before she had thought of establishing her boutique there and encouraging others to join her. In this sense Dastkar's location in Hauz Khas village can be considered to be independent of the spirit of later developments. This independence was clear from Dastkar's commitment to commissioning new craftwork from craftspeople which was sold at affordable prices without the pretentions of designer labels.

Fashion Fables of an Urban Village

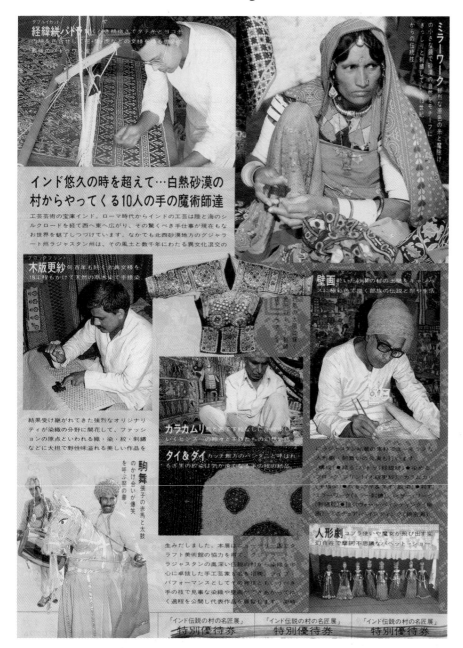

Fig. 9.6 A publicity leaflet for the Festival of India in Japan, showing the presentation of 'traditional India' to foreigners. Courtesy of the Ministry of Human Resource Development, Department of Culture, Government of India.

process as tourists do when they point their cameras at the most exotic and strange-looking Indian sights, ignoring the average man on a Delhi street with his tight-fitting trousers and synthetic shirt. To many of the boutique-owners, though by no means all, the village genuinely represented some kind of 'authentic' India which they had just discovered. And although they used this 'authenticity' to sell their products, this did not altogether detract from their own belief in it.[13] Many, like their customers, came to the village with a very romantic view of both the people and the place.[14] Just as Bina Ramani told me that 'villages are the real India' and 'villagers are really the only authentic people in India', so others said that 'villagers are so innocent' or that they are 'the most genuine people of India'. The woman whose fashion show I had attended explained:

'I had never visited the village before, but I knew most of the people with boutiques and they are all from very good families. So I visited the village and loved it and decided to have my boutique here. It has a very special atmosphere. The people are so friendly, though very slow to understand. You have to explain things to them over and over again. But they are kind. They always bring me tea. Actually, they are the closest people to nature, the closest you can get and that is really quite something. It says a lot for them.'

Another woman, explaining the appeal that Hauz Khas holds for Indian and foreign customers, said: 'People love the adventure of coming here. They are curious to know what a village is like. And they enjoy the experience and novelty of buying traditional dress in a real village setting. It's more authentic than the boutiques of South Delhi somehow.'

But the 'authentic' village atmosphere that the shopkeepers and customers enjoyed was not so much an enjoyment of the village itself as an enjoyment of their idea of how a village should be. They were not content to accept the villagers' tastes in furnishings or interiors, but instead imported their own hand-crafted items from all over India to decorate the walls and to

13 Although a number of boutique-owners bought and sold Gujarati embroidered textiles, most were entirely unaware that Gujarati villagers were themselves rejecting such clothes. This was because they tended to buy directly from itinerant traders or merchants.

14 There were, of course, some exceptions (usually male). In particular, there was one designer, Sunit Varma, who despised the romanticisation of village life. He had recently refused to have his photograph taken in a 'typical village setting' and told journalists that he had moved to Hauz Khas for purely financial reasons. He was sceptical about the ethnic revival in general and felt that it was largely a good excuse for anyone to set up as a designer without experience or knowledge of fashion. It was noticeable that men were on the whole more sceptical about the development than women.

Fashion Fables of an Urban Village

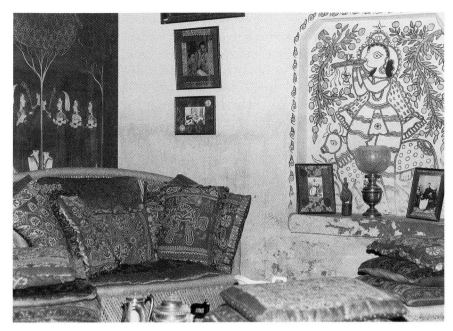

Fig. 9.7 Some 'ethnic' interiors of Hauz Khas boutiques, 1989, featuring Bihari wall-paintings, Gujarati embroidery and woodwork and South Indian brass and wickerwork.

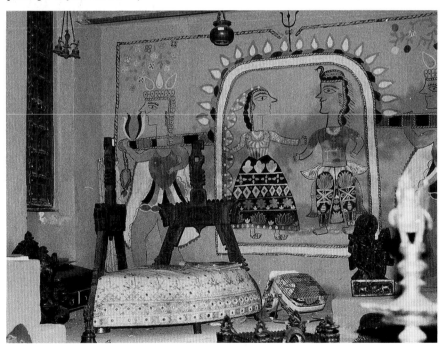

give the 'authentic village look' (see fig. 9.7). In short, they were striving to create some kind of super-village, in which various aspects of 'Village India', taken from different ages and regions, were brought together in one place under the banner of 'ethnic tradition'.[15] Although the explicit aim of the Hauz Khas Creative Arts Village Association was to 'preserve' the village atmosphere, what this actually entailed was 'creating' the village atmosphere. For as far as many boutique-owners were concerned, the village was not nearly 'villagey' enough.

In December 1989 the main preoccupations of the Association were the following: to 'preserve' the village atmosphere, to keep each shop as unique as possible, to choose where possible harmonious architecture and ethnic interiors, to keep the village small and exclusive, to keep the rents low, to build a large parking lot, to cobble the streets to prevent people getting their high-heeled shoes stuck in the mud, and to stop the villagers leading their buffaloes down the main shopping street while customers were still in the village. This last request was initiated after an almost tearful customer complained that a dirty buffalo had flicked its tail over her best coat. In other words, what they desired was some kind of sterilised village which they could fill with the most aesthetically appealing features of village life, and which displayed only the decorative aspect of 'tradition' without any of its associated hardship or discomfort – a village, in other words, that was beautiful and encouraged sales.

In some contexts, villagers were prepared to go along with this idealised presentation of the village. The village headman, in particular, whose family was making money from letting out rooms, seemed pleased to appear as the 'authentic Indian villager' when required. If a customer wanted to take his photograph, he brought out his hookah, put a turban on his head and sat on a string bed, creating a classical Indian village scene.[16] Similarly, when a coach-load of foreign tourists arrived in the village through Bina Ramani's arrangement, he presented each new arrival with a garland of flowers and explained the essence of village life. On another occasion extra genuine 'village features' were brought in, such as a horse and cart and a Rajasthani musician in 'traditional dress' (see fig. 9.3b). But there were other

15 As Brian Durrans pointed out in his critique of the Festival of India, 'Tradition is the unifying factor only as an abstraction; in detail, most traditions are particular and regional or local' (Durrans 1982: 16).

16 In Jalia, too, there were a few individuals who deliberately cultivated a *deshi* look to satisfy their audience. There was, for example, an old *Koli* man who, instead of wearing Western clothes to visit his son in Bombay, deliberately retained his *kediyun* and *chorni*, resulting in numerous tourists taking his photograph and giving him free cigarettes. But he was unusual. Most men were too anxious to be rid of the *deshi* look to recognise its marketability.

Fashion Fables of an Urban Village

times when villagers were not prepared to go along with the boutique-owners' perceptions of their life and were not entirely happy to see 'village life' enacted by outsiders within their own village. As a result, a number of misunderstandings resulted, with considerable disillusionment on both sides.

Village fashion versus village as fashion
When Bina Ramani first walked into the village and decided to open a workshop, the family from whom she rented the space were delighted. They soon turfed out the existing tenants who had been paying a nominal rent, and let out two rooms to this fashionable outsider. Soon she was renting part of the ground floor, the whole of the first floor and two rooms in the house next door. Her landlord was pleased to be receiving good money, and she was equally pleased since her rents were far below normal Delhi rates. When she encouraged her friends to join her in the village, they too found properties to rent with relative ease. The low village-style rents were undoubtedly a powerful incentive to newcomers, but they soon escalated. The landlords' wives, who used to bring tea to these auspicious new tenants, soon noticed the price tags on Ramani's clothes. If just one outfit could sell for 5,000 rupees, surely they could charge more rent? The early phase of these rent increases did not worry the boutique-owners too much, since rents were still very reasonable by South Delhi standards, but they began to cause considerable resentment among the villagers themselves. Those landlords who had let out their properties first became jealous of their neighbours who, realising what they could charge, increased their demands.

The new money that came flowing into the wealthier section of the village created in general a favourable response from the *Jat* villagers to the arrival of the boutiques. This was further highlighted by the novelty they experienced when they saw customers, especially the Hindi film-stars who had begun to be frequent visitors to this previously ignored village. This provided great entertainment for all the villagers. But the economic and architectural development of the village quickly became unstable. Many of the *Jat* landlords decided that, if they increased the size of a property and divided it up, then they could rent out each section and live off the proceeds without even having to go to work. Some therefore raised the height of their buildings from two to four floors, thereby renting out the first three floors and settling themselves on the fourth. Pleased with the opportunity to build themselves new modern apartments, they chose to add concrete extensions on top of their original brick houses. This of course horrified the boutique-owners since it ruined the 'village atmosphere' of the street. But there was more to come. An interesting case was that of Aruna.[17]

Aruna worked for an airlines company and decided to sell ethnic clothes when she realised how much they were appreciated by foreigners. Unlike the first boutique-owners who were exceptionally wealthy and well-connected, she belonged to the second wave of owners who came from moderately wealthy upper-middle-class families but were not part of the international Delhi élite. She and her partner were selling mainly cotton ethnic clothes from Rajasthan at fairly affordable prices, hoping to attract those clients who could not afford top designer labels.

Aruna needed her shop to be a financial success but, when I met her after it had been open for only two weeks, she was already extremely anxious. First there was the problem of the building. Aruna described its appearance when she first came to the village: 'I loved it instantly. It had real village atmosphere. It was small and intimate with little windows looking out towards the lake [empty reservoir]. It had lots of sunlight and was full of nooks and crannies. I was going to do the whole thing up in bamboo and make it really ethnic.' What she was describing were two rooms, situated in a deep but narrow two-storey house owned by five brothers. The two rooms were on the ground floor and she agreed to pay 4,000[18] rupees a month in total, thereby establishing the only boutique in that particular alleyway. Her landlord agreed and threw out his previous tenants, from whom he received only 100 rupees a month for each room. But he then decided that he could get even more rent if he demolished the building and built a new four-storey structure. His brothers, who had previously been opposed to the idea of letting out space to shops, agreed and before long the whole structure was razed and rebuilt in the form of uniform concrete blocks, each four storeys high and without any windows facing the reservoir. Aruna suddenly found herself shelved in a concrete precinct, surrounded by new shops selling similar things to her own, and without any of the 'village atmosphere' that had attracted her in the first place. Not only this, but her landlord decided to double her rent, arguing that she was now occupying high-quality accommodation. Faced with the option of agreeing or leaving, Aruna agreed to pay the increased rate for she knew that rents were soaring throughout the village and it would be impossible to find another space. But she was disillusioned and disappointed.

In an attempt to re-impose some of the lost 'village atmosphere' on the place, she turned to her landlady and appealed to her to plaster the inside

---

17 This is a pseudonym.
18 All of the figures quoted above were mentioned in conversation and have not been verified.

walls with mud and cow dung paste to give them a more ethnic look. Her landlady was amazed, and remarked with humour (in Hindi): 'Well, I thought that with all these changes in the village, at least I would never have to plaster a wall or a floor again. I thought that was the end of the custom. And then you turn to me and ask me to plaster your walls!' But mud looks strange on a flat concrete surface and the village effect does not take long to wear thin. Furthermore, changes in the village were not merely aesthetic but pervaded every aspect of village life. Aruna, who had been observing these changes ever since she first signed her contract some six months earlier, felt genuinely anxious:

'To be honest, I am really disappointed. I thought villagers were such innocent people. But they are very shrewd, real business people. In fact they have completely lost their innocence and become very commercial.... The effects of the sudden changes on the village are terrible. My landlord has become a drunkard. He gave up his job as a car mechanic and just sits and drinks and plays cards all day. He earns nothing and spends all his money on videos. All the villagers have TVs and videos now.... My landlord does not actually live in this building. His house is the one on the corner of the street, the only old house left, but even that is going to be pulled down. Already he has forced all his family to live in the cramped upper floor so he can rent out the ground floor. He used to keep two cows and sell their milk, but now he has got rid of them because he can rent out his cow shed for 8,000 rupees a month. He has also sold his *chakki* for grinding wheat. Last week he was so drunk that he beat up his wife with an iron rod and I had to take her to the hospital for stitches. The situation is getting out of hand. The villagers just want more and more money.

The experience of contact with the villagers was undoubtedly leading boutique-owners to reconsider their image of the innocent villager who bows down in respect and awe at the social élite. As an astute boutique-owner put it:

'Basically, we are all used to having servants and being able to boss them about. But here we are the tenants. We cannot treat our landlords as servants. Such an attitude creates hostility. In our [CAVA's] last meeting with the village council, we were trying to stress that any more development should stop now before the whole village becomes a building site and loses all its charm. But one of the villagers turned to Bina and said: "You just want to fill your own stomach. You don't care about anybody else's." ... There has been one case of hostility. That was in the *Harijan* quarter. A woman decided to open a boutique there but the other *Harijans* resented the money that one family was getting. They tried to attack the woman and break into her shop. But the situation is unclear and we don't know exactly what happened. There was one more incident when a salesman employed to work in one of the shops was beaten up for staring too much at the village girls. These developments are worrying. The villagers are very good people on the whole but they don't understand anything about the artistic side of the village. They just want money and they believe in muscle power.'

Just as the villagers could not understand the townspeople's nostalgia for those features of the village which they themselves sought to eliminate, so they found it difficult to understand the new fashions that were being marketed in the village. Part of this confusion revolved around the fact that some of the clothes on sale in the village were actually the cast-offs of the villagers themselves. Aruna, for example, was selling some of the old sequined veils and *lehngas* of her landlady, much to the latter's surprise. She, being a modern *Jat* woman, had not worn a *lehnga* for the past fifteen or twenty years and could not believe that anyone would want to buy the old trousseau things that had lain stashed away in her trunk:

> 'I never even thought of trying to sell them', she admitted. 'Who would want such things? But now I cannot help but laugh and laugh, that what we have cast away, these smart people begin to wear. To us, these *lehngas* are nothing but waste. You know, before these fashion shops came, I was using such cloth to wipe the floor or for putting under a baby's bottom or for stuffing a quilt. But I was happy to sell them and get some money.'[19]

As for the Rajasthani labourers, who were charging people 10 rupees for taking their photograph, they were quite incredulous at the prices of *lehngas* in the boutiques. As yet they had not sold any of their own clothes, perhaps

---

19   The fact that one person's rubbish can become another person's treasure has been brilliantly articulated by Michael Thompson. He shows how people assign goods to the categories of 'durable' and 'transient'. Durable goods increase in value over time while the transient decrease in value and eventually become rubbish. This rubbish can, however, be reconverted into durables after lying redundant in the rubbish category for some time. Hauz Khas village is a perfect example of the urban élite converting the rubbish of the village peasant into exclusive durables. Thompson's description of the transformation of a working-class Georgian slum in Islington into a paradise for the rising 'frontier middle class' bears uncanny resemblance to the architectural battles in Hauz Khas (see M. Thompson 1979).

Fashion Fables of an Urban Village

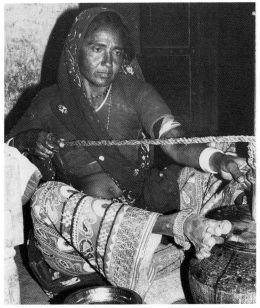

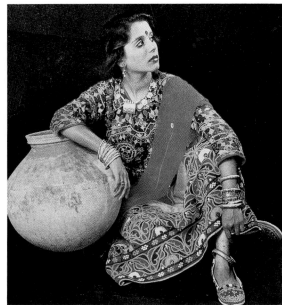

Fig. 9.8(a) A *Kharak* woman from Jalia churning curd, 1989.

Fig. 9.8(b) An ethnic chic cover girl from the teenage magazine *Teen Talk*, Nov. 1988.

because, like the semi-itinerant *Bharwads*, they relied on dress as a means of retaining their group identity wherever they travelled. But these women enjoyed peering inside shop windows and laughing because wealthy people would pay up to ten times the usual price for a simple cotton skirt.

Just as the village houses were not quite ethnic enough for the boutique-owners' purposes, so too village clothes often required a few ethnic alterations. Plastic buttons, for example, were frequently replaced by colourful string fastenings that look more authentic. Figs 9.8a and 9.8b highlight the differences between 'ethnic chic' fashion and the village fashion it seeks to emulate. The first shows a *Kharak* woman in Jalia, hard at work churning buttermilk. She wears a *ghaghro*, embroidered in the mango design, and a plain *kapdu*. She has retained her *boloya* (ivory bangles), but has adopted a synthetic half-sari and no longer wears heavy bands of silver round her ankles. The second shows, by way of contrast, an ethnic chic cover-girl. She too sports a *ghaghro* of the type worn in the Larabad district, this time embroidered in the parrot and fish design. But the similarities belie the fact that in the second picture many of the functional aspects of Saurashtran dress have been replaced by merely decorative equivalents: the cover-girl's feet are adorned in pretty embroidered slippers while the village woman goes bare-foot; the cover-girl's scarf is decorative while the village woman's is a head covering and veil. Even the earthenware pot used for churning buttermilk has become a mere prop in the creation of the village look. And if one examines the cover-girl's *ghaghro* itself, it becomes clear that even this has been subtly transformed: the machine-made border has been totally removed, thereby preserving the garment's ethnic quality, but at the same time the open flap has been stitched up, thereby preventing the garment from looking 'too ethnic' and indecent. By the same token, the *kapdus* on sale in Hauz Khas village were often given cloth backs to make them more decent and presentable in an urban setting. Designing ethnic clothes, then, involved processing elements of village dress into a new acceptable form before selling them as 'ethnic dress' to the urban élite. While some Hauz Khas stylists designed radically new collections in which they revealed their personal creativity, many simply rearranged elements of existing village dress into new acceptable forms.

While the older generation of Hauz Khas villagers stared in bewilderment at these developments, some of the younger generation were more influenced by them. Although at first young village women did not consider wearing cotton fabric (because of its backward connotations) or *deshi* styles, they did enter some of the cheaper shops and there were some cases of village girls bringing their own material to a boutique-owner and ordering replicas of *shalwar kamizes* on sale in the shop. Conversely, there were some boutique-owners who had formed direct contracts with village tailors in Rajasthan who now made up special tribal clothes expressly for the Delhi market. Just as boutique-owners selected the most 'traditional'-looking elements of village design, so villagers often favoured the least 'traditional'-looking styles when they emulated the Delhi élite. There were also a few cases of young girls in the village cutting their long hair in imitation of boutique-owners, tourists and film-stars. Young men meanwhile were beginning to take to designer jeans and sunglasses in a big way and were apparently much more self-conscious about their appearance than in the past.

But although villagers were willing to sell their old clothes to the boutique-owners and the headman was prepared to dress up and act the part of 'traditional village leader', this did not mean that villagers were willing to sell every aspect of their cultural environment. As Martinez has shown in the context of a Japanese tourist village, residents are selective about which aspects of their culture they choose to present to tourists and foreigners. Certain traditions may be carefully preserved and kept away from the tourist eye (Martinez 1990: 110). When the village headman came to the fashion show described at the beginning of this chapter, he left after the first ten minutes. When asked why, he replied:

> 'I was shocked and disgusted. Our women in this village have been doing *ghunghut* for generations and generations as a sign of respect and tradition. And now I see these women on the stage, playing with *ghunghut*, and then removing their veils, revealing their bodies and dressing and moving like prostitutes. It is a disgrace. I could not stay to see it here in my village. So I came home.'

Like the super-village that the boutique-owners tried to create, ethnic chic fashion took only the glamour of tradition with little consideration of its social and cultural context. Although most villagers had enjoyed the spectacular aspect of the fashion show, which they said was 'like a movie', there was a general consensus that the way the models used their veils and showed their bodies was shameful and disgraceful. This raises once again questions about the nature of the relationship between ethnic chic fashion and the fashion it seeks to imitate.

What is ethnic chic?

We have proceeded this far without any analysis of what is meant by 'ethnic chic' and the frequently used phrase 'going ethnic'. These phrases were so widely and loosely used that it seemed nobody quite knew what they meant. The term 'ethnic' in its original sense refers to the racial identity of a group – literally, their ethnic identity. But the word has developed a new meaning in the West where it is often used to refer to any mode of behaviour or a material artefact that seems 'exotic' or 'primitive' or merely non-Western. It was a popular term during the hippy period in the 1970s when many Westerners 'went ethnic' and wore 'ethnic clothes'. Its resurgence in India is curious at a time when at least some self-conscious Westerners are beginning to recognise that non-Western countries do not form a conglomerate mass that can be bracketed together by the term 'ethnic'. But the choice of the word to describe India's new fashion is significant in that it highlights the gap between the wearers of ethnic clothes and the ethnic groups whom they claim to emulate. If ethnically-clad modern women felt a close bond with peasant and tribal women, they would perhaps have chosen to describe the fashion as *'deshi'* or simply 'Indian'. But by chosing the international vocabulary of the 'ethnic' the wearers of ethnic chic have already defined themselves as outsiders fascinated by the 'exoticism' of the primitive other, just like foreigners. As for the 'chic', this too indicates that the ethnicity of clothing is more a question of international fashion than of identification with India's many ethnic groups.[20]

To clarify the matter, let us examine the case of Liveleen Sharma, a Delhi socialite, married to a wealthy executive in a multinational company, and see what she means by 'going ethnic'. She gave a long interview to the *Sunday Mail* in December 1989 about her dress and ideas. A photograph of her, ethnically adorned, graced the front cover under the headline 'The original ethnic chic' (fig. 9.9). The reader is told inside that Liveleen Sharma 'is a picture of the urban Indian woman trying to get back to her ethnic roots'. But what are these roots, and how did she return to them? Logically, her ethnic roots should be traced through her background and her return to these roots should be her personal biography. So what are we told of her life history?

Little is mentioned of the early stages except that she was born in Lahore into a wealthy family, and has 'Sikh, Hindu and a tinge of Muslim blood'. As a young woman she modelled in Paris, got married and raised a family. 'Then', we are told, 'she visited Rajasthan.' She recalls:

'I saw dark complexioned Rajasthani men in big turbans with rock hard bodies. I saw them oozing with sex. In comparison, the conventionally handsome guys I used to meet in London and Paris paled into insignificance. Even in Delhi, I would park my car near a construction sight and watch wide-eyed the village women with slush-filled baskets on their heads, more often than not a baby in an arm, walking down more gracefully than a model can ever imagine to do on a ramp.'

The result of this revelation, which could perhaps be more accurately described as visual seduction, was that Liveleen, who previously sported 'a very Western look', now 'turned ethnic with a vengeance'. Nowadays she

.... dresses up like a low caste *Bungri* woman, *natnis* (rope walker, acrobat) – either in a sari or a *lehnga*, with a long backless blouse and no bra .... her jewellery is always silver and chunky. Heavy earrings, a choker, a ring for every finger of her hennaed hands and an *arsi* (ring with a big mirror), bracelets and anklets. The arms from the wrists to the shoulders are studded with lac and silver bangles. A heavy make-up with an Om inscribed in the middle of her eyebrows completes the look.

20 In this sense the new wave of ethnic chic fashion should be distinguished from the more consistent attempts made by handicraft boards and development organisations to promote India's crafts, including textiles and dress. While the latter have devoted considerable time and attention to reviving indigenous forms of production and technique, the ethnic chic fashion designers were generally unconcerned about indigenous craft as long as they could obtain the desired ethnic effect. This meant that they often bought up and re-used secondhand textiles from street markets and itinerant traders rather than commissioning new work.

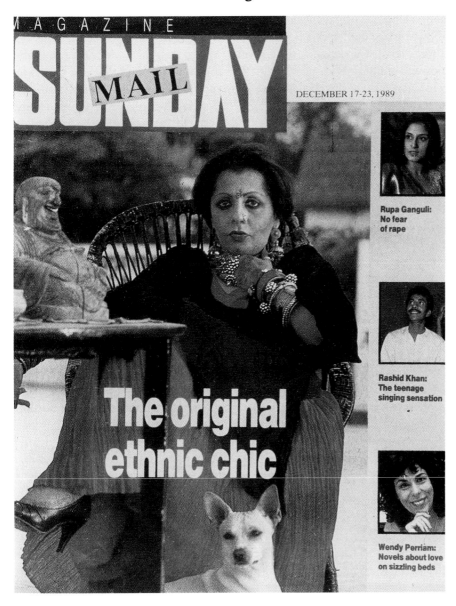

Fig. 9.9 Portrait of 'the urban woman trying to get back to her ethnic roots'. Reproduced from the *Sunday Mail Magazine*, Dec. 1989.

Liveleen's personal transformation was not, according to the *Sunday Mail*, 'a put-on job'; she altered not only her dress, but also her entire house and garden, which are now filled with 'bric-a-brac from villages in different parts of the country'. This, it is claimed, proves the sincerity of her conversion. The second proof is that she purports to hold traditional values concerning a woman's role and her natural inferiority to men (although it is not clear whether this is one of her new 'ethnic' ideas, or an idea she has always held). Certainly, at some level, Liveleen feels she has returned to tradition and announces prophetically: 'There is a wave around that will turn into a tornado. We will start taking pride in ourselves and our traditional values.'

But the question remains: why, coming from a wealthy Lahore family of mixed origin, did she choose to dress as a low-caste *Bungri* woman? Is this really a return to her 'ethnic roots'? Secondly, although she has adopted an 'ethnic' appearance (high-heeled shoes, make-up and plucked eyebrows excluded), her actual lifestyle seems far from 'ethnic'. While the beautiful Rajasthani bricklayers were labouring on building sites, she was watching them from the comfort of her car. And at one stage in the interview, she professes: 'Almost every working day in our married life, I've lunched with my husband Sunny in a classy restaurant.' Hardly an 'ethnic' lifestyle! Furthermore, for Liveleen an important part of looking 'ethnic' is that she gets noticed wherever she goes. Unlike the Rajasthani labourers who express their group identity through their dress, she expresses her individuality through emulating them. The idea that ethnic chic clothes allow a woman to look unique and glamorous, without *necessarily* being as expensive as they might look, has played an important part in the development of the fashion. Liveleen herself clearly enjoys this sensationalist aspect:

'I am the most popular unpaid model around. The way tourists click me! There was this photo-journalist from Japan, shooting our village belles. When he noticed me in a five-star hotel, he freaked out. . . . Other rich women shell out anything between 2,000 and 8,000 rupees on an outfit bought at a boutique. But they all look like sheep – indistinguishable from each other. . . . The women of the filthy rich will always have a diamond bigger than mine. So why compete?'

The *Sunday Mail* is understandably confused about how to interpret Liveleen Sharma and her 'ethnic' ways. In a series of rhetorical questions, it asks: 'Is she a model? Is she an actress? Is she one of the Shobha Dé socialites? [Shobha Dé is a Bombay socialite and author of raunchy popular fiction.] Is she a visual jingle for ethnic chic? Is she a danger to the emancipation of women? Is she just the frisky wife of Sunny Sharma, an executive with a multinational? Or is she all that is tender and nice about Indian womanhood?' Finally, it asks simply: 'Isn't she India, taking pride in its culture?'

This question is curiously difficult to answer. For while 'ethnic chic' is a return to Indianness, this return has been facilitated through a sense of foreignness in which foreign values and perceptions have played an essential part. Furthermore, the Indianness which ethnic chic venerates is so constructed that it has little relationship to any existing Indian tradition, however defined. As Hauz Khas controversies demonstrate, an 'ethnic chic' lifestyle and aesthetic rest uneasily with the realities of an Indian villager's life. Yet at another level 'ethnic chic' is a cultural revival even if its appreciation of India's heritage depends on breaking many of the traditions of which that heritage is composed. Liveleen Sharma is not so much 'India, taking pride in its culture' as India presenting an idealised image of its culture to a wealthy cosmopolitan élite. At an international level, then, 'ethnic chic' masquerades as *real* Indian dress from an 'authentic Indian village' even though, at a local level, it bears little relationship to the village aesthetic on which it is founded.

There are many outlets for ethnic clothes in India, but few embody as acutely as Hauz Khas the paradoxes on which 'ethnic chic' fashion is founded. For Hauz Khas is both a village and a super-village, with evolving, dissolving and invented traditions competing for space.[21] It contains villagers building concrete apartments and urbanites replastering the walls with mud; villagers clad in nylon and rayon and boutique-owners in hand-spun cotton and silk; villagers struggling to distance themselves from the natural environment, and urbanites putting 'nature' back into the village where they think it belongs. Such battles of cultural and aesthetic values are not unusual in themselves, but the particular feature of Hauz Khas village is that these battles are all being waged at the same time and in the same place.

In the museum, the very 'temple of authenticity' (Handler 1986: 4), images of India are controllable and contained. In the Craft Emporium, that mecca of 'traditional arts', tokens of India are selected and arranged expressly for sale. At international festivals, 'Indian tradition' is staged and marketed to suit a chosen international consumer. But in Hauz Khas, despite concerted efforts, not a single person or group is capable of controlling the image of 'traditional Indian village life', for this image is being negated as fast as it is being created. At Hauz Khas, both village and city, past and present, 'tradition' and 'modernity' juggle for expression in a single arena where history is remade as fast as it is rejected, and new developments are rapidly repainted with a traditional village gloss. Hauz Khas acts simultaneously as both the proof and refutation of the romance of the Indian

---

21 For a discussion of the notion of invented traditions, see Hobsbawm and Ranger (eds) 1983.

village. It is a suitable environment for selling 'ethnic' clothes because ethnic chic embodies precisely the same set of paradoxical relations.

The romanticisation of the village and its products is not, of course, unique to Hauz Khas, or indeed to India. It is a phenomenon that typically arises in rapidly industrialising societies in situations where people are sufficiently removed from 'village life' to mourn its loss (cf. Dewey 1972); it comes to represent some sort of ideal existence, closer to nature and beauty than its urban equivalent. But, as Brian Moeran has pointed out, people tend to idealise nature most when they are not directly involved with it in a struggle for survival. Furthermore, 'the aesthetic ideal which associates the quality of traditional arts and crafts with closeness to nature derives primarily from urbanisation, which itself usually – though not necessarily – depends on industrialisation' (Moeran 1990a: 223). It is perhaps no coincidence that the boutique-owner who told me that villagers 'are the closest people to nature, the closest you can get' was the daughter of one of India's leading industrialists. Just as the romance of the village is venerated by those outside it, so 'traditional village dress' and hand-woven fabrics are often appreciated most by those who do not have to wear them but can choose to do so.

The question remains: what is 'traditional dress'? It is of course impossible to answer, for the term 'traditional' does not refer to any particular features of a garment but only to the fact that that garment is perceived as something that was worn and accepted by people in the seemingly timeless past. And just as 'the past' refers as much to last year as it does to the last millennium, so the term 'traditional' may describe the dress of any epoch. Hence the pink scarf of *Bharwad* men in Jalia is regarded as an important part of 'traditional *Bharwad* dress', even though it has only been adopted in the past ten years. Traditions do not have to pass an age-test in order to be valid, although age does lend them credibility and often encourages us to accept them as 'traditional'.

While it is entirely unconstructive to search for the physical components of 'traditional Indian dress', it is helpful to examine how a garment is designated as 'traditional' and what this designation actually means. In Hauz Khas the *lehnga*, bodice and veil combination was the most common outfit worn by the Hindu women of the village before independence. Urbanites refered to it as 'traditional' or 'ethnic', while villagers refered to it literally as 'stuff of the past'. Both groups agreed to identify the same outfit as the dress of a past era. But while for the boutique-owners the age of the dress lent it charm and authenticity, for the villagers it made it old-fashioned and unappealing. And while the veil was the only aspect of

316

the outfit which fashionable urbanites discarded as superfluous, it was that which villagers retained as the most important. In other words, each group selected those aspects of the outfit which they regarded as significant in the process of preserving traditions. While the boutique-owners kept the aesthetic aspect but dismissed veiling as an old-fashioned custom, the villagers dismissed the *lehnga* and bodice as old-fashioned, but maintained veiling.

The process by which we categorise things as 'traditional' and 'old-fashioned' is the process by which the 'stuff of the past' is divided into the categories of relevant and irrelevant. The 'traditional' is that stuff of the past (real or imagined) that we consider relevant to our present and our future, while the 'old-fashioned' is that stuff of the past which we dismiss as irrelevant to our contemporary life. Thus while the term 'old-fashioned' is used to invalidate the relevance of things of the past to the present, the term 'traditional' is often used to legitimise things of the present by reference to the past. Designating things as 'traditional' is therefore a means of implying their authenticity and justifying their continued existence (cf. Picton 1990).

The boutique-owners and followers of ethnic chic often accused villagers of failing to appreciate their own artistic traditions. Yet what these fashionable urbanites failed to acknowledge was that when they themselves dressed in ethnic clothes, they looked not only 'traditional' but also 'modern', since the idea of dressing like villagers was part of a national urban and, to some extent, international fashion trend. But if villagers, either in Hauz Khas or Jalia, donned the same 'ethnic clothes', they did not participate in contemporary urban fashion in the same way for, living within a village environment, they found themselves classified as backward and uneducated by local standards. They seemed to feel trapped in a time-warp from which many wished to escape. By designating Hauz Khas as 'traditional' and trying to preserve the 'village atmosphere', boutique-owners were in effect denying villagers a right to manage their own future. Meanwhile, by replacing mud and brick houses with concrete apartments, villagers were denying the boutique-owners access to the village's past. The irony of the situation is that it is the boutique-owners themselves who gave the villagers the means with which to rebuild their village and hence 'destroy' its 'village atmosphere'. Similarly, ethnic chic is at once the destruction and rebuilding of India's clothing traditions.

10 Dressing for Distinction: A Historical Review

Any exploration of the processes whereby individuals and groups define their identity through their clothes must highlight the two elements of choice and constraint which form the conceptual framework within which the problem of what to wear is situated. However great the constraints, some element of choice is always possible. Even in situations where the very idea of individual action appears submerged by social convention, there is always the possibility of defying convention and breaking the rules. When Gandhi wore his *dhoti* to Buckingham Palace and Hansaben wore her cardigan in the kitchen in Jalia, both were using clothes to challenge the foundations of the hierarchical relations which oppressed them, even though they could not reverse those hierarchical norms with a single gesture (the authority of the King, as of Hansaben's father-in-law, remained undisputed).

If material culture is the primary object of our study, then human agency is the subject, for people manipulate objects such as clothes in defining themselves. But material culture is not merely the *object* here for, despite being produced and consumed by human beings, it has a way of taking on a subjectivity of its own. For, in the same way that we define ourselves through the objects we consume, so our consumption defines us and we become the objects of a categorisation process in which the world of material culture is the subject (cf. Miller 1985, Bourdieu 1984, Douglas and Isherwood 1980). So our clothes define us as much as we define ourselves through our clothes, and differences in dress do not merely suggest that 'we' are different from 'them', but also naturalise these differences and thereby become the very basis and proof of difference itself (cf. Hodder 1982).

Understanding the dual processes of differentiation and identification is central to understanding the development of any clothing tradition, for clothes are literally a means of classification – whether of individuals, groups, castes, classes, regions or nations. And in the same way that clothes draw boundaries which *exclude* those dressed differently, so they encompass and *include* those dressed in the same way. This is the process of identification. While individuals and groups are not necessarily motivated by the desire to differentiate themselves from others, differentiation none the less results from their actions. And similarly, while individuals are not necessarily seeking to

Dressing for Distinction: A Historical Review

identify with others when they share the same dress, they are none the less interpreted as identifying with them. Hence differentiation and identification are the unavoidable, though sometimes intended, consequences of the choices we make. What Bourdieu argues for 'taste' is equally true for dress:

> Taste classifies, and it classifies the classifier. Social subjects, classified by their classification, distinguish themselves by the distinctions they make, between the beautiful and the ugly, the distinguished and the vulgar, in which their position in the objective classifications is expressed or betrayed (Bourdieu 1984: 6).

Many scholars, from the nineteenth century to the present, have highlighted the importance of clothes as a means of identification and differentiation in India (cf. Johnson 1863–6, Watson 1868–75, Dongerkery 1960, Elson 1979, J. Jain 1980, Chishti and Sanyal 1989). But their models are often rigid and therefore obscure the existence of the problem of what to wear. But if differentiation and identification are defined as *processes*, then that problem emerges from obscurity. For, if too many diverse groups begin to identify with the same type of dress, then one group (often consisting of those who first wore the dress) will eventually differentiate themselves by wearing something else. Viewed within this framework, the recent history of Indian dress may be interpreted as a series of 'strategies of distinction' (cf. Bourdieu 1984) which form patterns of differentiation both between India and the West and between different groups within Indian society. The dominant strategies, which are summarised below, have been led largely by the Indian élite, but have in turn become the strategies of middle and lower sections of society as they follow. In each phase there are certain individuals and groups who do not fit the pattern, but this does not alter the structure of the historical processes themselves.

Phase 1: the appeal of European dress[1]
During the period of British rule in India, European dress gradually gained popularity among the Indian upper classes. This was not a simple case of Indians blindly following the West. On the contrary Indian people were fairly resistant to Western clothes, often refusing to allow them entry into their houses even when they allowed their use in the workplace. But with the spread of the British education system and, to some extent, the value system that went with it, European dress gradually came to be regarded

---

1 Bourdieu's notion of 'strategies of distinction' could of course be applied equally to the history of dress in Moghul and pre-Moghul India.

by the educated few as a sign of the wearer's progress and success.

Through wearing European styles, upper-class Indians dissociated themselves from the uneducated Indian majority while at the same time associating themselves with the ruling British élite. This apparent quest for integration was not so much motivated by admiration for the British as by acceptance of the idea that India's development could be brought about through cooperation with European values and ideas of progress. This cooperation was predominantly male. Indian women remained largely shielded from both the British and their clothes. However, élite women did adopt selected features of European dress, such as voluminous petticoats and lacy blouses, which distinguished them from other Indian women.

The response of British men to Indian men's strategy of identification was to further the process of differentiation, both by trying to prevent Indians from wearing European styles and by tightening their own sartorial codes and thereby making them less accessible to Indians. Motivated by anything from feelings of racial superiority to a more humble desire to respect Indian traditions, British men wanted to keep differences apparent. Differences between Indian and European dress were used not only to mark out racial difference, but also to justify racial discrimination.

During the early twentieth century, a large proportion of Indian villagers remained in Indian styles but took to wearing machine-manufactured cloth, imported from the West. This was not only cheaper than most Indian manufactures but also finer, and was therefore associated with higher levels of refinement. By the mid-twentieth century a considerable proportion of village men were turning first to Western-style shirts and then to shirts and trousers. They were not so much following the British – with whom they had little or no contact – as following the Indian élite who were following the British. Women, as we have seen, were more conservative in their dress, owing partly to ideas of female modesty and partly to the fact that Indian men were anxious to preserve their women from the tainting influence of the West.

Phase 2: responding with khadi
The spread of *khadi*, so successfully propagated by Gandhi, was a deliberate step away from the increasing Westernisation of Indian dress. Gandhi recognised that dress was a concrete symbol to which everybody could relate, and portrayed his disillusionment with the British through his gradual shedding of Western garments. This was not merely a rejection of Western values but a reassertion of Indian values as morally superior as well as socially, politically and economically more appropriate to India.

Dressing for Distinction: A Historical Review

Not content with merely breaking the link between the dress of the Indian and Western élite, Gandhi chose as his image for India the clothing and lifestyle most antithetical to the British and to their ideas of progress. He tried to encourage all Indians to identify with the plight of the poorest villager, not merely through wearing the latter's clothes but also through sharing his labour. All men and women were to spin their own thread and so participate in the production of their own garments. In short, Gandhi invited Indians, whatever their background, religion or caste, to be like villagers, thereby providing an alternative model of modernisation to the prevalent European model. He also sought to wipe out social and religious differentiation within his own society, masking all distinctions under a *khadi* blanket which was to unite Indians against the West.

The response to Gandhi's efforts was mixed, but throughout the freedom struggle a number of educated Indians did take to wearing *khadi*, often motivated by their recognition of its effectiveness as a strategic move against the British. Yet those who did adopt it simultaneously found alternative means of differentiation beneath this seemingly egalitarian sartorial mask. Differences of design, texture, colour and style were developed both to express and reveal social, religious, economic and cultural differences.

The overall effect of the *khadi* movement on the clothes of the uneducated majority is more difficult to gauge. Though principally an upper-class movement, it did incorporate various groups who felt that *khadi* represented their interests. These included both wealthy peasant landlords and *Harijan* weavers. While some villagers wore *khadi* for political reasons, others did so because it was their habitual dress. But a large proportion of the female village population remained either in the cheaper, finer mill-cloth they had recently adopted or, like Saurashtran peasant women, in other forms of regional dress. Just as the Westernisation of dress was essentially male-dominated, so was the re-Indianisation of dress through *khadi*. It did, however, incorporate a number of women from élite families (including rural élites) who began for the first time to participate in Indian politics.

Phase 3: post-independence modernisation

After independence Indian politicians were placed in a difficult position politically and sartorially. Having defined Indian identity in terms of *khadi*, they could not simply reject such dress the moment the British turned their backs. The problem was that Gandhi had woven into *khadi* an entire notion of an ideal craft-based society which, though convenient as an alternative to British society, did not at all conform to the vision of the majority of Indian politicians. They resolved this conflict by pursuing their own

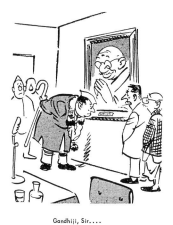

Gandhiji, Sir....

Fig. 10.1 Courtesy of R. K. Laxman in the *Times of India*.

policy of modernisation (including industrialisation), but at the same time continuing to dress in hand-woven clothes and Indian styles. By wearing the *sherwani pyjama* Nehru, India's first prime minister, managed to avoid looking Western while simultaneously avoiding looking like the Hindu peasant in his *dhoti*. From the 1950s onwards, *khadi dhotis* and Gandhi caps became increasingly confined to important political occasions and removed from Gandhian ideas (see fig. 10.1).

But independent India, despite its industrial policy, did not entirely neglect the pre-independence veneration for village life. Nor did politicians forget the need to show their affiliation with Indian villagers. The Nehru family, as we have seen, decided to express their personal affiliation by adopting temporary tokens of the dress of the diverse peoples of India when on political tour. They also encouraged the establishment of an institutional framework through which Indian handicrafts and textiles could be 'supported' and 'revived'. In 1952 the All India Handicraft Board was established with the idea that urban Indians had a moral duty to support Indian handicrafts, although they no longer needed to become craftspeople themselves. Many of the people involved in this movement were highly dedicated individuals with a genuine interest in appreciating and reviving indigenous craft skills. In particular it was prominent women like Kamaladevi Chattopadhyaya and Pupul Jayakar, not to mention Indira Gandhi herself, who tried to popularise hand-loom fabrics of different regions by actually wearing them. Most of the people involved in this craft revival no longer advocated a minimalist Gandhian approach to Indian dress, but they did reiterate the need for India to differentiate itself from the dominant stream of Western culture. Women in particular were praised for their loyalty to Indian dress, and encouraged to become the patrons and keepers of Indian clothing traditions which were now opposed to Western dress in aesthetic, rather than political, terms. Kamala Dongerkery, one of the women involved in this revival, wrote:

> It is for the Indian woman to think out and utilise every item of artistic excellence whether it be the fisherman's cap, the decorated Lucknow kurtha, silver or ivory ornaments of Kashmir or Saurashtra. . . . The point to be remembered is the attractiveness of the article and the artistic value rather than the finery and grandeur and the cost of the article. . . . An adaptation of Indian designs and colours, incorporated in the fashions of teenagers, would be in harmony with the general costume of the people and would, perhaps, transform India into an oriental fairyland. Western clothes, however beautiful, comfortable and useful, do not as

Dressing for Distinction: A Historical Review

a rule fit into the picturesque pattern of Indian life.... We must be able to utilise simple and common materials to aesthetic advantage in order that we may feel at one with the multitude (Dongerkery 1960: 77).

Dongerkery's appeal was, of course, directed towards educated urban women who had lost touch with their local sartorial traditions. But such women, some of whom had only recently differentiated themselves from 'the multitude', did not necessarily wish to identify with the common people. Nor did they necessarily share the same vision of India as an 'oriental fairyland' with a 'picturesque' pattern of life. Furthermore, this romanticisation of the village through craft rested uneasily with the government's attempts to 'develop' and 'modernise' the technology and living standards of villagers. This was an era in which India's primary political and economic aim was to 'develop'.

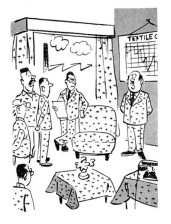

In spite of all our efforts there's still a large stock of unsold cloth with us!

Fig. 10.2 Courtesy of R. K. Laxman in the *Times of India*.

Most urbanites (politicians, academics and artists excluded) quickly switched their affiliations back to mill-cloth. Men returned to trousers and women were attracted to enticing new varieties of synthetics both from India and from abroad. Some young women even adopted European styles, such as skirts, blouses and later trousers and denim jeans. Well-to-do families contented themselves with buying the odd hand-made Indian tablecloth from a cottage emporium and feeling they had fulfilled their duty to India. The result was that most government-backed handloom projects ran at a loss and the enthusiastic production of handloom textiles rarely met with the same enthusiastic levels of consumption (see fig. 10.2).

In general, independent India showed a return to the modernisation of dress in the form of machine-made fabrics and foreign styles. In the cities, the development of the film industry popularised certain images, in particular the hero in jeans and sunglasses and the heroine in a variety of shapes and guises. So powerful was the appeal of the movie image that some girls would even take their tailors to the cinema so that they could copy dress designs from films (Chaudhuri 1976: 137). Disgusted by what he sees as an ever-increasing tendency towards eroticism and cheapness, Chaudhuri calls this era 'the age of Ugliness' and accuses Indian women of falling prey to it: 'If I might be frank in the expression of my opinion, for the most part our women are going to hell, for me an aesthetic hell though for many it is also a moral one, down a path spread with nylon and paved with imitation gold' (*ibid.*: 109).

Since most Indian women do not share Chaudhuri's perception of what constitutes an 'aesthetic hell', there are indeed many who are following the 'nylon path'. Quite apart from the fact that synthetic saris and *shalwar*

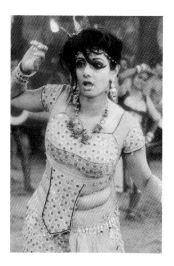

Fig. 10.3 Postcard of the actress
Sri Devi, dressed in a film star
version of village embroidery.
By Jain Picture Publishers.

kamizes are relatively cheap and easy to maintain, there is also the fact that
for many women their adoption is part of a process by which they can
distance themselves from the backward associations of local dress and join
the ranks of the 'progressive'. Adopting such clothes becomes one of the
many strategies through which a social group is able to upgrade itself. So
in Jalia it was wealthy high-caste women who were the first to adopt synthetic saris. This differentiated them from the peasant women who still
wore backless bodices and hand-embroidered clothes. Yet today *Kanbi*
women are themselves anxious to differentiate themselves from the category
of village farmer, and are leaving *ghaghro*-wearing to *Kharak* women who
probably adopted the dress from the *Kanbis* in the first place. In areas where
cinema, television and videos are easily accessible, there are no doubt many
village women who, like urban women, are influenced by the fashions of
Hindi film-stars.[2] Yet just at the time when the middle classes in towns
and villages seemed to be formulating a shared sartorial image in which
the synthetic sari and *shalwar kamiz* had a central place, the women of the
Indian élite, including many Hindi film-stars, chose to branch away from
the 'nylon path' and return down a muddy side-street back to the village.

Phase 4: ethnic chic – return to roots?
Ethnic chic, the fourth phase in this historical progression, is one of the
means by which the élite educated minority has redefined its position and
taste to the Indian masses and to the West. It is a circular step, for the
élite are literally stepping into village dress at the very moment when the
majority of villagers are stepping out of it. By doing this they can differentiate themselves from the increasing mass of the sari-wearing, denim jeans-
wearing middle classes, who still follow the earlier example of the Indian
élite.

Ethnic chic is a means of asserting one's membership of a high social
sphere by dressing in peasant and tribal fabrics and/or styles which for most
of the century have been associated with a low social sphere. Its exclusivity
is safeguarded by the 'tribals' and 'peasants' who are themselves rejecting
these clothes while the provincial middle classes, who recently rejected
them, are far too close to their real implications to return to them. If a
young woman in a provincial city like Larabad were to dress herself in an

2   In Jalia televisions were still in very limited supply, and going to the cinema in the city was
    predominantly a male activity; I only once heard women's clothes referred to in terms of
    films – when an itinerant trader arrived in the village, claiming to sell the types of sari worn
    by Sita in the television version of the *Ramayana*. I am not aware that he obtained any sales.

Dressing for Distinction: A Historical Review

embroidered *ghaghro* and *kapdu*, she might be confused with the *real* village peasant, and that would sully her reputation. For her, village clothes are associated with backwardness, illiteracy, a tough farming life, restrictive rules for women and a general lack of taste and refinement. It is only through being at a sufficient distance (socially and to some extent geographically) from these implications that the Indian élite can choose to dress themselves in peasant and tribal clothes.

This return to ethnic dress is very different from the return to *khadi* in the nationalist period, although ethnic fashion relies to some extent on *khadi* philosophy to give it credibility.[3] Gandhi's romanticisation of the village involved the idea of the simplicity and morality of village life, and identification and participation with the villager. But ethnic chic relies merely on the hollow idea of identification without any real attempt at participation. This theme is exemplified in the many Hindi films in which the heroine changes in and out of different regional outfits without being affiliated either to the region or to the groups who traditionally wear such clothes. These films focus on the spectacular and romantic aspects of village life which are generally divorced from the social context of the village. This extraction of the aesthetic and marketable elements of peasant and tribal India has played an essential part in the Festival of India, in *Apna Utsav* (our festival) and in numerous stagings of folk dances now so popular in India's major cities. Fig. 10.4 shows a politician watching a folk dance in a village and assuming that villagers have taken the idea from the city. It reveals the actual distance between the urban élite and the tribal performers. It is that same distance which, in the field of fashion, has enabled the 'ethnic' to become the 'chic'.

Yet ethnic chic, despite its distance from the people it imitates, poses as – and to some extent *is* – a cultural revival in that it venerates an Indian aesthetic above a Western one. It is a means by which the Indian élite distinguishes itself not only from the Indian masses but also from the West. Many people describe their personal choice of ethnic clothes as part of a sudden realisation that the West does not hold all the answers; it is a sort of anti-modern, anti-Western approach to dress. On the other hand, the fashion of ethnic chic and the new appreciation of Indian culture that accompanies it is, as we have seen, very much linked to the West and to

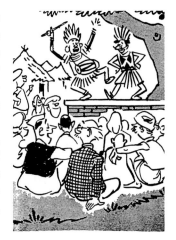

This village must be pretty advanced—they have folk dances here for entertainment just as we have in the city!

Fig. 10.4 Courtesy of R. K. Laxman in the *Times of India*.

3   For example, Bina Ramani employed refugee tailors in her workshop in Hauz Khas village. In this sense she perpetuates the Gandhian association between craft and social welfare. But, unlike Gandhi, she did not participate in the menial work herself. Rather she designed clothes which were made by the poor and sold to the rich, keeping in line with the fashion industry's characteristically capitalist organisation.

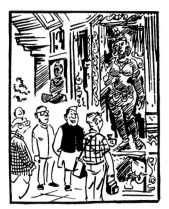

I developed an interest in these things in America when I went there recently for the festival.

Fig. 10.5 Courtesy of R. K. Laxman in the *Times of India*.

the West's appreciation of India's art and craft heritage (see fig. 10.5). It is also stimulated by Indian people's sense of foreignness in relation to India, and this sense of foreignness is due to the nature of their close historical association with the West. Furthermore, in criticising Western ideas of progress ethnic chic at the same time participates in the anti-modernist ideas which are themselves part of Western culture. Fashions 'went ethnic' in the West before doing so in India, and few years pass without some mention of a new 'ethnic' wave hitting the fashion houses of Paris, New York and London. Can ethnic chic separate itself from the more international trend of ethnic fashion? And is it even intended to? Returning to the fashion show at Hauz Khas, it was noticeable that the most definitively Western clothes in the show were modelled first, seeming to indicate that the ethnic clothes were to be viewed as designer fashion garments and not as traditional handicraft or even as genuine peasant clothes. Ethnic chic is, therefore, not only a means of differentiation from other Indians and from the West, but also a means of identification with an increasingly cosmopolitan 'global élite' who share common tastes. As Bina Ramani put it, her designs were for 'international people'; such an international élite, bound together through shared tastes, to some extent transcends mere cultural boundaries (cf. Appadurai and Breckenridge 1988).

Thus ethnic chic is a 'fashion' as much as it is a cultural revival. And this concept of fashion, incorporating as it does the constant need for changing clothes, has been developed principally in the West. This is not to say that Indian clothes remained unchanged; indeed the whole of this book has tended to show the opposite to be true. But the point is that people can only change their clothes within the accepted limits of their social situation, and as we can see from the many examples in Jalia, the constraints in an Indian village are many and the opportunities for change comparatively few, especially for women. Constrained by both caste and veiling restrictions, few village women have more than one style of clothing from which to choose at any given time. Fashion, on the other hand, relies on people's ability to play with image, to select one image one day but be able to abandon it later if required. It offers the potential for transforming identities rather than trying to fix an identity definitively in time and space. A fashionable Delhi student can dress like an American sportswoman one day and like a Gujarati peasant the next, and no one will fix her to these images unless she chooses to fix herself to them by wearing the same style constantly. And then, sooner or later, she will be 'out of fashion'. Fashion is the veneration of the ephemeral (cf. Wilson 1987). It also goes hand in hand with the notion of individualism. We are constantly told by magazines that it is through fashion that we can express 'ourselves'. Ethnic chic has appropriated all these notions. By rearranging elements of village dress, women of the urban élite, like Liveleen Sharma, can express their individuality and their exclusivity.[4]

Yet ethnic chic as an exclusive fashion faces two main problems. First, it alienates those who wore hand-made Indian clothes before the 'ethnic revival'. These are the women, and to a less extent the men, who have consistently advocated the appreciation of Indian handicrafts since the 1950s. They have long worn textiles woven, dyed and embroidered by hand. Having selected these on a mixture of aesthetic and moral grounds, many now balk at the new ethnic fashion:

> Those who have always dressed traditional look at this fashion wave suspiciously – they don't know whether to love it or hate it. . . . As the fashion spreads it becomes vulgar and defies its own ends. Or as Martand Singh[5] put it: 'Ultimately a god becomes an ashtray' (*India Today* 30 Apr. 1988: 78).

This perspective is felt particularly by those directly involved in both governmental and non-governmental craft organisations. While on the one hand they are pleased that at last the public is showing more interest in indigenous designs, on the other hand they are often dubious about the quality and longevity of this new wave of enthusiasm. Some feel that it is born out of ignorance rather than the appreciation of Indian handiwork. They complain that status-conscious people, with little aesthetic sense but keen to keep up with the fashion, end up mixing and matching garments and textiles from different parts of India without any understanding of how they should be worn or how they should be combined. Furthermore, many feel that there is now a vulgar surfeit of ethnic exoticism, with people trying to outdo each other with their degrees of ethnicness.[6]

The very popularity of ethnic chic is debasing its reputation, among not only the arts and crafts lovers but also those who took to ethnic chic as

---

4 The spread of fashion in India from the early 1980s onwards has been facilitated by increasing social mobility, the rapid expansion of a new middle-class category of consumers, the development of an industry dedicated to the production of fashion, and the new but increasing separation of the roles of designer and producer. These factors have been boosted by the spread of the film industry and television, which market a number of images to people all over India, including romantic portraits of Indian villagers in regional styles of dress. The development of the Indian fashion industry is too large a subject to be covered in this book.

5 Martand Singh is the secretary of the Indian National Trust for Art and Cultural Heritage (INTACH). He was also involved in the organisation of the Festival of India.

6 One fashion designer in Ahmedabad, a woman who has long appreciated Indian crafts,

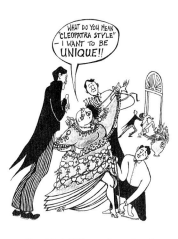

Fig. 10.6 'Like snakes, Bombay's
nouveau riche is shedding old
wardrobe in search of the
exclusive identity'. Courtesy of
Manjula Padmanabhan.

a symbol of exclusivity and uniqueness. For so rapidly has the fashion spread
down the social hierarchy, with machine-made replicas of ethnic clothes
readily available for the more popular consumer, that it can no longer be
termed 'exclusive'. New methods need to be found by which the fashionable
élite can separate itself from the burgeoning middle-class consumer
(fig. 10.6). Such methods were beginning to emerge in the late 1980s with
the development of a new cult of exclusivity, best exhibited in the so-called
'Artwear' fashion. This is a fashion so exclusive and so expensive that, like
all *haute couture*, it is worn only by a minute wealthy minority.

Phase 5: beyond ethnic chic to Artwear exclusivity

Artwear is one of the latest 'strategies of distinction' in Indian fashion. Ethnic
chic was exclusive through combining tribal and peasant dress with the
Western concept of fashion. Artwear is like ethnic chic without the ethnic;
it is really a new form of Indian chic. It consists of garments composed not
merely by designers, but by a two-person team consisting of a designer and
an artist. The result is 'not-to-be-repeated, once-only outfits' (*India Today* 30
June 1989). The man who organised the get-together of artist/designer
teams[7] in Bombay described what it means to wear an Artwear garment:
'When you wear artwear you become part of a painting – not everyone has
the courage to be so bold. You are making a statement, isn't it? You wear
it because you know that nobody else is also wearing it' (*ibid.*). The
assurance that no one else is wearing it is probably true, since the forty
or so outfits resulting from the artist – designer liaison cost up to 20,000
rupees (then the equivalent of £1,000) per dress.

With this new development of clothes as an artform has come the
attempt to rework the sari as new high fashion. In recent years it had
become increasingly threatened in fashionable circles by the emergence of
alternative clothes for women (including Western styles, ethnic chic outfits
and the *shalwar kamiz*). Furthermore, the synthetic sari is now so popular
as to have entirely lost its exclusivity for the urban élite, while the handloom sari is associated more with 'tradition' and sometimes with wealth
(if made from extravagant materials), but not usually with high fashion,

---

explained that in 1988, tired of the glare of too much Gujarati mirror-work and embroidery,
she tried to market a collection of more subtle and simple clothes. But her customers complained. They wanted the really exotic tribal look, and she ultimately conformed to their
demand in order to preserve her sales.

7 Bina Ramani, of Hauz Khas fame, was among the designers selected to work with artists to
produce Artwear garments. Some of the other designers selected also sell their work in Hauz
Khas.

328

Dressing for Distinction: A Historical Review

Fig. 10.7 The progressive eroticisation of the sari. Courtesy of Prakash and Penguin Books India.

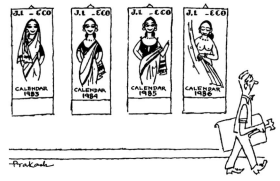

glamour and exclusivity. As *India Today* put it, the sari was considered by many as 'staid, standard and almost sacred' (15 Dec. 1990). Now, however, it is re-emerging as an erotic wrap which can expose as much as it conceals. The blouse is being discarded[8] and the sari itself is changing its size, altering its form and being tied in a variety of new ways – with a ruffle in the front, a bustle behind, and even as a woman's turban (fig. 10.8). Experimentation with the sari is one of the latest means by which a woman can be elegant, exclusive, Indian, unconventional, sexy and expensive all at the same time.

It is yet to be seen how much this latest sari fashion will develop. Needless to say, it is encountering considerable opposition from traditionalists who see any tampering with the sari form as sacrilege (*ibid.*). But if it is well marketed through advertising and, more important, through films, it may be the look of the future in India. For our purposes it is irrelevant whether it succeeds or not; it is included here simply to illustrate one of the latest developments in the long and arduous search for an Indian dress which is both non-Western and fashionable, a search which began in the late nineteenth century but has since taken many a diverse path.

The problem of what to wear remains

Bourdieu's concept of 'strategies of distinction' has been a useful tool for understanding the emergence and resurgence of various clothing trends in India. But it is not sufficient for comprehension of the full magnitude, or indeed the full triviality, of the problem of what to wear. For this is a personal problem that is integral to the particular lived experience of individuals, groups and nations. It is not enough simply to locate a person's

---

8 Like ethnic chic fashion, this mode of wearing the sari without a blouse plays on earlier Indian traditions long rejected by the Indian élite but still practised to some extent in remote rural areas, such as the hills of Orissa.

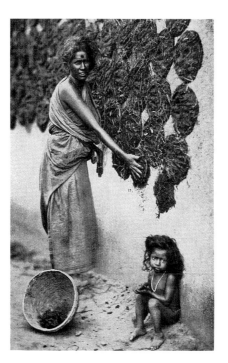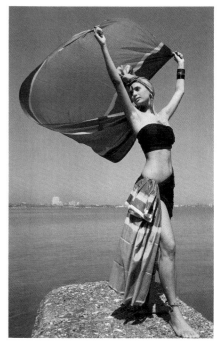

Fig. 10.8 *Left*: A photograph of a woman drying cow-dung cakes in the 1920s.
Reproduced from H. V. Glasenapp's *Indien*, 1925. Courtesy of SOAS. The woman wears
a sari without a blouse. *Right*: The 1980s fashion version of the sari without a blouse.
Reproduced from the magazine *Glad Rags*, 1989, vol. 2, no. 2.

position within a historical trend without attempting to comprehend how
that person arrived where he or she now stands, and how he or she feels
about other trends. For, despite participating in 'strategies of distinction',
people are not necessarily conscious of the implications of their choice of
clothes (Lurie 1992), or motivated by a desire to be distinctive (although
some clearly are). Indeed some, like the *Harijans* of Jalia, actually seek to
escape classification rather than reveal their identity through their dress,
and yet others are concerned less with identity than with the practical problems of price and availability. Despite the varying degrees of seriousness
and consciousness with which the problem is treated, and although fashion
magazines define the problem in largely aesthetic and economic terms, I
would argue that the problem of what to wear is not merely mundane but
also a social, cultural and political dilemma.

At its broadest, the problem of what to wear is formulated within the
framework of the specific historical development of a culture. In India this
problem has for the past century been inextricably linked to the colonial

encounter and its after-effects. The question arises whether the educated urban Indian can today look 'Indian' without looking too self-consciously so. For women this is not a problem. They have never abandoned Indian styles on a mass scale, and have successfully adapted Indian outfits such as the *shalwar kamiz* to the whims of contemporary fashion. But for men the situation is more complex. So much have European styles been incorporated into their wardrobes that most now consider them part of Indian dress. But while broadening the category of Indian dress to accept European styles, Indian men have simultaneously down-graded indigenous forms of dress so drastically that it now becomes difficult for a professional man to wear a *kurta pyjama*, let alone a *dhoti*, to his place of work.[9] To do so would seem too self-consciously Indian, suggesting the image of the hypocritical politician.

Part of the problem lies perhaps in the formulation of the question, since the very idea of 'looking Indian' seems to have emerged only through the Indian's encounter with the non-Indian. In his book *We Indians* (1982), Khushwant Singh describes the evolution of his own personal awareness of 'being Indian'. As a small child he lived in a village in Western Punjab (now Pakistan), and when people asked him who he was, he replied by giving the name of his subcaste and family. When his family moved to live in a neighbouring town, he left his subcaste out of the description and defined himself as a Sikh, mentioning his caste only to those of his own religious persuasion. By the time he was twelve, his family had moved to Delhi, and when he met people from other linguistic regions of India, Kushwant Singh described himself to his new schoolmates as a 'Sikh from Punjab'. Finally, on reaching England, he began to describe himself as Indian. He records:

> The first time I became conscious of being Indian was when I went to university in England. This was not very surprising since only Englishmen who had been to India could recognise me as a Sikh or a Punjabi. For others I was just an Indian. Like other foreigners living in England, we Indians tended to herd together. We preferred to live in the same boarding houses; joined Indian clubs and forgathered at Indian religious festivals. By then we also started taking an interest in our freedom movement. To present a united front against the English, we suppressed our

---

9 Exceptions are found among artists, photographers and left-wing intellectuals who often wear *khadi kurta pyjamas* or *kurtas* with trousers to work. It is noticeable that these are usually made from flecked or coloured rather than white *khadi*, perhaps in a desire to deflect from the possible association with the *khadi*-clad politician.

religious and linguistic separateness and insisted that we were Indians (Singh 1982: 11–12).

Yet by conforming to this notion of 'the Indian', partly out of necessity (he was defined as such by the English) and partly out of choice (he embraced a category through which Indians could present a united image against the British), Khushwant Singh was not only helping to validate the category of 'Indian' but also expressing his relationship to the West. Probably the single most penetrating analysis of how this identity dilemma has manifested itself in India is by Ashis Nandy, who points out that there can be no such thing as 'the Indian', since 'the West is now everywhere, within the West and outside; in structures and in minds' (Nandy 1983: xi). For him any attempt to get outside the West is inextricably bound to the West since it sets itself up in opposition to the West. He writes: 'The pressure to be the obverse of the West distorts the traditional priorities in the Indian's total view of man and universe and destroys his culture's unique gestalt. In fact it binds him even more irrevocably to the West' (Nandy 1983: 73). Nandy's point, perhaps influenced by Edward Said's *Orientalism* (1978), is that people born within the historical construction of colonialism are all co-victims of colonialism, whether they are born of the West or the non-West. If one applies his arguments to the clothing of both the British and Indian élite during the *Raj*, it is clear that the British were obliged to intensify their Britishness in the face of the alien Indian, and Indians were obliged to intensify their Indianness in the face of the alien British. In both cases a national and sartorial identity was reinforced through that encounter.

One of Gandhi's greatest achievements was his establishment of a new Indian dress. But the problem was that for those Indian men who had been born and educated directly under the British system, a *khadi dhoti* felt more foreign than a tailored suit. Furthermore, after independence, were these men to remain ossified in some apparently timeless 'traditional' Indian outfit while Indian peasants, less concerned with the implications of empire, put aside their rustic *dhotis* in favour of synthetic trousers? The answer was clearly 'no'. But the question remained. How could the Indian élite, conscious of its relationship to the West, look modern without appearing Western, and look Indian without appearing 'traditional'? In a sense it was a search for an Indian modernism, but since modernism had been defined in India in Western terms, any attempt to adopt modern dress risked and still risks being interpreted as an attempt to imitate Western dress.

This problem is specific to a certain educated milieu of Indian society.

Dressing for Distinction: A Historical Review

As Nandy points out, only a small group of Indians try to define Indianness while 'large groups live their lives as if such definitions were irrelevant' (Nandy 1983: 102). This is not to say that the vast majority of Indians, who continue to inhabit India's villages, are any less self-conscious about their presentation of self. As the Jalia example shows, there is just as much controversy in a village concerning the question of what to wear as there is in a town or city. But the question is framed differently. Nobody in Jalia discusses dress in terms of national identity or Indianness; indeed, most people tend not even to think in these terms. So a person dressing in styles that are clearly of Western origin is perceived as dressing in city styles, not Western ones. Hansaben's cardigan was controversial not because it crossed the boundaries of national Indian styles but because it crossed the sartorial limits of the village and was considered unacceptable dress for a married Jalia woman.

In Jalia, then, identity dilemmas tended to be framed within the geographical limits of the local area. To people of the village the terms *deshi* and 'foren' did not refer to the Indian and the Western, but rather to the Kathiawadi and the non-Kathiawadi. Even Ahmedabad, despite being situated in Gujarat, was often referred to as a 'foren' place. One of the major concerns of most groups in the village was how to modernise their dress without stepping outside the social system in which social relations in the village were defined. It was a question of how to bring in 'foren' elements without their seeming *too* 'foren' to other members of the caste and village. While for *Brahmans, Vaniyas, Harijans* and *Kanbis* this meant owning saris from as far away as possible, for *Kharaks* it meant incorporating new designs and motifs of desirable modern objects within the framework of their existing embroidered clothes. Constrained by their being uneducated and considered too unrefined to dress in saris, their particular form of modernisation was confined to the *deshi* medium of hand-embroidery which these women were becoming increasingly reluctant to wear. *Bharwads* were the exception to the dominant village trend since they sought actively to maintain a *deshi* look and to fend off 'foren' influences on the grounds that these were a threat to the caste. Within each different stratum of village society there was a concern to express, retain or change social identity through dress. But the idea of an 'Indian dress' was never even contemplated.

The fact that most of the population do not see the problem of what to wear as a national dilemma does not, of course, alleviate the problem for those who do. The Indian élite still have to wear something, even when they are highly aware of the symbolism of the various sartorial alternatives available to them. Politicians have remained faithful to the hand-spun look,

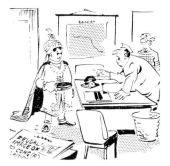

As a minister your indulging in a little luxury and extravagance is O.K. But giving up the old simple style of dress is really going too far!

Fig. 10.9 Courtesy of R. K. Laxman in the *Times of India*.

in public if not in private, for most realise their political obligation to look Indian and to appear humble (see fig. 10.9). But for those less directly concerned with their public image, the choice of what to wear is at once more personal, more free and, as a result, more difficult. The Indian intelligentsia are keenly aware of the sensitivity of this problem, which is much debated in the media along with other sensitive issues such as whether one should speak in Hindi or English or a regional language. Political cartoonists, like Ravi Laxman, provide a constant critical commentary on the appearance of Indian public figures and on the complexity of the relationship between India and the West (see fig. 10.10). And Indian journalists have reached a level of self-critical sarcasm concerning their own culture that is probably unmatched anywhere in the world. But this makes it no easier when it comes to deciding what to wear.

An advertisement for Vimal fabrics highlights the problems:

'No two persons can quite agree to what Indian culture is. But all agree it's unfathomably rich.'

'Vimal has always been reflecting the richness of Indian culture.'

By making 'richness' its referent, the Vimal advertisement carefully avoids trying to define what Indian culture is while at the same time claiming to reflect it. And it is perhaps in the recognition of the need for multifaceted interpretations of Indian culture that the problem of what to wear finds its resolution. For many educated Indians the answer lies not in settling for *khadi*, or for Western dress, or for ethnic chic, but in combining all these elements; and although this involves the risk of being associated with all of them, it at least avoids too close association with any single one of them. Few people want to present a definitively Western image, because this can be too easily interpreted as aping the West. But on the other hand, few people want to spend their lives wearing only white *khadi*,[10] which has become associated more with hypocrisy than with morality or Indianness. On the other hand ethnic chic, as a modern reworking of traditional elements, appeals to people for its Indianness but is criticised for being an expensive glamorisation of poverty through exploitation and ignorance. Few people settle for it permanently, though Liveleen Sharma appears to be an exception. For most women, including the boutique-owners of Hauz Khas, dressing in ethnic clothes is something you do from time to time, perhaps in the

10   What *khadi* actually is and how it is defined is becoming increasingly difficult to surmise. So keen have *khadi* organisations been to make this fabric appeal to different groups of people, that they are even marketing a product called 'polyester *khadi*'!

Dressing for Distinction: A Historical Review

evenings or when you want to look glamorous or are attending a wedding. It is not something for daily wear, since ethnic dress has a marginalising effect, masking (although it also secretly reveals) a person's internationality.

Being international and affiliating oneself to globally acceptable fashion trends is in fact a popular method of defining identity today, especially for men. Nationalism, as Jawaharlal Nehru used to argue, is enriching, but it is also limiting if it prevents progress and participation in world affairs. Fashionable men and women reveal through their dress that they are content to be Indian but that they also participate in trends that transcend national boundaries. Many advertisements play on this idea, such as the Dinesh 'Take the world in your stride' series, which shows an Indian man in Dinesh clothes appearing in a variety of different countries throughout the world. Similarly the Globetrotter and Benzer sequences of advertisements play on the same idea of international travel and encounter (fig. 10.11).

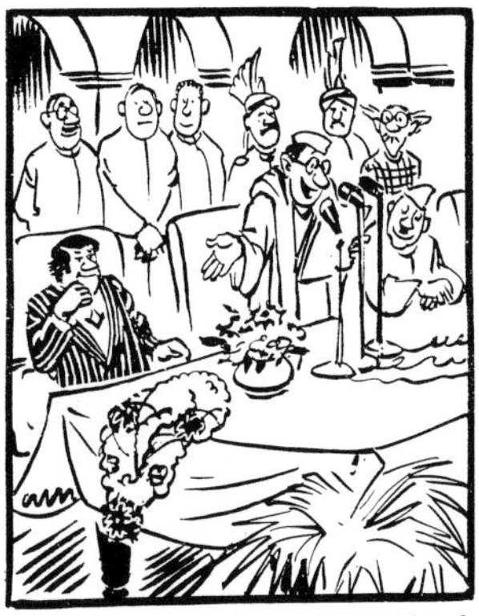

The development of a new mixed Indian wardrobe may be compared to the development of other new cultural formations, such as a national cuisine. Appadurai has shown how Indian cookery books include different regional dishes from all over India as 'cosmopolitan and parochial expressions enrich and sharpen each other by dialectical interaction' (Appadurai 1988: 22). And just as the new Indian diet consists of regional Indian dishes combined with occasional Western ones, so a balanced Indian wardrobe consists of a variety of regional styles, combined with a few Western ones. A fashionable urban woman's wardrobe might contain some clothes considered classically Indian, like the sari; some that are both modern and Indian, like the *shalwar kamiz*; some that are glamorously ethnic, like Gujarati embroidery; some that are chic in Western terms, and some leisurewear and at least one pair of denim jeans. Jeans are perhaps more popular than skirts among this sector of the population since they are associated with America and therefore escape colonial implications. Skirts and dresses, which have a deeper association with the imperial past, seem to be more popular in provincial towns and cities than in cosmopolitan ones.[11] A prosperous man's wardrobe generally contains an abundance of trousers and shirts, jeans, the odd suit and at least something Indian, usually a *kurta pyjama* and some *khadi* shirts, or perhaps even a smart silk *dhoti* for special occasions or a simple plain *lungi* for relaxing at home. Through mixing and matching these combinations for appropriate occasions, the educated, modern, fashionable Indian can find a solution to, and some enjoyment of, the problem of what to wear. And

...And he has the welfare and prosperity of our nation at heart. He is truly a patriot. He is no ordinary Indian. He is a non-resident Indian!

Fig. 10.10 Courtesy of R. K. Laxman in the *Times of India*.

---

11 For many these styles, when worn by adults, are still associated with Christians and Eurasians, although these are more or less universally accepted by young girls.

even if the end-result is somewhat eclectic, what does it matter? Perhaps Raj Kapoor had the answer when, back in 1955, he sang:

> *mera juta hai japani*
> *ye patlun inglistani*
> *sir pe lal topi rusi*
> *phir bhi dil hai hindustani.*

[My shoes are Japanese/These trousers are English/On my head is a Russian hat/But still my heart is Indian.]

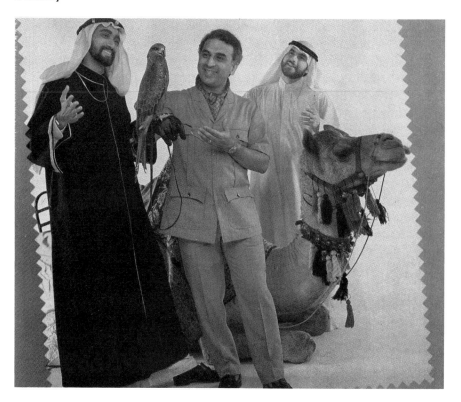

Fig. 10.11 An advertisement from the Dinesh 'Take the World in your Stride' series, 1989. The safari suit, relic of colonial shooting parties, is an example of men's dress that has passed from the British and Indian élite to the Indian middle classes.

Postscript
A Return Visit to India, 1993–1994

Coming back to Delhi five years later, I was struck immediately by the change of atmosphere. The opening up of India's previously tightly controlled trade barriers had encouraged a new wave of international spirit and an increased emphasis on things foreign, whether clothes, computers, luxury bathrooms or fast food. 'Global' was the buzz-word of the moment, ever present in advertisements, some of which actually featured foreign consumers as the main protagonists. The huge success of cable television, with its projection of images from all over the world, had clearly been influential in stimulating the taste for the 'foreign'. Debates in the press were no longer internally focused on questions of 'ethnic identity' but were externally oriented towards how best India should make its mark on the international stage.

This international focus was clearly present in the spread of the fashion industry, which no longer occupied an exclusive corner of the market place. Fashion designers had proliferated, and ready-made clothes of all styles were available on a much wider scale than ever before. The *shalwar kamiz* was still very much 'in', but seemed to be changing shape quicker than ever, sometimes going in at the waist and out at the hips, sometimes flaring from the chest downwards in a way reminiscent of earlier Moghul styles. It was with an awareness of these changes in the capital that I took the train and bus back to Jalia, wondering what I might find there. Stopping off in Larabad on the way I ambled through the main bazaar, noticing that many of the children's clothes and *shalwar kamizes* on sale contained inserts of Gujarati-style embroidery, albeit of a cheaply-made commercial type. The fashion wheel had clearly turned one more notch during the five years of my absence. The cosmopolitan sophisticates of Delhi were already tiring of mirror-work embroidery, but the very fact that they had worn it in the 1980s had been enough to remove its backward associations in a local city like Larabad. Here Gujarati women were beginning to buy cheap machine-made versions of the type of embroidery that they once made and wore.

The main purpose of my visit was to attend Leriben's wedding in Jalia. By the time I arrived, attention was focused on her trousseau, much of which was being packed away ready for transportation to her in-laws. I was told that it contained twenty-five saris from her parents, some 'sachi' (true) and some 'khotu' (false), symbolising the fact that as a wife she should be both glamorous and hardworking. She had also been given costly gold and diamond jewellery and a long list of other items including a fridge, cupboard, bed, fan, clock, folding chairs and a host of culinary equipment. The level of consumption had clearly risen. A fridge had taken up residence in the family house, and luxury items like plastic coffee sets and ice-cream sets had found their way into village cupboards. There was also a noticeable change in the status of different family members. Hansaben had grown large and assertive, tossing her sari about with noticeable authority. When in a quiet moment I asked her if relations with her in-laws were fine now, she answered with a meaningful smile: 'Have you seen my son?'

Yet Jalia had changed little. Most people still seemed to talk, eat, work and dress in much the same way as before. Cable television had not yet found its way to the village, and the feeling was one of familiarity more than surprise.

Two days after Leriben's departure to her in-laws, she returned to visit Jalia, triumphant and beaming about her first experience of married life. I was surprised that she was wearing her sari in the 'Bengali' style. When I inquired about this, she laughed and said that her in-laws were 'advanced'. They had told her that she need not perform *laj* when out of doors; she could simply cover her head with the border of her sari, and this was easy to do in the 'Bengali' style. Inside the home, however, she was to wear her sari in the Gujarati manner and to follow the normal *laj* procedures appropriate to senior male relatives. Her new home was in a town in a neighbouring district. She was proud of the fact that she had progressed from the village to a town, and took delight in recounting how everything was better in her new marital home. This was not the stereotypically timid and homesick weeping bride; she appeared radiantly happy. I found her endless talk of consumer luxuries rather depressing, but was pleased by her enthusiasm for the new life she was beginning.

Back in Delhi I returned to that other 'village' where change was of course more extreme. Wandering through the main street I realised the extent to which Hauz Khas village's 'ethnic transformation' had been characteristic of an era that was already in the past. Ethnic chic, though still visible in the architecture and presentation of some boutiques, was clearly no longer the dominant theme. It had been dwarfed by the general spread of rising concrete which made 'the village' look increasingly like any other shopping centre in South Delhi. And where an element of Indian exclusivity had been preserved, this was expressed less in rustic terms than in a yet more eclectic reworking of diverse Indian idioms which played on a range of historic and regional themes, interspersed and at times combined with the latest in international high-tech design. Most striking of all was the shell of a vast new 'state-of-the-art shopping complex', intended to house around 100 new boutiques and offices. Its base echoed the structure of the Turkish monument while the upper storeys were to be constructed in plate-glass and steel. The NRI (non-resident Indian) industrialist behind the development was aiming to construct a parking lot and a new approach road to the village. This would cut straight through the green zone that had prevented Hauz Khas village from merging with the dense urban mass of South Delhi.

Yet despite these commercial developments, parts of the village had an air of abandonment. Bricks and garbage littered alleyways, and occasional cows and buffaloes nosed at stray rubbish. Boutiques seemed to be closing down almost as fast as they were springing up, and the customers seemed comparatively few. Only twelve of the thirty-eight shops I had counted in 1989 still existed, although more than 100 new ones had sprung up to replace them. As for preserving the 'village atmosphere', the Creative Arts Village Association had collapsed in 1991 because of a mixture of disagreement among boutique-owners and lack of coordination from villagers. Some disillusioned ex-CAVA members now described the village as 'chaotic', 'characterless', 'purely commercial' and 'not a village any more'. Meanwhile, newcomers seemed to view the few remaining village features as more of a menace than an asset. They complained of poor construction, bad plumbing, irregular electricity and dirty buffaloes, not to mention 'ignorant villagers' who stood in the way of smooth commercial development. For them there was little question of exploiting the 'charm of village life'.

Fashion, like architecture, had gone through a period of intense diversification. The earlier peasant and tribal inspirations had not altogether disappeared, but now mingled more readily with new adaptations of historical forms of élite Indian dress, in which Moghul-inspired designs were conspicuous. Richly encrusted brocades and finely embroidered silks jostled for space among 'Artwear', skimpy black lycra and platform shoes. In furnishings, too, there seemed to be no limitations of style. Some boutiques sold modern designer furniture. Others sold old colonial and Indian models, while yet others sold a range of items typically associated with any ordinary tourist bazaar. Bina Ramani, who vacillated between calling Hauz Khas village a 'tremendous commercial success' and claiming to be 'totally appalled by what it had become', claimed that even in her worst dreams she could not have imagined that it would fall prey to the infamous

Kashmiri traders who haunt so many Indian shopping arcades with their crude tourist-trapping techniques.

But if the village was no longer as exclusive as it used to be, it had none the less made its mark on the map of Delhi. Not least, it had become the number-one spot for fashion shows, which were now fabulously staged in the monument grounds. The monument itself had been paved and floodlit, and now also functioned as a backdrop for business functions, marriage banquets and a nightly 'cultural show'. Meanwhile a well-known politician was drawing in the crowds with his vast new restaurant complex which attracted both South Delhiites and foreign diplomats as well as coachloads of foreign tourists. Exploiting the full range of marketable Indian idioms, his Village Bistro Complex offered 'theme nights' ranging from 'the Rajasthani landscape theme' to 'Ala-ud-Din-Khilji's tent theme'. Needless to say he also offered a 'village theme' in which he reconstructed that evasive commodity called 'village atmosphere' behind the restaurant walls, where it was safely tucked away from the intervention of potentially disruptive villagers.

But were there any villagers left? At first, among the proliferation of boutiques and restaurants, it was difficult to tell. But further inspection revealed that a few *Jat* families continued to live at the top of their buildings, although others had sold up and yet others came only to collect their rents. In the poorer section, the original inhabitants had mostly left the village or been pushed outside the original boundary, where a new slum-like compound had emerged. What those remaining felt about the developments was not easy to ascertain. The owners of substantial properties were inevitably the most favourable to the changes. The shops, which they now referred to as 'showrooms', had brought them vast amounts of money and propelled their village into prominence. Some did complain that the village had lost its old atmosphere; that children could no longer play in the streets or old men sit quietly out of doors. Others objected to the loud music and indecent behaviour of the bistro clients who corrupted their village youth and upset the elderly. But these were not people to sit about, counting their losses. As one old man put it, 'First it was the Muslim rulers, then it was the British, then the DDA (Delhi Development Authority), and now the showrooms – but we are still here living in our village.' The arrival of the boutiques was, after all, just one more event in the village's fragmented history.

I was not in Hauz Khas long enough to penetrate the subtler implications of relations between villagers, but there were some menacing signs that could not be ignored. Alcohol problems had escalated, unemployment continued, and rivalries seemed to have taken on an ugly hue. The village

Postscript

'headman' had been found dead down a well after a drinking session 'with friends' some two years before. Accident? Suicide? Murder? Everyone had their own interpretation, but whatever the reality, his death seemed somehow symbolic of the village's brutal transformation.

But life goes on, especially when there is money to be made. One more village becomes just one more shopping centre in South Delhi where politicians, exporters and NRI industrialists take over in the struggle for power. And Bina Ramani now looks back nostalgically to the gentle days of the late 1980s when she and a few exclusive friends established their boutiques in this seductively quiet place. Needless to say, she feels the village has lost its charm and the villagers their traditional values, and that the whole development has taken on a seedy commercial tone. Feeling a degree of sympathy, I ask her if she ever regretted having come to Hauz Khas. 'Oh God, no,' she replies, 'I've learned so much and I'm hoping to do the same sort of thing in other places in the future.' Asked how she would prevent the same scenario from being repeated elsewhere, she answers simply, 'Next time I won't rent, I'll buy!' And so ends the parable of Hauz Khas village.

A few months later I read in a Delhi magazine (*First City*, October 1994:56) that Bina Ramani is heading for Bangalore, where she has found another potential Indian paradise: 'A Wilderness area again. A fabulous place where I want to put together the best of India over the centuries – in arts, crafts, healing, spirituality. A holistic world. . . . Once it's a success we will have it outside every big city.'

And so another parable begins.

Bibliography

Oriental and India Office collections
L: P&J/7/27.
L:1/2/14.
Hopkinson Collection Mss.Eur.D.998: 26–36.

Books and articles
Abraham, A. (ed.), 1988, *The Penguin Book of Indian Cartoons*, Delhi: Penguin (India).
Ahluwalia, B. K., and S. Ahluwalia, 1981, *Tagore and Gandhi: The Gandhi Tagore Controversy*, Delhi: Pankaj.
Akbar, M. J., 1988, *Nehru: The Making of India*, London: Viking.
Alexander, M. (ed.), 1987, *Delhi and Agra: A Traveller's Companion*, London: Constable.
Ali, M., 1946 (1942), *My Life: A Fragment*, Lahore: Shaikh Muhammed Ashraf.
Alkazi, R., 1983, *Ancient Indian Costume*, Delhi: Art Heritage Books.
Allen, C. (ed.), 1985 (1975), *Plain Tales of the Raj*, London: Century Publishing.
Altekar, A. S., 1962, *The Position of Women in Hindu Civilization*, Delhi: Motilal Banarsidass.
Amin, S., 1984, 'Gandhi as Mahatma: Gorakhpur District, Eastern U.P., 1921–22' in R. Guha (ed.), *Subaltern Studies III*, Delhi: Oxford University Press.
Appadurai, A., 1988, 'How to Make a National Cuisine: Cookbooks in Contemporary India', *Comparative Studies in Society and History*, vol. 30, pp. 3–24.
—— (ed.), 1986, *The Social Life of Things: Commodities in Cultural Perspective*, Cambridge University Press.
—— and C. Breckenridge, 1988, 'Why Public Culture?', *Public Culture*, vol. 1, pp. 5–9.
Appasamy, J. (ed.), 1964, *Gogonendranath Tagore*, Delhi: Lalit Kala Akademi.
——, 1968, 'The Folk Inspiration in Modern Indian Painting' in *Indian Aesthetics and Art Activity*, Simla: Indian Institute of Advanced Society.
Ardener, S. (ed.), 1975, *Perceiving Women*, London: Malaby Press.
Baig, T. A., 1985, *Portrait of a Patriot: Sarojini Naidu*, Delhi: Congress Publications.
Baker, P. L., 1985, 'The Fez in Turkey: A Symbol of Modernisation?', *Costume*, no. 20, pp. 72–85.
Bakshi, S. R., 1987a, *Gandhi and Hindu-Muslim Unity*, Delhi: Deep and Deep.
——, 1987b, *Gandhi and the Ideology of Swadeshi*, Delhi: Reliance Publishing House.

Bibliography

Barley, N., 1983, 'The Warp and Woof of Culture', *RAIN* (Royal Anthropological Institute Newsletter), no. 59, pp. 7–8.

Barnes, R., and J. Eicher (eds), 1993 (1992), *Dress and Gender: Making and Meaning*, Providence, RI/Oxford: Berg.

Barot, K., 1977, *Gopal Darshan*, vol. 8 (Gujarati), Ahmedabad.

Barthes, R., 1973, *Mythologies*, London: Granada.

—— 1985, *The Fashion System*, London: Cape.

Barwell, M., 1960, *India Without Sentiment*, Calcutta: New Age Publishers.

Bayly, C., 1986, 'The Origins of Swadeshi (home industry): Cloth and Indian Society, 1700–1930' in A. Appadurai (ed.), as above.

—— (ed.), 1990, *The Raj: India and the British, 1600–1947*, London: National Portrait Gallery.

Bean S., 1989, 'Gandhi and Khadi: The Fabric of Independence' in A. Weiner and J. Schneider (eds), as below.

Ben-Ari, E., B. Moeran and J. Valentine (eds), 1990, *Unwrapping Japan: Society and Culture in Anthropological Perspective*, Manchester University Press.

Bernays, R., 1931, *Naked Fakir*, London: Gollancz.

Bernier, F., 1891, *Travels in the Moghul Empire (1656–68)*, London: Archibald Constable.

Berreman, G., 1972, 'Behind Many Masks: Ethnography and Impression Management', prologue to *Hindus of the Himalayas: Ethnography and Change*, Berkeley: University of California Press.

Billington, M. F., 1973 (1895), *Woman in India*, Delhi: Amarko Book Agency.

Birdwood, G., 1880, *The Industrial Arts of India*, repr. 1988 as *The Arts of India*, Calcutta: Rupa.

Bombay Gazeteer, 1901, vol. IX, part II: *Gujarat Population: Hindus*, Bombay: Government Central Press.

Bose, N., 1973, *Some Indian Tribes*, New Delhi: National Book Trust.

Bose, S. C., 1964, *The Indian Struggle, 1920–1942*, Bombay: Netaji Research Bureau.

—— 1984, *Distinction: A Social Critique in the Judgement of Taste*, London: Routledge and Kegan Paul.

Bourdieu, 1977, *Outline of a Theory in Practice*, Cambridge University Press.

Brailsford, H. N., 1943, *Subject India*, London: Gollancz.

Breckenridge, C. A., 1989, 'The Aesthetics of Politics and Colonial Collecting: India at World Fairs', *Comparative Studies of Society and History*, vol. 31, no. 2, pp. 195–216.

Briggs, J., 1828, *Letters Addressed to a Young Person in India; Calculated to Afford Instruction for his Conduct in General, and More Especially in his Intercourse with the Natives*, London: John Murray.

Bright, 1945, *Verdict on Britain*, Lahore: Dewan's Publications.

Brijbhushan, J., 1976, *Kamaladevi Chattopadhyaya: Portrait of a Rebel*, Delhi: Abhinav Publishers.

Brown, J., 1990, *Gandhi: Prisoner of Hope*, Delhi: Oxford University Press.

Buhler, A. and E. Fischer, 1979, *The Patola of Gujarat: Double Ikat in India* (2 vols), Basle: Museum of Ethnography.

Burke, N., 'The Raj: India 1890–1920, a Story in Photographs', unpubl., O.I.O.C.

Callaway, H., 1993, 'Dressing for Dinner in the Bush: Rituals of Self-definition and British Imperial Authority' in R. Barnes and J. Eicher (eds), as above.

Cardew, M., 1978, 'Design and Meaning in Preliterate Art' in M. Greenhalgh and V. Megaw (eds), *Art in Society*, London: Duckworth.

Census of India 1961, vol. 5: *Gujarat*, part 6: Village Survey Monographs, no. 4; part 7A: nos 4 and 21, Delhi: Central Government Publications.

Chatterjee, P., 1984, 'Gandhi and the Critique of Civil Society' in R. Guha (ed.), *Subaltern Studies*, as below.

Chattopadhyaya, K., 1964, 'Origin and Development of Embroidery in Our Land', *MARG*, vol. 17, no. 2, pp. 5–10.

Chaturvedi, B. K., n.d., *Dresses and Costumes of India*, Delhi: Diamond Pocket Books.

Chandra, B., 1966, *The Rise and Growth of Economic Nationalism in India: Economic Policies of Indian Nationalism Leadership*, 1880–1905, Delhi: People's Publishing House.

Chandra, M., 1973, *Costumes and Textiles, Cosmetics and Coiffure in Ancient and Medieval India*, Delhi: Orient Longmans.

Chaudhuri, N., 1976, *Culture in the Vanity Bag*, Bombay: Jaico.

——, 1987 (1951), *The Autobiography of an Unknown Indian*, London: Hogarth Press.

Chishti, R. K. and A. Sanyal, 1989, *Saris of India* (Madhya Pradesh volume), Delhi: Amr Vastra Kosh.

Cohn, B., 1955, 'The Changing Status of a Depressed Caste' in M. Marriott (ed.), *Village India: Studies in the Little Community*, University of Chicago Press.

——, 1983a, 'Cloth, Clothes and Colonialism', extended unpublished version of 1989 publication below, delivered at a symposium at Troutbeck, New York.

——, 1983b, 'Representing Authority in Victorian Britain' in E. Hobsbawm and T. Ranger (eds), *The Invention of Tradition*, Cambridge University Press.

——, 1987, *An Anthropologist among the Historians and Other Essays*, Delhi: Oxford University Press.

——, 1989, 'Cloth, Clothes and Colonialism: India in the Nineteenth Century' in A. Weiner and J. Schneider (eds), as below.

Coomaraswamy, A. K., 1908, *The Message of the East*, Madras: Ganesh.

—— 1909, *Essays in National Idealism*, notably 'Swadeshi True of False', repr. 1981, Delhi: Munshiram Manoharlal.

——, 1911, *Art and Swadeshi*, Madras: Ganesh.

Copland, I., 1982, *The British Raj and the Indian Princes: Paramountcy in Western India, 1857–1930*, Bombay: Orient Longman.

Cousins, F., 1984, 'Choix des matériaux et identification sociale. Evolution de vêtement féminin du Rajasthan', *L'Ethnographie*, pp. 153–60.

Crill, R., 1985, *Hats from India*, London: Victoria and Albert Museum.

Crooke, W., 1906, *Things Indian: Being Discursive Notes on Various Subjects Connected with India*, London: John Murray.

——, 1926, *Religion and Folklore in Northern India*, Oxford University Press.

Dalton, E. T., 1872, *Descriptive Ethnology of Bengal*, Calcutta: Asiatic Society of Bengal.

Bibliography

Dar, S. N., 1969, *Costumes of India and Pakisthan: Historical and Cultural Study*, Bombay: D. P. Taraporevala.

Darling, M. L. 1934, *Wisdom and Waste in a Punjab Village*, Oxford University Press.

Das, D. (ed.), 1970, *Gandhi in Cartoons*, Ahmedabad: Navajivan Trust.

Das, K. 1976, *My Story*, Delhi: Sterling Publishers.

Datta, M. M., 1963, *Kavi Madhusudan o tar patravali* (collection of Madhusudan's letters in Bengali and English), ed. K. Gupta, Calcutta: Grantha Nilaya.

Desai, I. P., 1976, *Untouchability in Rural Gujarat*, Bombay: Pupular Prakashan.

Desai, M., 1968, *Day to Day with Gandhi*, vol. 3, Varanasi: Sarva Seva Sangh Prakashan.

Dewey, C., 1972, 'Images of the Village Community: A Study in Anglo-Indian Ideology', *Modern Asian Studies*, vol. 6, no. 3, pp. 291–328.

Dey, M., 1948, *Portraits of Mahatma Gandhi*, Calcutta: Orient Longmans.

Dhamija, J., 1964, 'The Survey of Embroidery Traditions', *MARG*, 17, 2, pp. 11–67.

—— (ed.), 1985, *Crafts of Gujarat*, Ahmedabad: Mapin International.

——, 1988, 'Embroidery', *The Indian Magazine*, vol. 8, pp. 32–8.

Diwakar, 1949, *Glimpses of Gandhiji*, Bombay: Hind Kitabs.

Doke, J., 1967 (1909), *Mr Gandhi: An Indian Patriot in South Africa*, Madras.

Dongerkery, K., 1951, *The Romance of Indian Embroidery*, Bombay: Thacker.

——, 1960, *The Indian Sari*, Delhi: All India Handicrafts Board.

Douglas, M., and B. Isherwood, 1978, 1980, *The World of Goods: Towards an Anthropology of Consumption*, Harmondsworth: Penguin Books.

Dube, Leacock, Ardener (eds), 1986, *Visibility and Power: Essays on Women in Society and Development*, Delhi: Oxford University Press.

Dumont, L., 1970, *Homo Hierarchicus*, London: Weidenfeld and Nicolson.

Durrans, B., 1982, 'Handicrafts, Ideology and the Festival of India', *South Asia Research*, vol. 2, no. 1, pp. 13–22.

Dwarkadas, J., 1969, *Political Memoirs*, Bombay: United Publishing House.

Eco, U., 1986, 'Lumbar Thought' in *Travels in Hyper Reality*, San Diego, CA: Harcourt Brace Jovanovich.

Edwardes, M., 1986, *The Myth of the Mahatma: Gandhi, the British and the Raj*, London: Constable.

Ehrenfels, O.R., 1948, 'Kadan – Clothes and Culture Change', *Man in India*, 4, XXVIII, pp. 209–21.

Eicher, J., and M. E. Roach-Higgins, 1993, 'Definition and Classification of Dress: Implications for Analysis of Gender Roles' in Barnes and Eicher (eds), as above.

Elder, C., and R. W. Cobb, 1983, *The Political Uses of Symbols*, New York: Longman.

Elson, V., 1979, *Dowries from Kutch: A Women's Folk Art Tradition in India*, Los Angeles, CA: Museum of Cultural History.

Elwin, E. F., 1907, *Indian Jottings: From Ten Years' Experience in and around Poona City*, London: John Murray.

Elwin, V., 1932, *Mahatma Gandhi*, London: Golden Vista Press.

——, 1959, (1957), *A Philosophy for NEFA*, Shillong: Sachiu Roy.

Encyclopaedia of Islam, 1971, vol. 3, London: Luzac.

Enthoven, 1914, *Folklore Notes*, vol. 1: Gujarat, Bombay: British India Press.

——, 1920–2, *The Tribes and Castes of Bombay* (3 vols), Government of Bombay.

——, 1924, *The Folklore of Bombay*, Oxford: Clarendon Press.

Evans-Pritchard, E. E., 1967 (1940), *The Nuer*, Oxford: Clarendon Press.

Fabri, C., 1960, *Indian Dress*, Delhi: Orient Longmans.

Fischer, E. and H. Shah, 1970, *Rural Craftsmen and their Work*, Ahmedabad: National Institute of Design.

Frater, J., 1975, 'The Meaning of Folk Art in Rabari Life', *Textile Museum Journal*, vol. 4, no. 2, pp. 47–60.

Fruzzetti, L., 1982, *The Gift of a Virgin: Women, Marriage and Ritual in Bengali Society*, New Brunswick, NJ: Rutgers University Press.

Fürer-Haimendorff, C. von, 1939, *The Naked Nagas*, London: Methuen.

——, 1976, *Return to the Naked Nagas*, Delhi: Vikas.

Gaikwad, 1967, *The Anglo-Indians: A Study in the Problems and Processes Involved in Emotional and Cultural Integration*, London: Asia Publishing House.

Gandhi, M. K., 1946, *To the Women* (Gandhi series, vol. II), Karachi: Anand T. Hingorani.

——, 1989 (1927), *An Autobiography or Stories of my Experiments with Truth*, Ahmedabad: Navajivan Publishing House.

——, *Collected Works of Mahatma Gandhi*, vols: 1 (1958), 8 (1958), 10 (1963), 12 (1964), 13 (1979), 15 (1965), 16 (1965), 17 (1979), 18 (1979), 19 (1979), 20 (1966), 21 (1966), 22 (1979), 24 (1967), 25 (1979), 26 (1979), 27 (1979), 28 (1979), 29 (1968), 30 (1968), 31 (1979), 32 (1969), 33 (1969), 34 (1969), 35 (1969), 41 (1970), 47 (1971), 48 (1971), 75 (1979), 89 (1983), 90 (1984), Ahmedabad: Navajivan Press.

——, 1959, *Khadi: Why and How*, Ahmedabad: Navajivan Press.

Gangoli, O. C., n.d., *The Humorous Art of Gogonendranath Tagore*, Calcutta: Birla Academy of Art and Culture.

Gauba, K. L., 1945, *Verdict on England*, Lahore: Lion Press.

Gazetteer of the Bombay Precidency, 1884, vol. 8: Kathiawar.

Gell, A., 1986, 'Newcomers to the World of Goods: Consumption among the Muria Gonds' in A. Appadurai (ed.) as above.

Ghurye, G. S., 1951, *Indian Costume*, Bombay: Popular Book Depot.

Gillow, J. and N. Bernard, 1991, *Traditional Indian Textiles*, London: Thames and Hudson.

Glasenapp, H. V., 1925, *Indien. Der Indische Kulturkries*, Munich: Georg Müller.

Goffman, E., 1969, *The Presentation of Self in Everyday Life*, New York: Doubleday.

Gold Grodzins, A., 1988, *Fruitful Journeys: The Ways of Rajasthani Pilgrims*, Berkeley: University of California Press.

Goody, E. (ed.) 1982, *From Craft to Industry: The Ethnography of Proto-industrial Cloth Production*, Cambridge University Press.

Goody, J., and S. J. Tambiah, 1973, *Bridewealth and Dowry*, Cambridge University Press.

Goswamy, B. N., 1993, *Indian Costumes in the Collection of the Calico Museum of Textiles*, vol. 5: *Historical Textiles of India at the Calico Museum*, Ahmedabad: D. S. Mehta for the Calico Museum.

Bibliography

Graburn, N. (ed.), 1976, *Ethnic and Tourist Arts: Cultural Expressions from the Fourth World*, Berkeley: University of California Press.

Greenberger, A. 1969, *The British Image of India: A Study of the Literature of Imperialism, 1880–1960*, London: Oxford University Press.

Gross, N. D., and F. Fontana, 1981, *Shisha Embroidery*, Dover Publications.

Guha, R. (ed.), 1982–9, *Subaltern Studies: Writings on South Asian History and Society*, vols 1–6, Delhi: Oxford University Press.

Gujarat State Gazetteer, Amreli District District, 1972, and Bhavnagar District, 1969, Ahmedabad: Government of Gujarat.

Handler, R., 1986, 'Authenticity', *Anthropology Today*, vol. 2, no. 1, pp. 2–4.

Hardiman, D., 1981, *Peasant Nationalists of Gujarat*, Delhi: Oxford University Press.

Harrison, A., 1945, '88 Knightsbridge Road' in C. Shukla (ed.), 1945, as below.

Havell, E. B., 1912, *The Basis for Artistic and Industrial Revival in India*, Madras: Theosophist Office.

Haynes Holmes, J., 1945, 'What I Saw in Gandhi' in C. Shukla (ed.), 1945, as below.

Hebdige, D., 1979, *Subculture: The Meaning of Style*, London: Methuen.

Hitkari, S. S., 1980, *Phulkari: The Folk Art of Punjab*, New Delhi: Phulkari Publications.

——, 1981, *Ganesha Sthapana*, New Delhi: Phulkari Publications.

Hobsbawm, E., 1983, 'Inventing Traditions' in E. Hobsbawm and T. Ranger (eds), *The Invention of Tradition*, Cambridge University Press.

Hobson, S., 1978, *Family Web: A Story of India*, London: John Murray.

Hodder, I., 1982, *Symbols in Action: Ethno-archaeological Studies of Material Culture*, Cambridge University Press.

Hoffman, H.-J., 1984, 'How Clothes Communicate', *Media Development*, vol. 31, no. 4, pp. 7–11.

Hunt, J. D., 1978, *Gandhi in London*, New Delhi: Promilla.

Hürlimann, M., 1928, *Indien. Baukunst, Landschaft und Volksleben*, Berlin: Ernst Wasmuth.

Hutton, J. H., 1946, *Caste in India: Its Nature, Functions and Origins*, Cambridge University Press.

Imperial Gazetteer of India: Bombay Presidency, 1909 (2 vols), Calcutta: Government Publication.

Inden, R., 1990, *Imagining India*, Oxford: Basil Blackwell.

Irwin, J., and M. Hall, 1971, *Indian Painted and Printed Fabrics*, Ahmedabad: Calico Museum of Textiles.

——, 1973, *Indian Embroideries*, Ahmedabad: Calico Museum of Textiles.

Irwin, J., and P. Schwartz, 1966, *Indo-European Textile History*, Ahmedabad: Calico Museum of Textiles.

Iwatate, H., 1989 (1984), *Desert Village, Life, Crafts: Gujarat, Rajasthan*, Tokyo: Yoshiba.

Jacobson, D., 1970, 'Hidden Faces: Hindu and Muslim Purdah in a Central Indian Village', unpubl. Ph. D. thesis, Columbia University.

——, 1976, 'Women and Jewellery in Rural India' in G. R. Gupta (ed.), *Family and Social Change in Modern India*, Delhi: Vikas.

——, 1986 (1977), *The Women of North and Central India: Goddesses and Wives*, Delhi: Manohar.

Jain J., 1980, *Folk Art and Culture of Gujarat*, Ahmedabad: Shreyas Prakashan.

——, 1982, 'The Visual Vocabulary of Craft' in C. Kagal (ed.), *Shilpakar the Craftsman*, Bombay: Vasant Hanavar for the Crafts Council of India.

Jain, L. C., 1986, 'A Heritage to Keep: The Handicrafts Industry, 1955–1985', *Economic and Political Weekly*, vol. 21, no. 20, pp. 837–87.

Jaitly, J., 1985, 'Embroidery' in J. Dhamija (ed.) as above.

—— (ed.), 1990, *Crafts of Jammu and Kashmir*, Ahmedabad: Mapin.

Jawaharlal Nehru: A Memorial Album, 1964, Delhi: Popular Prakashan.

Jay Gopal 2, 1989 (Shepherd newsletter in Gujarati), Ahmedabad.

Jog, N. G., 1945, *Judge or Judas?*, Bombay: Thacker.

Johnson, W., 1863–6, *The Oriental Races and Tribes, Residents and Visitors of Bombay* (2 vols), London: W. J. Johnson.

Johnstone, J., 1896, *My Experiences in Manipur and the Naga Hills*, London: Sampson Low, Marston and Co.

Joshi, O. P., 1993, 'Continuity and Change in Hindu Women's Dress' in R. Barnes and J. Eicher (eds), as above.

Joshi, V. H., 1989, 'Modern Politico-economic Change and Rural Social Transformation: A Saurashtran Case-study', unpubl.

Kalarthi, M. 1960, *Anecdotes from Bapu's Life*, Ahmedabad: Navajivan Trust.

—— 1962, *Ba and Bapu*, Ahmedabad: Navajivan Trust.

Kalelkar, K., 1950, *Stray Glimpses of Bapu*, Ahmedabad: Navajivan Trust.

Kalhan, P., 1973, *Kamala Nehru: An Intimate Biography*, Delhi: Vikas.

Kashyap, S. P. and R. S. Tiwari, 1987, *Shaping Diamonds in Surat: Some Passas* [Facets], Ahmedabad: Sardar Patel Institute.

Kelker, N. C., 1949, 'My Contact with Mahatma Gandhi' in Shukla, C. (ed.), 1949, as below.

Kennedy, M., 1908, *Criminal Classes in the Bombay Presidency*, Bombay: Government Central Press.

Khan, A. G., 1969, *My Life and Struggle*, Delhi: Hind Pocket Books.

Kishwar, M., 1985, 'Gandhi on Women', *Economic and Political Weekly*, vol. 20, no. 40, pp. 1691–1702, and no. 41, pp. 1753–8.

Kripalani, J. B., 1938, *The Gandhian Way*, Bombay: Vora.

—— 1949, 'Pratham Darshan' in C. Shukla (ed.), 1949, as below.

Krishnadas, 1928, *Seven Months with Mahatma Gandhi: Being an Inside View of the Non-Co-operation Movement (1921–22)*, Madras: S. Ganesan.

Kumar, 1984, 'Gandhi's Ideological Clothing', *Media Development*, 31, no. 4, pp. 19–21.

Kumar, N., 1988, *The Artisans of Benares: Popular Culture and Identity 1880–1986*, Princeton University Press.

Kumria, R. R., 1941, *New Values for a New India*, Lahore: Minerva Bookshop.

Kuper, H., 1973, 'Costume and Identity', *Comparative Studies in Society and History*, 15, pp. 348–67.

Bibliography

Lal, C., 1969, *Laugh with Gandhi*, Switzerland: Chaman Lal.

Laver, J., 1963, *Costume*, London: Cassell.

Laxman, R., 1961–89, *You Said It*, vol. 1: 1987 (1961), vol. 2: 1998 (1971); vol. 3: 1989 (1968), vol. 4: 1989 (1970), vol. 5: 1989 (1974), vol. 7: 1989 (1984), Bombay: India Book House.

Laxman, R., 1988, *The Eloquent Brush*, Delhi: *Times of India*.

Leslie, J., 1993, 'The Significance of Dress for the Orthodox Hindu Woman' in R. Barnes and J. Eicher (eds) (as above).

Lester, M., 1932, *Entertaining Gandhi*, London: Ivor Nicholson and Watson.

Lipsey, R., 1977, *Coomaraswamy: His Life and Works*, vol. 3, Princeton University Press.

Lurie, A., 1992 (1981), *The Language of Clothes*, London: Bloomsbury.

Luschinsky, M., 1962, 'The Life of Women in a Village in North India', unpubl. Ph. D. thesis, Cornell University.

Maloney, C., 1976, *The Evil Eye*, New York: Columbia University Press.

Martinez, L., 1990, 'Tourism and the Ama: The Search for the Real Japan' in Ben-Ari *et al.* (eds) as above.

Masani, M., 1946 (1940), *Our India*, Bombay Oxford University Press.

Masani, R. P., 1960, *Dadabhai Naoroji*, Delhi: Government of India.

Masselos, J., n.d., 'The Artist as Patron: Women's Embroidery in Gujarat', Working Papers no. 1, Sydney Centre for Asian Studies.

Mehta, G., 1949, 'Meeting Gandhiji. C. Shukla, (ed.), 1949, as below.

Mehta, R., 1976, 'From Purdah to Modernity' in B. R. Nanda (ed.), *Indian Women from Purdah to Modernity*, Delhi: Vikas.

Miller, D., 1983, 'Things Ain't What They Used To Be', *RAIN*, no. 59, pp. 5–7.

—— 1985, *Artefacts as Categories: A Study of Ceramic Variability in Central India*, Cambridge University Press.

Minault, G., 1982, 'The Khilafat Movement: Religious Symbolism and Political Mobilization in India', New York: Columbia University Press.

Moeran, B., 1984, *Lost Innocence: Folk Craft Potters of Onta, Japan*, Berkeley: University of California Press.

—— 1990a, 'Japanese Ceramics and the Discourse of Tradition', *Journal of Design History*, vol. 3, no. 4, pp. 213–25.

—— 1990b, 'Rapt Discourses: Anthropology, Japanism and Japan' in E. Ben Ari *et al.* (eds), as above.

Mohan, J., 1979, 'Ananda K. Coomaraswamy', Delhi: Ministry of Information and Broadcasting.

Mohanty, B. C., and J. P. Mohanty, 1983, *Block Printing and Dyeing in Bagru, Rajasthan*, Ahmedabad: Calico Museum.

Morton, E., 1953, *The Women in Gandhi's Life*, New York: Dodd, Mead.

Murphey, R., 1964, 'Social Distance and the Veil', *American Anthropologist*, vol. 66, pp. 1257–73.

Murphey, V., and R. Crill, 1991, *Tie-dyed Textiles of India: Tradition and Trade*, London: Victoria and Albert Museum.

Nabholz-Kartaschoff, M. L., 1986, *Golden Sprays and Scarlet Flowers: Traditional Indian Textiles*, Kyoto: Shikosha Publishing.

Nanavati, J., M. Vora and M. Dhaky, 1966, *The Embroidery and Beadwork of Kutch and Saurashtra*, Baroda: Museum Monograph Series.

Nanda, B. R., 1972, *Gandhi: A Pictorial Biography*, Delhi: Government Publications Division.

—— (ed.), 1976, *Indian Women from Purdah to Modernity*, Delhi: Vikas.

——, 1989 (1958), *Mahatma Gandhi*, Delhi: Oxford University Press.

Nandy, A., 1983, *The Intimate Enemy: Loss and Recovery of Self under Colonialism*, Delhi: Oxford University Press.

Narendra, R., 1989, 'Hauz Khas Village, New Delhi: An Approach towards Redevelopment', unpubl. B. Arch. thesis, School of Planning and Architecture, Delhi.

Nehru, J., 1972, *Selected Works of Jawaharlal Nehru*, vol. 1, Delhi: Orient Longman.

Nehru, M., 1982–8, *Selected Works of Motilal Nehru* (4 vols) ed. R. Kumar, Delhi: Vikas.

Nichols, B., 1944, *Verdict on India*, London: Cape.

Nicholson, J., 1988, *Traditional Indian Arts of Gujarat*, Leicester Museum (England).

Owens, V. S., 1984, 'Camouflaged at the Costume Ball', *Media Development*, vol. 31, no. 4, pp. 17–19.

Paine, S., 1990, *Embroidered Textiles: Traditional Patterns from Five Continents*, London: Thames and Hudson.

Pakvasa, 1949, 'Dandi March and After' in C. Shukla (ed.), 1949, as below.

Papanek, H., 1973, 'Purdah: Separate Worlds and Symbolic Shelter', *Comparative Studies in Society and History*, vol. 15, pp. 289–325.

—— and G. Pollock, 1981, *Old Mistresses: Women, Art and Ideology*, London: Routledge and Kegan Paul.

Parker, R., 1986, *The Subversive Stitch: Embroidery and the Making of Femininity*, London: Women's Press.

Parkin, D., 1982, Introduction to *Semantic Anthropology*, London: Academic Press.

Parmar, K., 1969, *Saurashtra nu lok bharat* (Gujarati = The folk embroidery of Saurashtra), Ahmedabad: Gujarat Rajay Loksahitya Samiti.

Parry, J., 1986, 'The Gift, the Indian Gift, and the "Indian Gift" ', *Man*, vol. 21, pp. 453–73.

Phelan, J., 1984, 'Surfaces in the Media World of Political Fashion', *Media Development*, vol. 31. no. 4, pp. 12–14.

Picton, J., 1990, 'Transformations of the Artefact: John Wayne, Plastic Bags and the Eye-that-surpasses-all-other-eyes' in C. Deliss (ed.), *Lotte, der Katalog*, London: Gräfin.

—— and J. Mack, 1979, *African Textiles*, London: British Museum Publications.

Pinney, C., 1990, 'Colonial Anthropology in the "Laboratory of Mankind"' in C. Bayly (ed.), as above.

Pocock, D., 1972, *Kanbi and Patidar*, Oxford: Clarendon Press.

—— 1973, *Mind Body and Wealth: A Study of Belief and Practice in an Indian Village*, Oxford: Basil Blackwell.

Polak, M. G., 1950 (1949), *Mr Gandhi: The Man*, Bombay: Vora.

Bibliography

Polak, S. L., 1959, 'Some South African Reminiscences' in C. Shukla (ed.), 1949, as above.

Postans, M., 1838, *Cutch, or Random Sketches of Western India*, London: Smith, Elder.

——, 1839, *Western India in 1838*, vol. 1, London: Saunders and Ottley.

Pyarelal, 1965, *Mahatma Gandhi, the Early Phase*, vol. 1, Ahmedabad: Navajivan.

Radice, C. W., 1986, 'Tremendous Literary Rebel: The Life and Works of Madhusudan Datta (1824–73)', unpubl. Ph. D. thesis, Faculty of Oriental Studies, Oxford University.

Rai, G., 1945, *Gandhi and Kasturba: The Story of their Life*, Lahore: Kasturba Memorial Publications.

Ramanujan, M., 1984, 'The Language of Clothes: An Indian Perspective', *Media Development*, 4., pp. 30–3.

Ray, S., 1977, 'Michael Madhusudan Datta: The First Modern Poet of India' in S. Ray (ed.), *Apartheid in Shakespeare and other Reflections*, Melbourne.

Raychaudhuri, T., 1988, *Europe Reconsidered: Perceptions of the West in Nineteenth Century Bengal*, Delhi: Oxford University Press.

Risley, H., 1908, *The People of India*, London: Thacker.

Rudolf, L., and S. Rudolf, 1987 (1969), *The Modernity of Tradition: Political Development in India*, Chicago: Orient Longman.

Russell, R. V., 1916, *The Tribes and Castes of the Central Provinces of India*, London: Macmillan.

Said, E., 1985 (1978), *Orientalism*, Harmondsworth: Penguin Books.

Salvador, M., 1976, 'The Clothing Arts of the Cuna of San Blas, Panama' in N. L. Graburn (ed.), as above.

Saraf, D. N., 1982, *Indian Crafts: Development and Potential*, Delhi: Vikas.

Sarkar, S., 1984, 'The Conditions and Nature of Subaltern Militancy: Bengal from Swadeshi to Non-co-operation, 1905-22' in R. Guha (ed.), as above, vol. 3.

—— 1985 (1983), *Modern India, 1885–1947*, Madras: Macmillan India.

Schlaginweit, E., 1880, *Indien in Wort und Bild*, Leipzig: Heinrich Schmidt and Carl Gunter.

Schneider, J., 1980, 'Trousseau as Treasure: Some Contradictions of Late 19th Century Change in Sicily' in E. Ross (ed.), *Beyond Myths in Culture*, London: Academic Press.

—— J., and A. Weiner, 1989, Introduction to A. Weiner and J. Schneider (eds), as below.

Sengupta, P., 1966, *Sarojini Naidu: A Bibliography*, London: Asia Publishing House.

Seth, S., 1980, 'The Arts of the Kharak', unpubl. Ph.D. thesis, Baroda University (Fine Arts Dept).

Shah, A. M., 1988, 'The Rural-Urban Networks in India', *South Asia*, vol. 11, no. 2, pp. 1–27.

Shah, G., 1983, 'Socio Economic Stratification and Politics in Rural Gujarat', in Lakdawala (ed.), *Gujarat Economy, Problems and Prospects*, Ahmedabad: Sardar Patel Institute of Economic and Social Research.

Shah, S. M., 1987 (1969), 'Rural Class Structure in Gujarat', in A. R. Desai, *Rural Sociology in India*, Bombay: Popular Prakashan.

Shankar, P., n.d., *Shankar's Cartoons of Nehru*, Delhi.

Sharar, A. H., 1975, *Lucknow: The Last Phase of an Oriental Culture* (reprint), London: Paul Elek.

Sharma, U., 1978a, 'Segregation and its Consequences in India: Rural Women of Himachal Pradesh' in P. Caplan and J. Bujra (eds), *Women United, Women Divided*, London: Tavistock.

——, 1978b, 'Women and Their Affines: The Veil as a Symbol of Separation', *Man*, 13, pp. 218–33.

——, 1980, 'Purdah and Public Space' in A. de Souza (ed.), *Women in Contemporary India and South Asia*, Delhi: Manohar.

——, 1984, 'Dowry in India and its Consequences for Women' in R. Hirschon, *Women and Property, Women as Property*, London: Croom Helm.

Shore, F. J., 1837, *Notes on Indian Affairs*, vol. 1, London: J. W. Parker.

Shukla, C. (ed.), 1945, *Gandhi as We Knew Him*, Bombay: Vora.

—— (ed.), 1949, *Incidents in Gandhiji's Life*, Bombay, Vora.

Singh, K., 1982, *We Indians*, Delhi: Orient Paperbacks.

Slade, M. (Mirabehn), 1984 (1960), *The Spirit's Pilgrimage (Mirabehn)*, Arlington, VA: Great Ocean Publishers.

Solvyns, B., 1799, *A Collection of Two Hundred and Fifty Coloured Etchings Descriptive of the Manners, Customs and Dresses of the Hindoos*, Calcutta.

Spodek, H., 1976, *Urban-Rural Integration in Regional Development: A Case Study of Saurashtra, India, 1800–1960*, University of Chicago Press.

Srinivas, M. N., 1956, 'Sanskritization and Westernization' in A. Aiyappant and L. K. Bala Ratnam (eds), *Society in India*, Madras: Social Science Association.

——, 1968, *Social Change in Modern India*, Berkeley: University of California Press.

——, 1976, 'The Changing Position of Women', T. H. Huxley Memorial Lecture, London: Royal Antiropological Institute.

Steevan, C., 1876, *The Archaeological and Monumental Remains of Delhi*, Delhi: Ashish Publishing House (reprint, n.d.).

Steevens, G. W., 1899, *In India*, London: Thos. Nelson.

Stuart, C., 1809, *The Ladies Moniter: being a series of letters published in Bengal on the subject of female apparel*, London.

Swallow, D., 1982, 'Production and Control in the Indian Garment Export Industry' in E. Goody (ed.), *From Craft to Industry*, Cambridge University Press.

Swayne-Thomas, A., 1981, *Indian Summer: A Mem-sahib in India and Sind*, London: New English Library.

Tagore, G., 1917, *Virup Vajra: Realm of the Absurd*, Calcutta: Vichitra Press.

Tagore, R., 1917, *My Reminiscences*, London: Macmillan.

——, 1921, *Glimpses of Bengal: Selected Letters of Rabindranath Tagore, 1885–1895*, London: Macmillan.

——, 1945, *My Boyhood Days*, Calcutta: Vishva Bharati.

——, 1960, 'Coat or Chapkan', *Rabindra Rachanavali*, XII, Calcutta: Vishva Bharati, pp. 223–9.

Tambiah, 1973, 'Dowry and Bridewealth and Property Rights in South Asia' in S. J.

Bibliography

Tambiah and J. Goody (eds), *Bridewealth and Dowry*, Cambridge University Press.

Tambs-Lyche H., 1992, 'Power and Devotion: Religion and Society in Saurashtra' (3 vols), unpubl. Ph.D. thesis, University of Bergen, Norway.

Tarlo, E., forthcoming, 'Traders as Trendsetters: The Marketing of Village Embroidery in Gujarat'. Paper presented at the conference 'Cloth, the World Economy and the Artisan', Dartmouth College, NH, 1993. To be published under the same title in a book edited by D. Haynes and J. Byfield.

Tarrant, N., 1994, *The Development of Costume*, London: Routledge.

Tavernier, J. B. 1889, *Travels in India* (original French edition 1676), 2 vols, London: Macmillan.

Templewood, Viscount, 1954, *Nine Troubled Years*, London: Collins.

——, 1967, *Abdul Ghaffar Khan: Faith Is a Battle*, Bombay: Popular Prakashan.

Tendulkar, D. G., 1952–4, *Mahatma*, vol. 3 (1952), 5 (1952) and 8 (1954), Bombay: Vithalbhai K. Jhaverji and D. G. Tendulkar.

Thompson, C., 1981, 'A Sense of Sharm: Some Thoughts on Its Implication for the Position of Women in a Village in Central India', *South Asia Research*, vol. 2, pp. 39–54.

Thompson, M., 1979, *Rubbish Theory: The Creation and Destruction of Value*, Oxford University Press.

Urwick, W., 1891, *Indian Pictures Drawn with Pencil*, London: Religious Tract Society.

Vadgama, K., 1984, *India in Britain*, London: Robert Royce.

Van der Veen, K. W., 1972, *I Give Thee My Daughter: Marriage and Hierarchy among Anavil Brahmans of South Gujarat*, Assen: Van Gorcum.

Vatuk, S., 1975, 'Gifts and Affines in North India', *Contributions to Indian Sociology*, vol. 9, no. 2, pp. 155–96.

Veblen, T., 1925, *The Theory of the Leisure Class*, London: Geo. Allen and Unwin.

Vijayatunga, J., 1970 (1935), *Grass for my Feet*, London: Howard Baker.

Vittachi, T., 1987, *The Brown Sahib Revisited*, Delhi: Penguin Books.

Walsh, J. E., 1983, *Growing up in British India: Indian Autobiographers on Childhood and Education under the Raj*, New York: Holmes and Meier.

Waterbury, 1989, 'Embroidery for Tourists: A Contemporary Putting-out System in Oaxaca, Mexico' in A. Weiner and J. Schneider (eds), as below.

Watson, J. F., 1866, *The Textile Manufactures and the Costumes of the People of India* (with 18 vols of textile samples), London: G. E. Eyre and W. Spottiswood.

—— J. W. Kaye, 1868–75, *The People of India* (8 vols), London: India Museum.

Watts, N. A., 1970, *The Half-clad Tribals of Eastern India*, Calcutta: Orient Longman.

Weiner, A. and J. Schneider (eds), 1989, *Cloth and Human Experience*, Washington: Smithsonian Institution Press.

Weir, S., 1989, Palestinian Costume, London: British Museum Publications.

Werbner, P., 1990, 'Economic Rationality and Hierarchical Gift Economies: Value and ranking among British Pakistanis', *Man*, vol. 25, no. 2, pp. 266–86.

Wilberforce-Bell, H., 1980 (1916), *The History of Kathiawad from Earliest Times*, Delhi: Ajay Book Service.

Wilson, E., 1987 (1985), *Adorned in Dreams: Fashion and Modernity*, London: Virago.

Wiser, C., and W. Wiser, 1930, *Behind Mud Walls*, New York: R. R. Smith.

Woodruff, D., 1955, *The Men Who Ruled India*, vol. 1: *The Founders*, London: Cape.

Younger, C., 1983, 'Racial Attitudes to the Anglo-Indian's perceptions of a Community before and after Independence', *South Asia*, vol. 6, no. 2.

Yule, H., and A. C. Burnell, 1903 (1886), *Hobson-Jobson*, London: John Murray.

Zutshi, G. L., 1970, *Frontier Gandhi*, Delhi: National Publishing House.

Newspapers, journals, magazines

Anthropology Today (London)

Bombay (Bombay)

Comparative Studies in Society and History (London)

Costume (Journal of the Costume Society)

Debonair (Bombay)

Economic and Political Weekly (Bombay)

L'Ethnographie (Paris)

First City (Delhi)

Flair (Bombay)

Frontline (Madras)

Glad Rags (Bombay)

The Guardian (London)

Harijan (Ahmedabad)

Hindi Punch (Bombay)

The Hindu (Madras)

Hindustan Times (Delhi)

Illustrated Weekly (Bombay)

The Independent (London)

The India Magazine (Delhi)

India Today (Delhi)

India Worldwide

Indian Art (London, 1884–92; later became *Journal of Indian Art and Industry*)

Man (London)

Man in India (Ranchi)

MARG: A Magazine of the Arts (Bombay)

Media Development (Journal of the World Association for Christian Communication, London)

Modern Asian Studies (Cambridge)

Movie (Bombay)

Public Culture (Philadelphia)

RAIN (*Royal Anthropological Institute Newsletter*, London)

Show Time (Bombay)

Society (Bombay)

Bibliography

South Asia (Australia)
South Asia Research (London)
Star and Style (Bombay)
Statesman (Calcutta)
Sunday Mail (Delhi)
Sweet Sixteen (fashion catalogue, Bombay)
Teen Talk (Ahmedabad)
The Times (London)
Times of India (Bombay)
Whiteaway, Laidlaw & Co. Ltd., Bombay, catalogue

Index

Index